STUDEN

ILLUSTRATED
Dental Embryology, Histology, AND Anatomy

Copyright © 2026 by Elsevier Inc. All rights are reserved, including those for text and data mining, AI training, and similar technologies.

STUDENT WORKBOOK FOR

ILLUSTRATED

Dental Embryology, Histology, AND Anatomy

SIXTH EDITION

M. J. FEHRENBACH, RDH, MS

Oral Biologist and Dental Hygienist,
Past Adjunct Instructor, Bachelor of Applied Science Degree Dental Hygiene Program,
Seattle Central College, Seattle, Washington
Educational Consultant and Dental Science Technical Writer,
Seattle, Washington

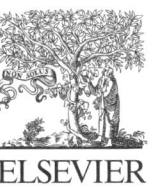

ELSEVIER

Copyright © 2026 by Elsevier Inc. All rights are reserved, including those for text and data mining, AI training, and similar technologies.

Elsevier
3251 Riverport Lane
St. Louis, Missouri 63043

STUDENT WORKBOOK FOR ILLUSTRATED DENTAL EMBRYOLOGY,
HISTOLOGY, AND ANATOMY, SIXTH EDITION

ISBN: 978-0-443-10425-1

Copyright © 2026 by Elsevier Inc. All rights are reserved, including those for text and data mining, AI training, and similar technologies.

For accessibility purposes, images in electronic versions of this book are accompanied by alt text descriptions provided by Elsevier. For more information, see https://www.elsevier.com/about/accessibility.

Publisher's note: Elsevier takes a neutral position with respect to territorial disputes or jurisdictional claims in its published content, including in maps and institutional affiliations.

No part of this publication may be reproduced or transmitted in any form or by any means, electronic or mechanical, including photocopying, recording, or any information storage and retrieval system, without permission in writing from the publisher. Details on how to seek permission, further information about the Publisher's permissions policies and our arrangements with organizations such as the Copyright Clearance Center and the Copyright Licensing Agency, can be found at our website: www.elsevier.com/permissions.

This book and the individual contributions contained in it are protected under copyright by the Publisher (other than as may be noted herein).

Although for mechanical reasons all pages of this publication are perforated, only those pages imprinted with an Elsevier Inc. copyright notice are intended for removal.

Notice

Practitioners and researchers must always rely on their own experience and knowledge in evaluating and using any information, methods, compounds or experiments described herein. Because of rapid advances in the medical sciences, in particular, independent verification of diagnoses and drug dosages should be made. To the fullest extent of the law, no responsibility is assumed by Elsevier, authors, editors or contributors for any injury and/or damage to persons or property as a matter of products liability, negligence or otherwise, or from any use or operation of any methods, products, instructions, or ideas contained in the material herein.

Previous editions copyrighted 2022, 2016, 2011, 2006 and 1997

Content Strategist: Kelly Skelton
Content Development Specialist: Deborah Poulson
Publishing Services Manager: Deepthi Unni
Project Manager: Gayathri S
Design Direction: Gopalakrishnan Venkatraman

Printed in India

Last digit is the print number: 9   8   7   6   5   4   3   2   1

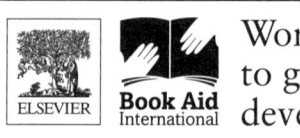

PREFACE

This innovative student workbook serves as a companion to the associated textbook in its latest sixth edition, *Illustrated Dental Embryology, Histology, and Anatomy* (Fehrenbach and Popowicz, Elsevier, 2026). It provides a wide range of knowledge-building activities in an engaging format to strengthen the student dental professional's understanding of the structures, terminology, and concepts of oral biology discussed in the textbook.

Thus this fully updated student workbook features activities such as structure identification exercises, terminology exercises, tooth drawing exercises, and concept exercises. Clinical observation of extraoral and intraoral structures, dentition, and occlusion has been added to include the related clinical aspects of dentistry. Case studies with questions are also included, along with removable flashcards using the original illustrations of the permanent dentition from the textbook. These materials go beyond just being busy work and create a sound bridge of understanding for the future dental professional between the written materials and the day to day dental care of the patient.

Additional material for students purchasing the associated textbook can be found online on the associated Student Evolve Resources website, such as review and assessment concepts, enhanced core concepts, and review quizzes with answers.

It is hoped that these materials will help students integrate basic dental science with clinical dental coursework and prepare the student dental professional for both competency examinations and future clinical situations.

M. J. Fehrenbach

CONTENTS

Structure Identification Exercises 1
Clinical Identification Exercises 73
Terminology Exercises 83
Tooth Drawing Exercises 121
Concept Exercises 207
Case Study Exercises 225
Flashcards 263

ILLUSTRATION CREDITS

Chapter 1

1.1 (Modified from Fehrenbach MJ, Herring SW. *Illustrated Anatomy of the Head and Neck*. 6th ed. St. Louis: Elsevier; 2021.)

1.2 A and B (From Fehrenbach MJ, Herring SW. *Illustrated Anatomy of the Head and Neck*. 6th ed. St. Louis: Elsevier; 2021.)

1.5 (Modified from Fehrenbach MJ, Herring SW. *Illustrated Anatomy of the Head and Neck*. 6th ed. St. Louis: Elsevier, 2021.)

1.7 (From Fehrenbach MJ, Herring SW. *Illustrated Anatomy of the Head and Neck*. 6th ed. St. Louis: Elsevier; 2021.)

1.10 (Modified from Fehrenbach MJ, Herring SW. *Illustrated Anatomy of the Head and Neck*. 6th ed. St. Louis: Elsevier; 2021.)

1.11 (From Fehrenbach MJ, Herring SW. *Illustrated Anatomy of the Head and Neck*. 6th ed. St. Louis: Elsevier; 2021.)

1.12 (From Fehrenbach MJ, Herring SW. *Illustrated Anatomy of the Head and Neck*. 6th ed. St. Louis: Elsevier; 2021.)

Chapter 2

2.1 (From Fehrenbach MJ, Herring SW. *Illustrated Anatomy of the Head and Neck*. 6th ed. St. Louis: Elsevier; 2021.)

2.2 (From Fehrenbach MJ, Herring SW. *Illustrated Anatomy of the Head and Neck*. 6th ed. St. Louis: Elsevier; 2021.)

2.9 (From Fehrenbach MJ, Herring SW. *Illustrated Anatomy of the Head and Neck*. 6th ed. St. Louis: Elsevier; 2021.)

2.10 (From Fehrenbach MJ, Herring SW. *Illustrated Anatomy of the Head and Neck*. 6th ed. St. Louis: Elsevier; 2021.)

2.11 (From Fehrenbach MJ, Herring SW. *Illustrated Anatomy of the Head and Neck*. 6th ed. St. Louis: Elsevier; 2021.)

2.12 (From Fehrenbach MJ, Herring SW. *Illustrated Anatomy of the Head and Neck*. 6th ed. St. Louis: Elsevier; 2021.)

2.14 (From Fehrenbach MJ, Herring SW. *Illustrated Anatomy of the Head and Neck*. 6th ed. St. Louis: Elsevier; 2021.)

2.16 (From Fehrenbach MJ, Herring SW. *Illustrated Anatomy of the Head and Neck*. 6th ed. St. Louis: Elsevier; 2021.)

2.17 (From Fehrenbach MJ, Herring SW. *Illustrated Anatomy of the Head and Neck*. 6th ed. St. Louis: Elsevier; 2021.)

2.18 (From Fehrenbach MJ, Herring SW. *Illustrated Anatomy of the Head and Neck*. 6th ed. St. Louis: Elsevier; 2021.)

Chapter 6

6.27 (Courtesy M. J. Fehrenbach, RDH, MS.)

Chapter 7

7.6 (From Lowe JS, Anderson PG. *Stevens and Lowe's Human Histology*. 5th ed. St. Louis: Elsevier; 2020.)

Chapter 8

8.10 A (From Applegate EJ. *The Anatomy and Physiology Learning System*. 4th ed. St. Louis: Elsevier; 2011.)

Chapter 11

11.7 A and B (From Fehrenbach MJ, Herring SW. *Illustrated Anatomy of the Head and Neck*. 6th ed. St. Louis: Elsevier; 2021.)

11.16A (Modified from Fehrenbach MJ, Herring SW. *Illustrated Anatomy of the Head and Neck*. 6th ed. St. Louis: Elsevier; 2021.)

11.19 (From Fehrenbach MJ, Herring SW. *Illustrated Anatomy of the Head and Neck*. 6th ed. St. Louis: Elsevier; 2021.)

11.21 (Modified from Fehrenbach MJ, Herring SW. *Illustrated Anatomy of the Head and Neck*. 6th ed. St. Louis: Elsevier; 2021.)

Chapter 14

14.14 (Courtesy M. J. Fehrenbach, RDH, MS.)
14.16 (Courtesy M. J. Fehrenbach, RDH, MS.)

Chapter 19

19.1 (From Fehrenbach MJ, Herring SW. *Illustrated Anatomy of the Head and Neck*. 6th ed. St. Louis: Elsevier; 2021.)

19.5 (From Fehrenbach MJ, Herring SW. *Illustrated Anatomy of the Head and Neck*, 6th ed. St. Louis: Elsevier; 2021.)

19.6 (From Fehrenbach MJ, Herring SW. *Illustrated Anatomy of the Head and Neck*. 6th ed. St. Louis: Elsevier; 2021.)

19.8 A and B (From Fehrenbach MJ, Herring SW. *Illustrated Anatomy of the Head and Neck*. 6th ed. St. Louis: Elsevier; 2021.)

Fill in the labeled areas to allow for **structure identification** using the figures from the associated textbook *per chapter*. This will be one of the initial steps in learning about these structures in more depth as a student dental professional. The **correct answers** can be obtained from comparing your answer fill-ins to the labels on numbered figures from the textbook. Feel free to add additional labeling and other notes as needed.

UNIT 1: OROFACIAL STRUCTURE

Chapter 1: Face and Neck Regions

1. Figure 1.1

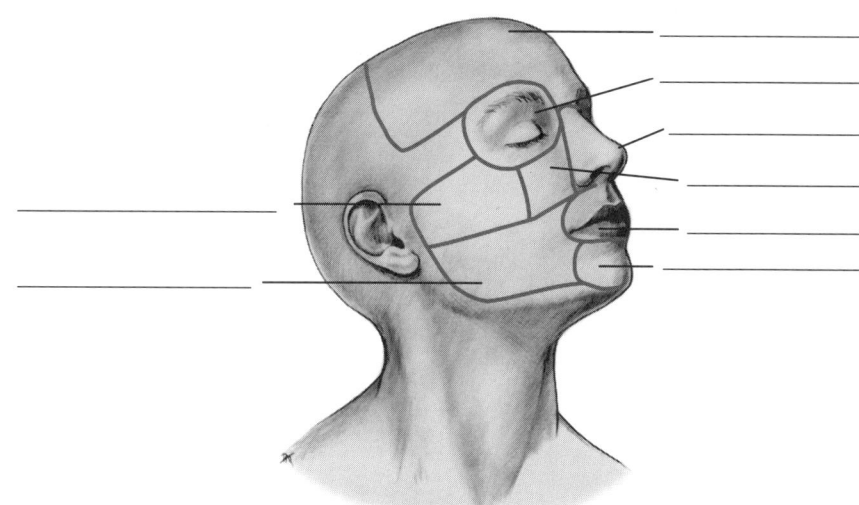

2. Figure 1.2, *A, B*

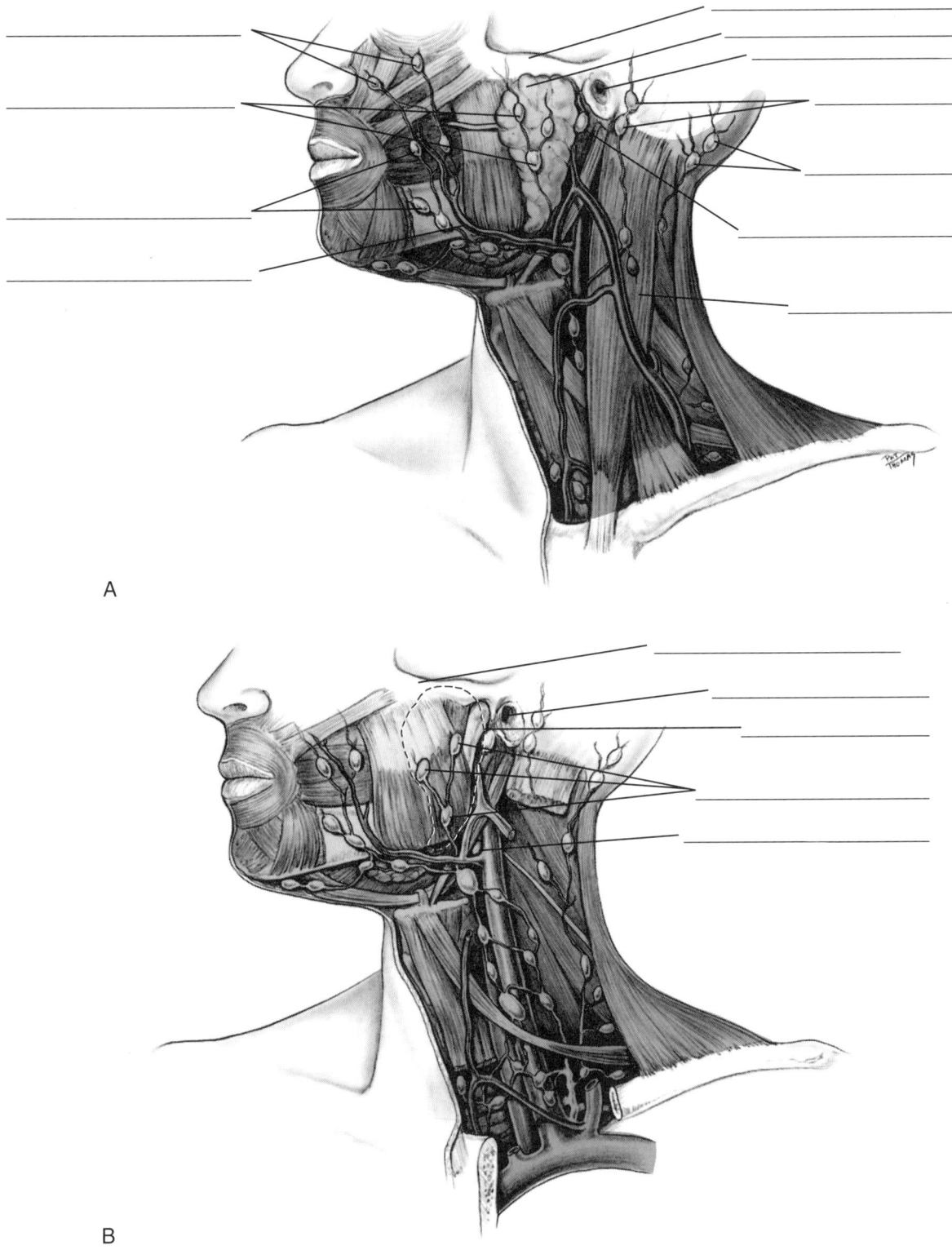

A

B

3. Figure 1.5

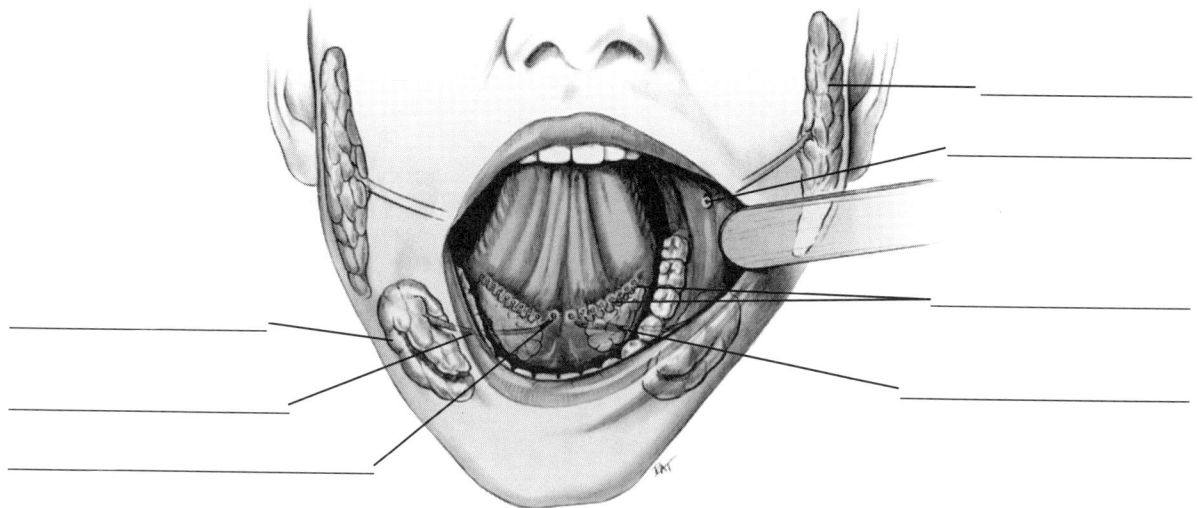

4. Figure 1.7, *A, B*

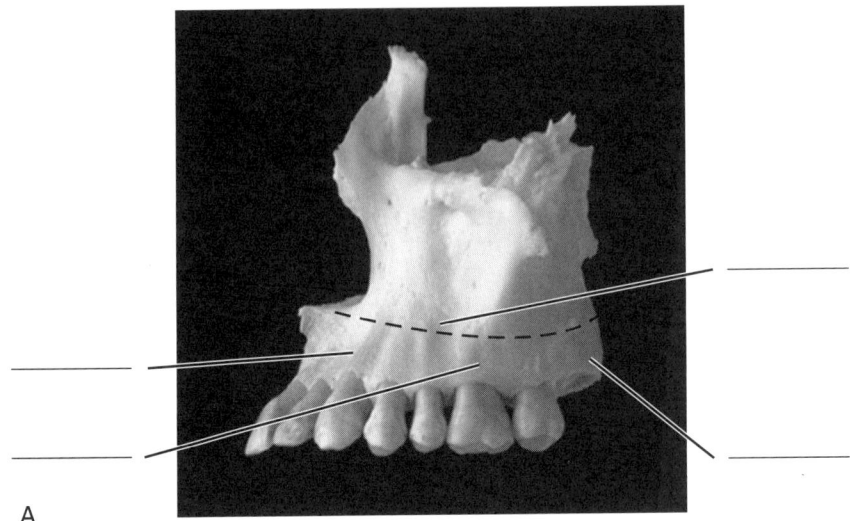

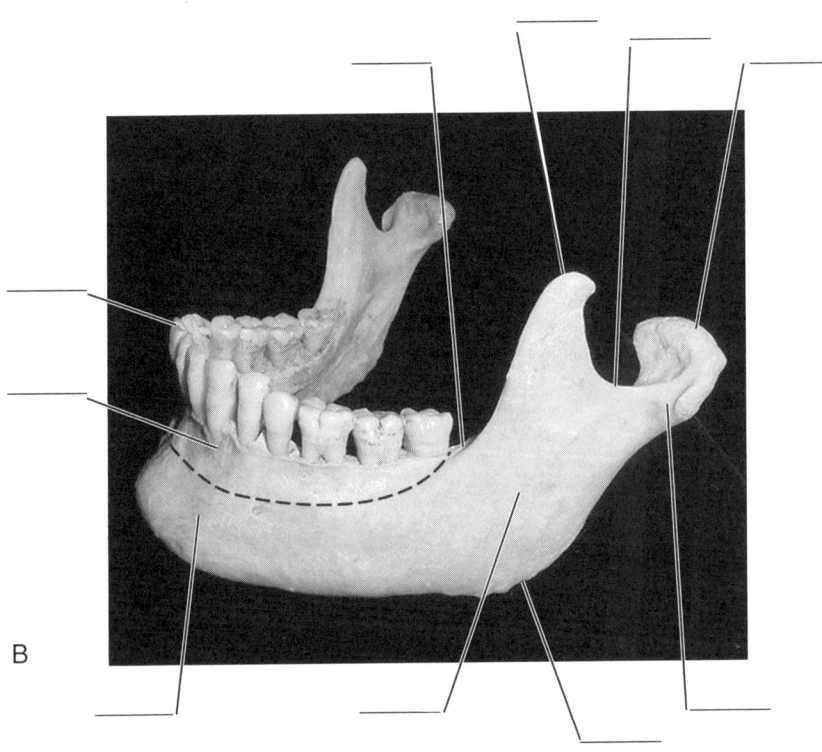

5. Figure 1.10

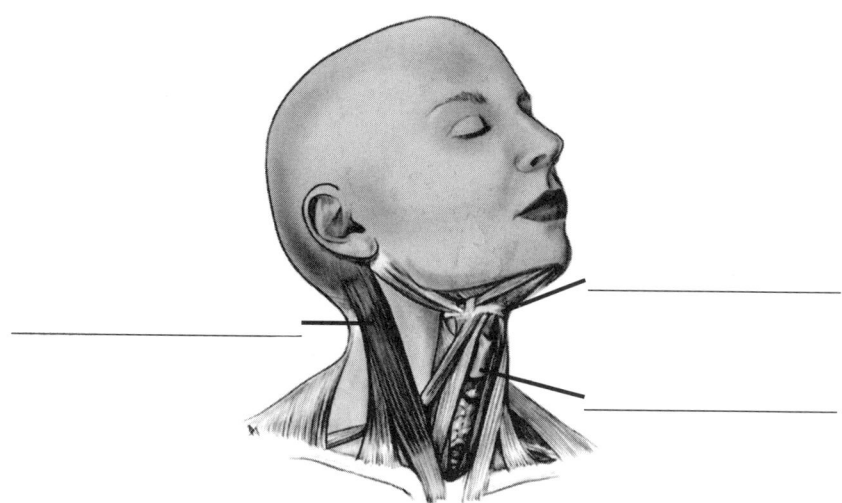

6. Figure 1.11, *A, B*

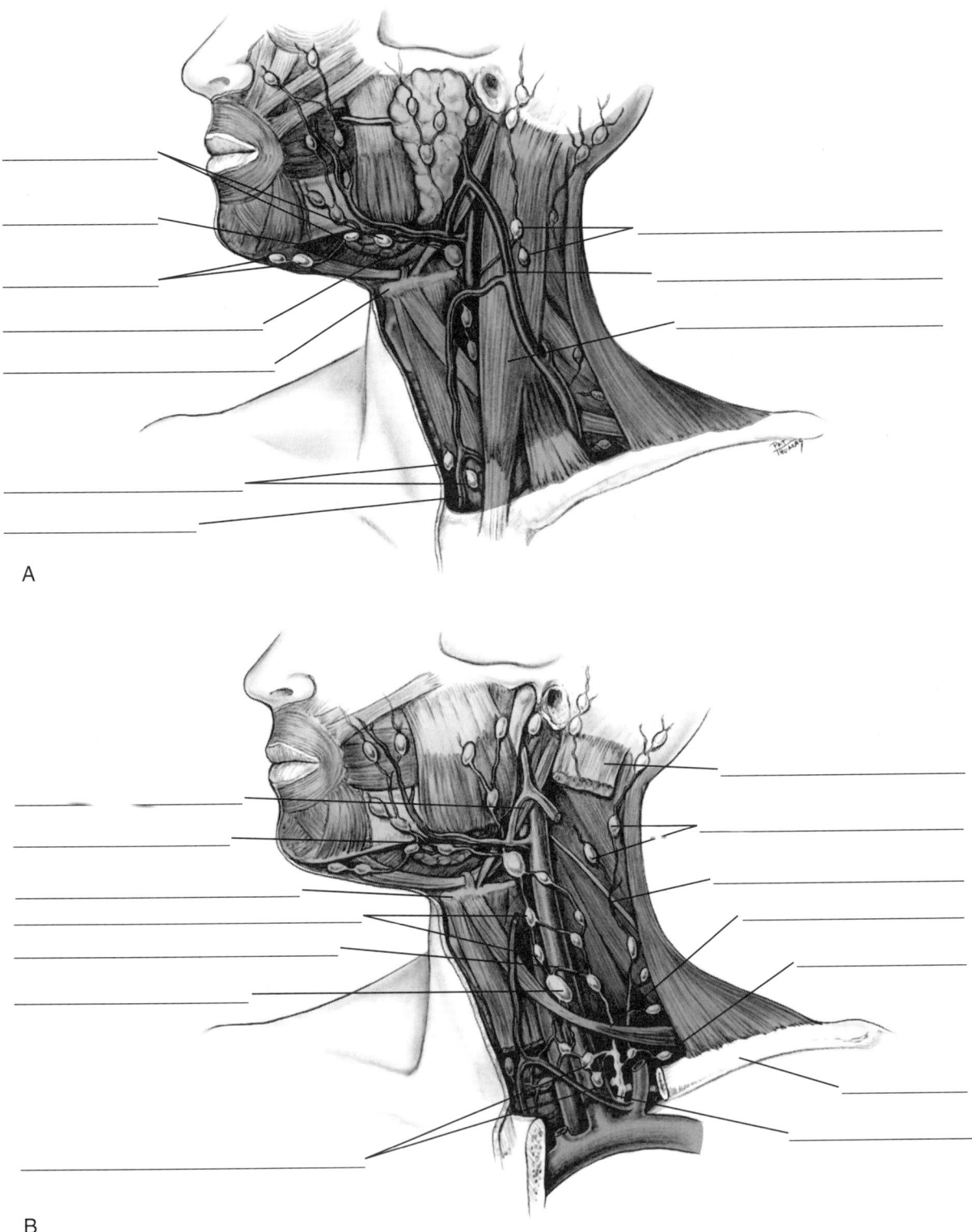

7. Figure 1.12

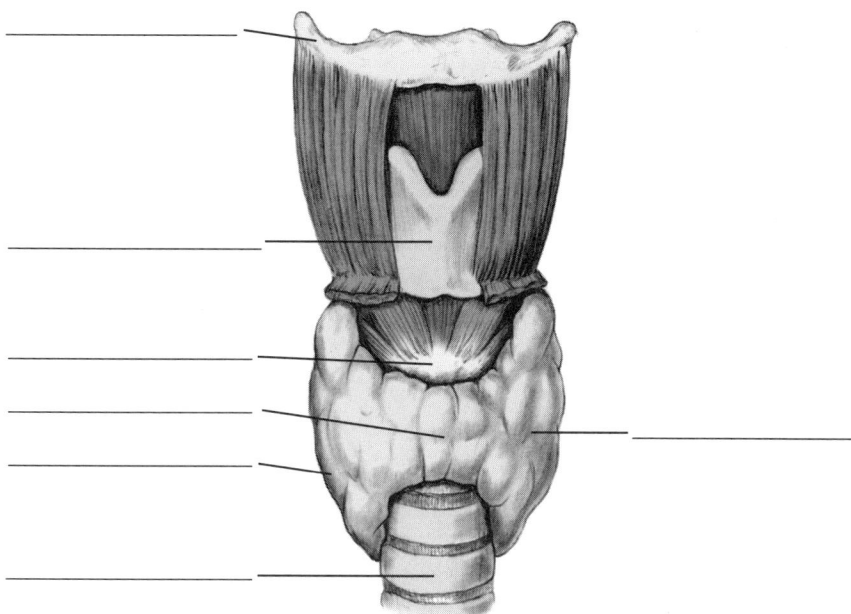

Chapter 2: Oral Cavity and Pharynx

8. Figure 2.1

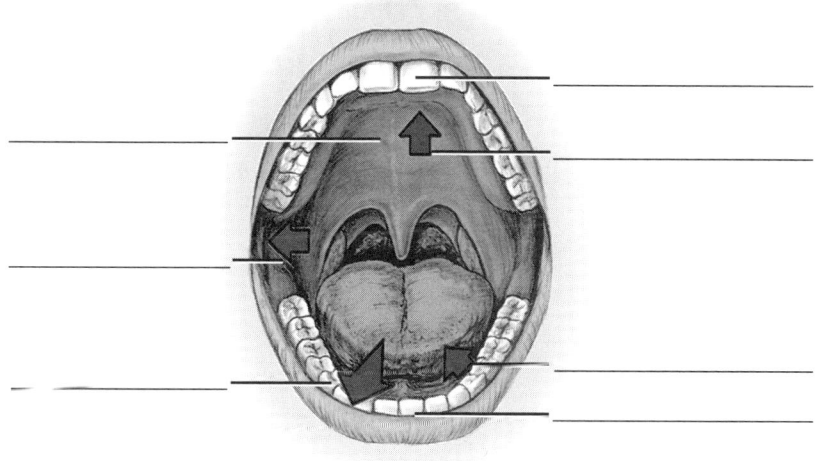

9. Figure 2.2

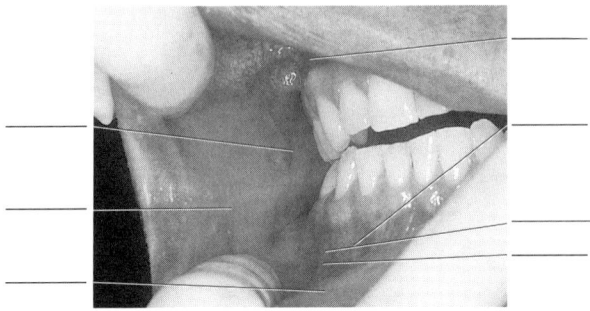

10. Figure 2.4

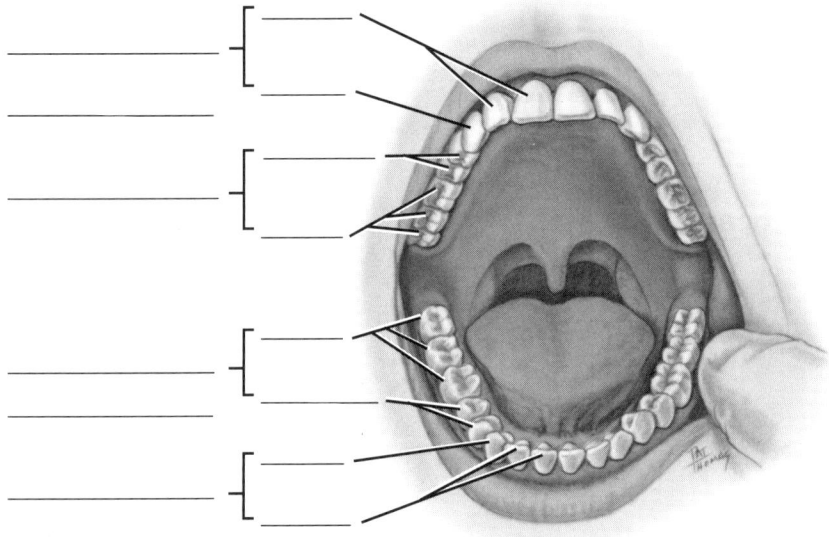

11. Figure 2.6

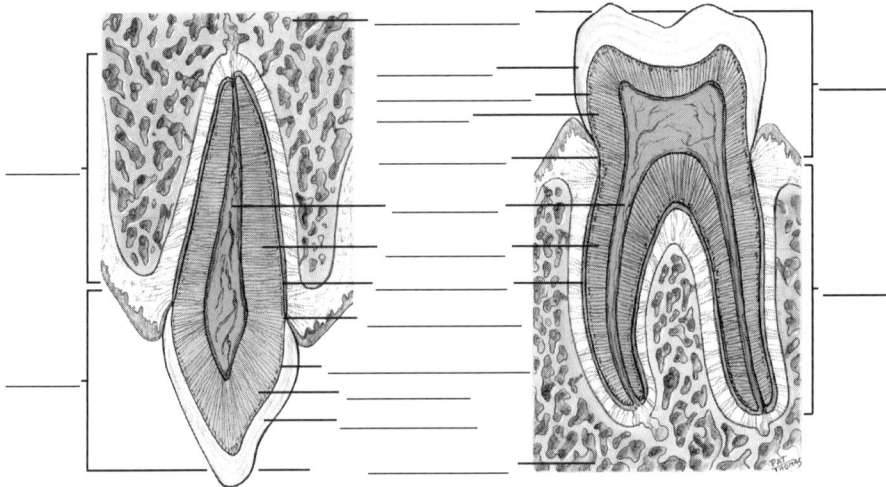

12. Figures 2.9 and 2.10

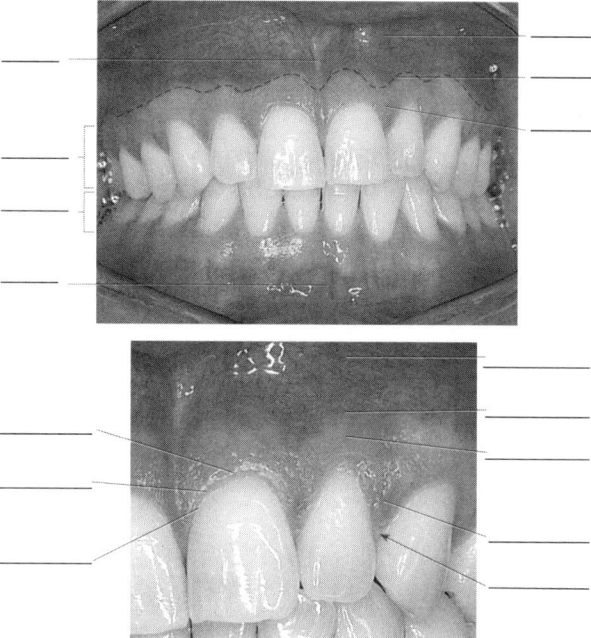

13. Figure 2.11

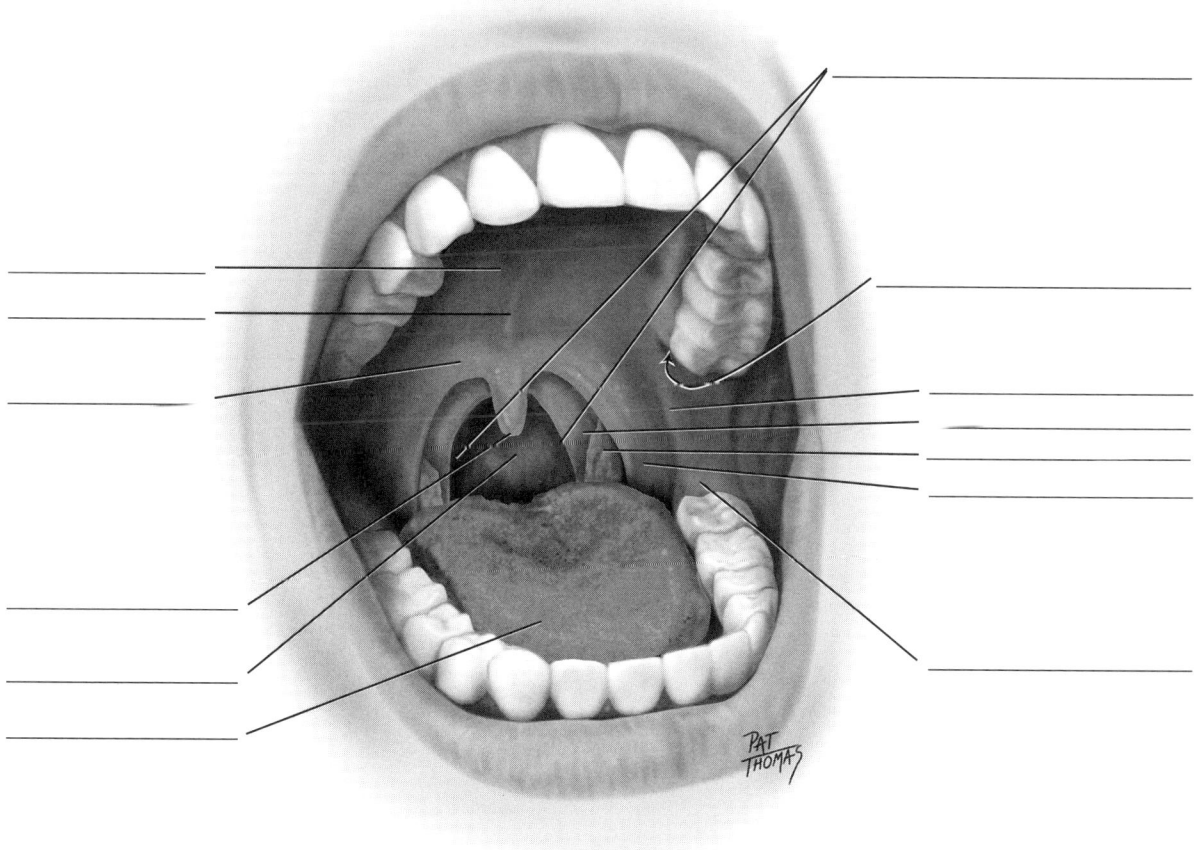

14. Figure 2.12

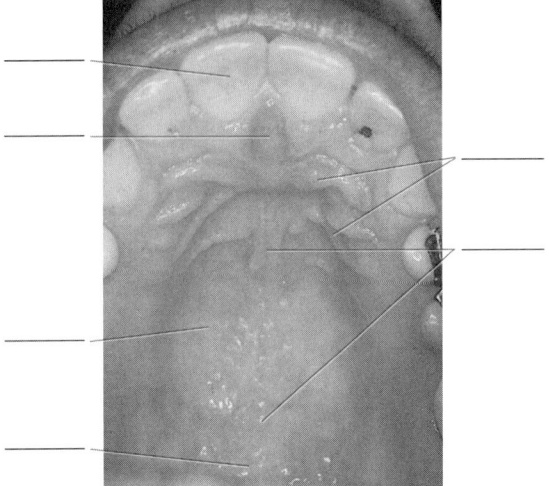

15. Figure 2.14

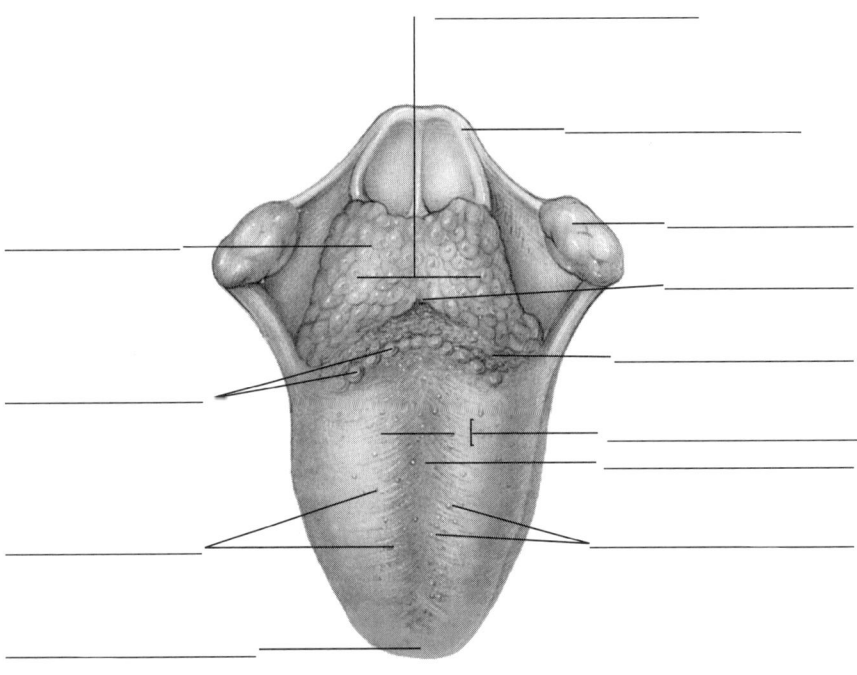

16. Figure 2.16

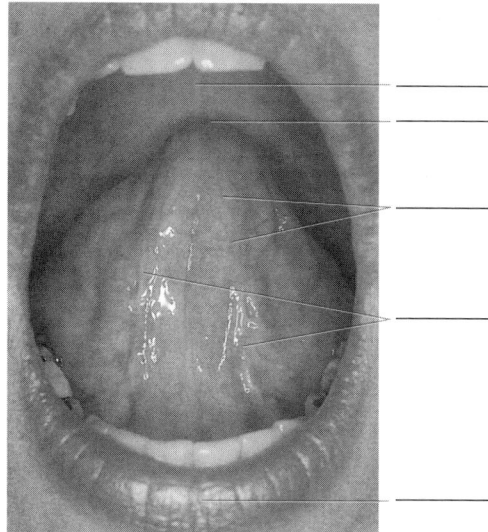

17. Figure 2.17

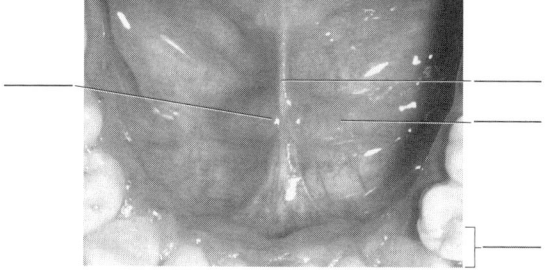

18. Figure 2.18

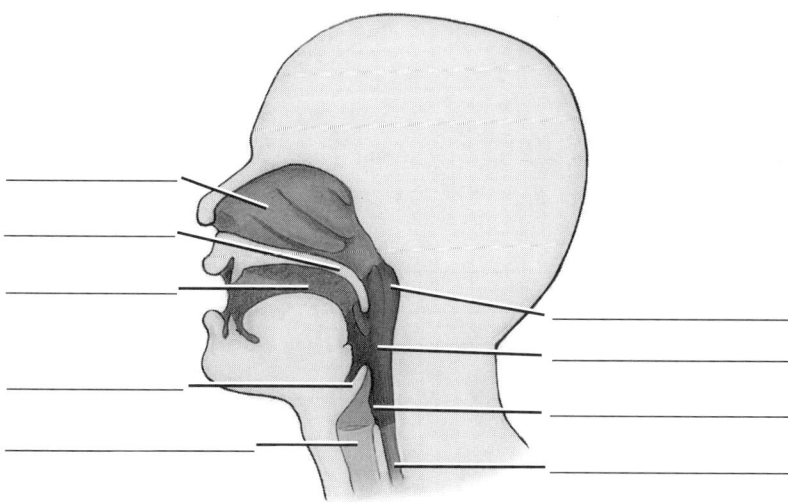

UNIT 2: DENTAL EMBRYOLOGY

Chapter 3: Prenatal Development

1. Figure 3.4, *B*

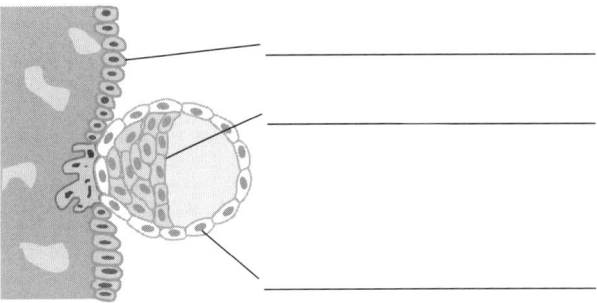

2. Figure 3.6, *A*

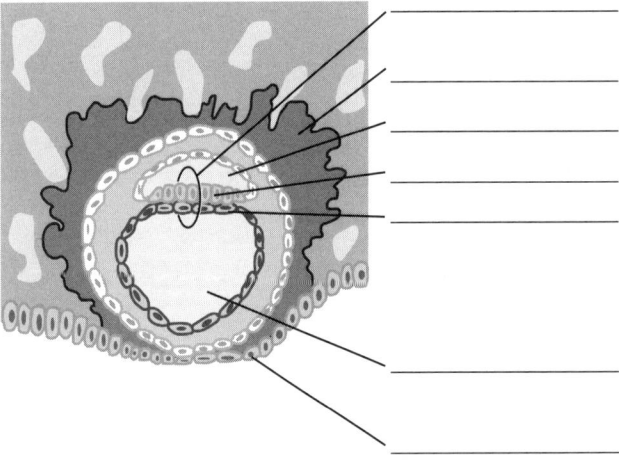

3. Figure 3.7, *C*

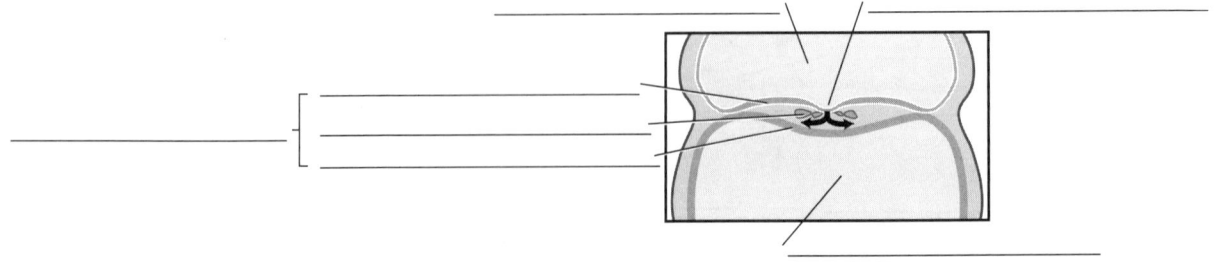

4. Figure 3.8

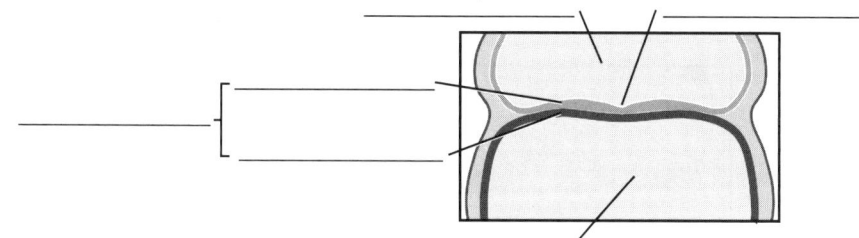

5. Figure 3.9

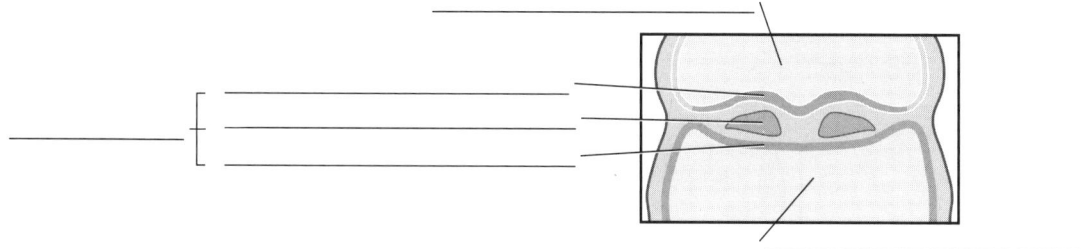

6. Figure 3.10, *A, B, C*

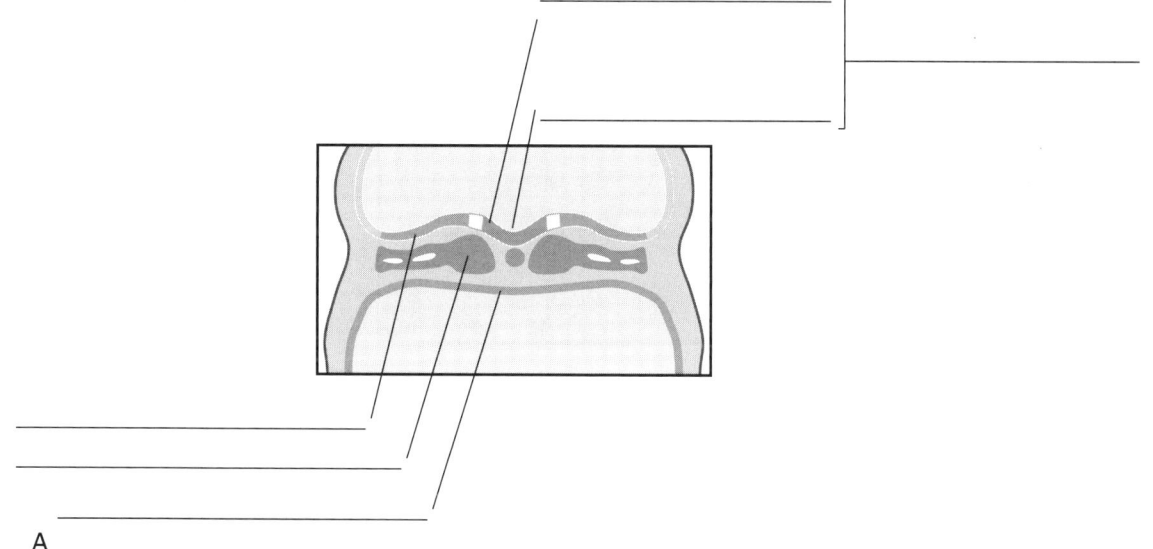

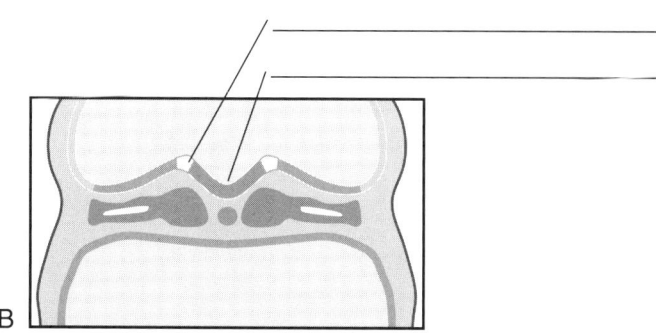

6. Figure 3.10, *A, B, C* (continued)

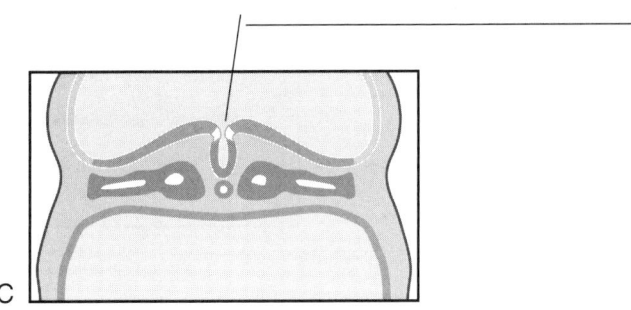

7. Figure 3.12, *A, B*

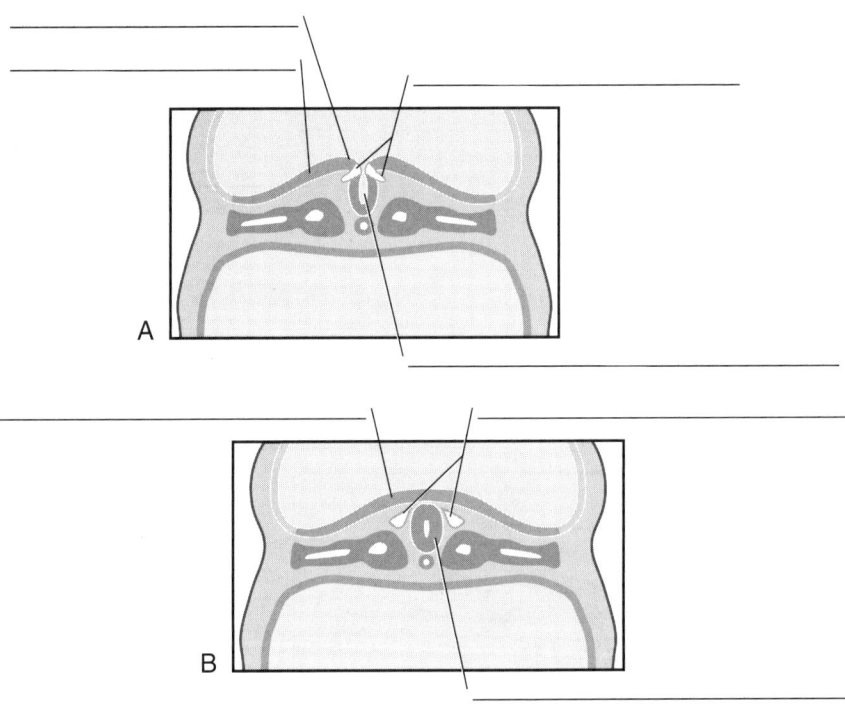

8. Figure 3.13, *A, B*

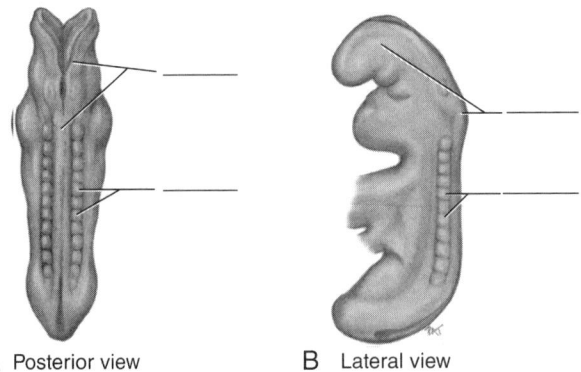

9. Figure 3.14, *B, C*

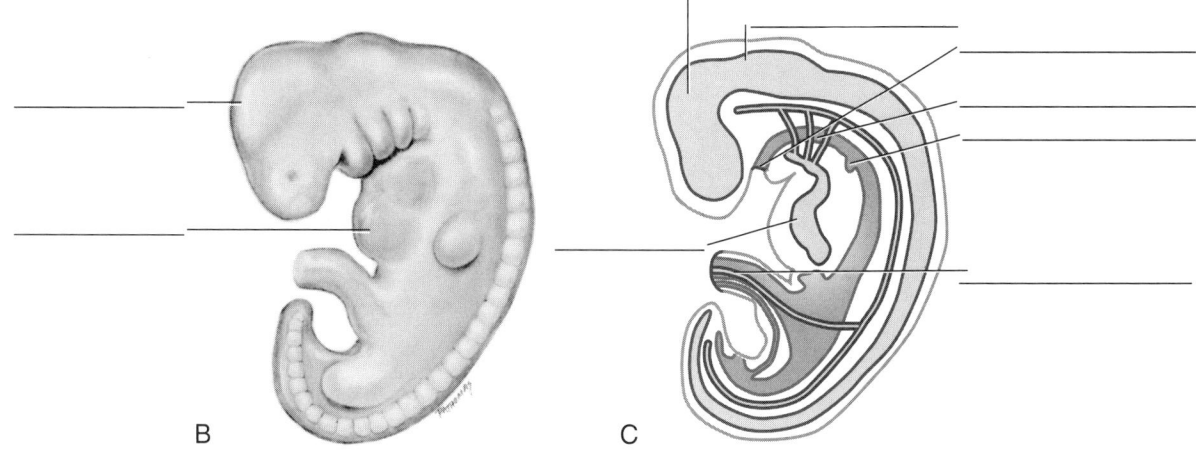

Chapter 4: Face and Neck Development

10. Figure 4.2

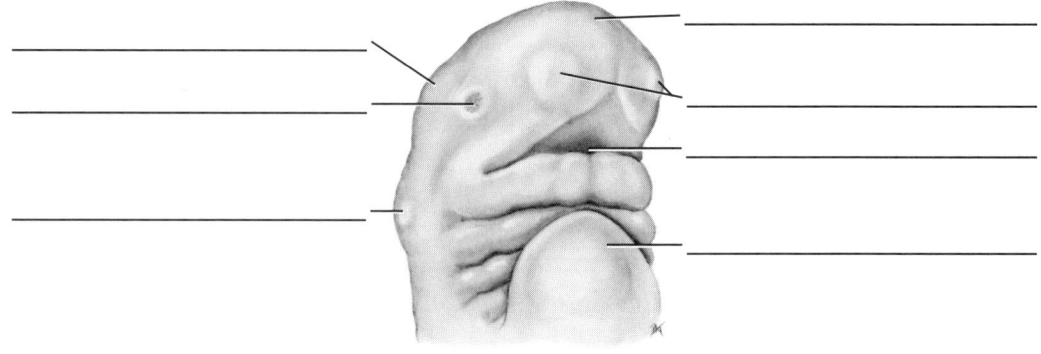

11. Figure 4.3

Embryonic derivatives

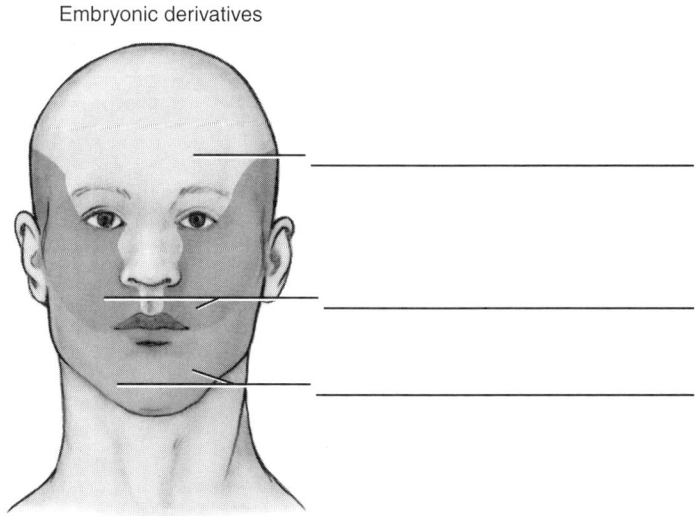

12. Figure 4.5

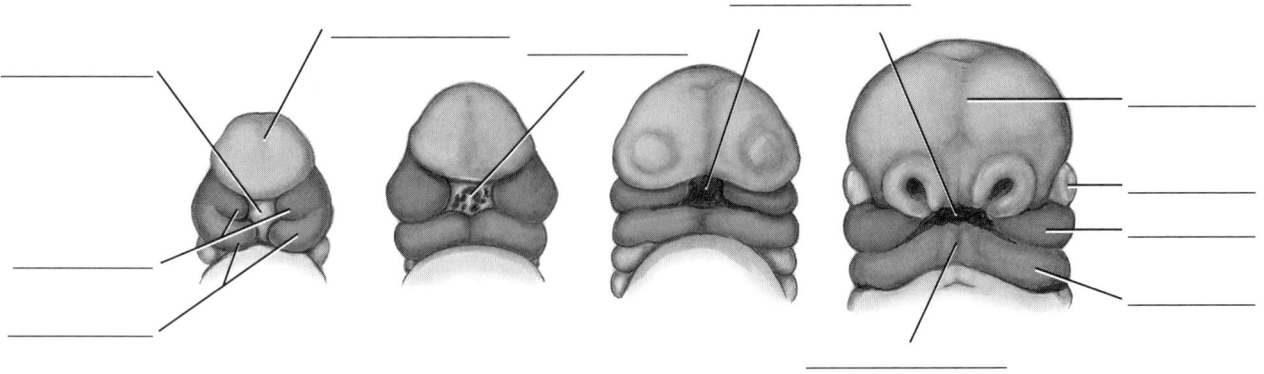

13. Figure 4.6

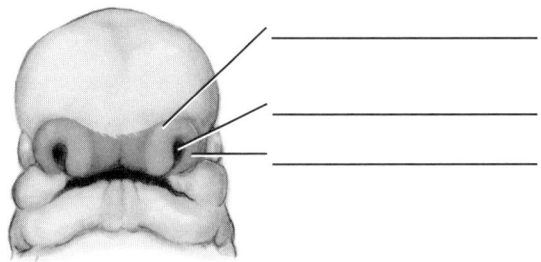

14. Figure 4.7, *B, C*

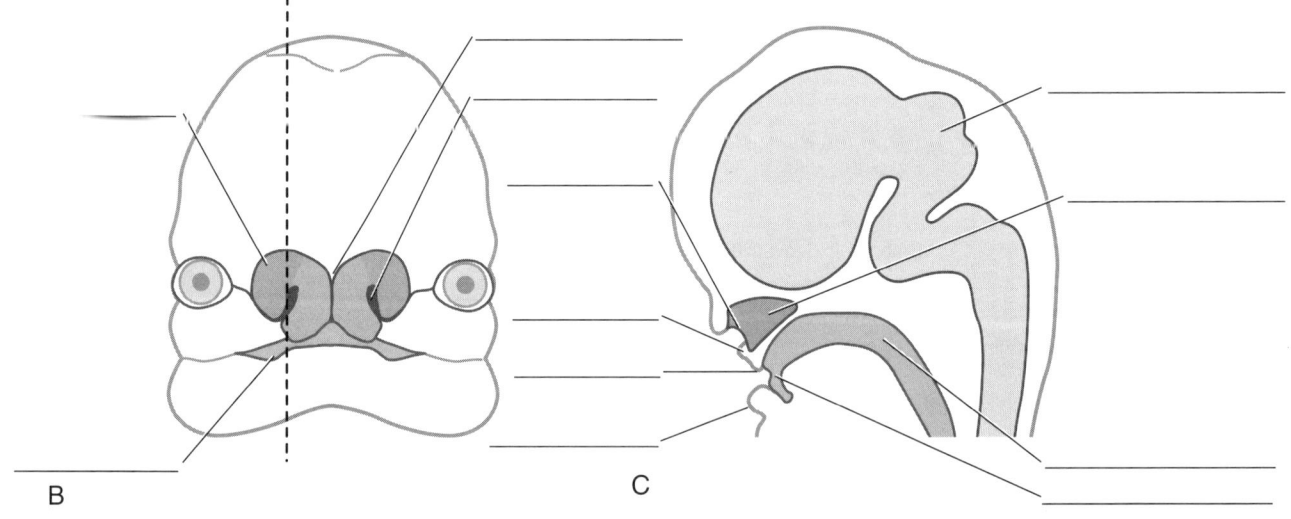

15. Figure 4.9, *B*

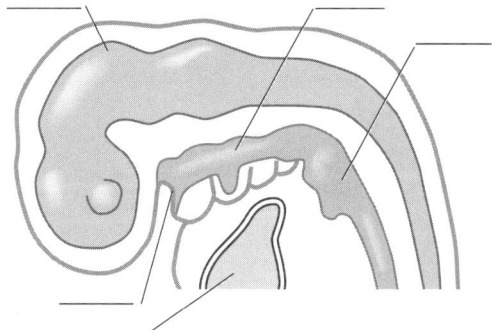

16. Figure 4.10, *B, C, D*

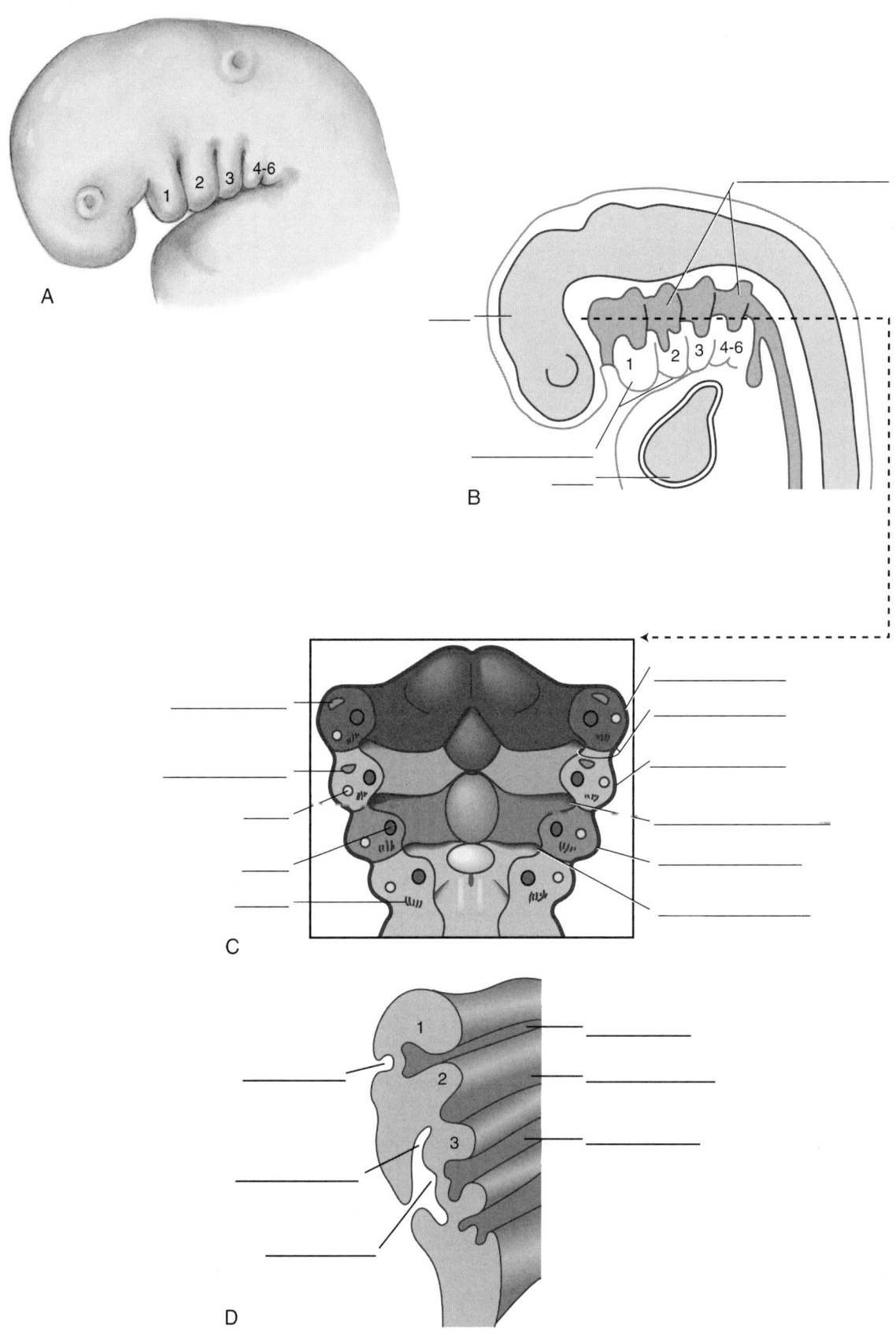

Chapter 5: Orofacial Development

17. Figure 5.1, *A, B*

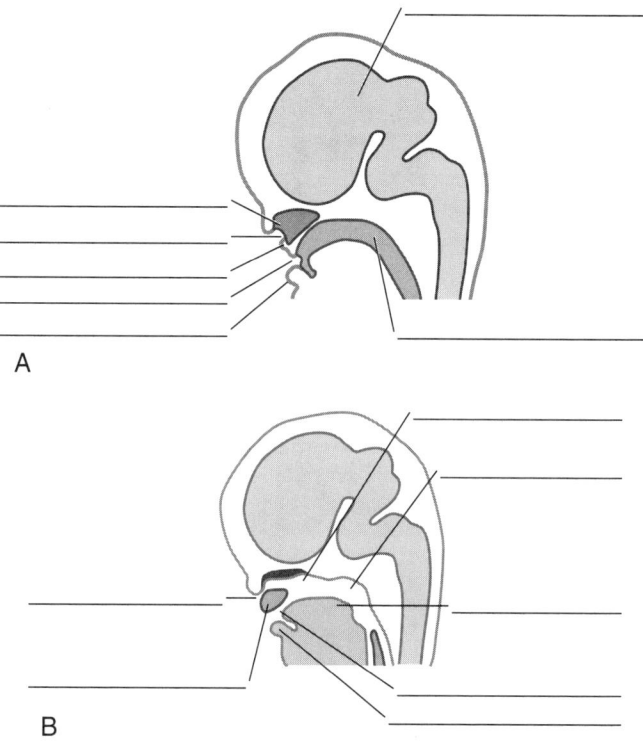

18. Figure 5.2, *A, C*

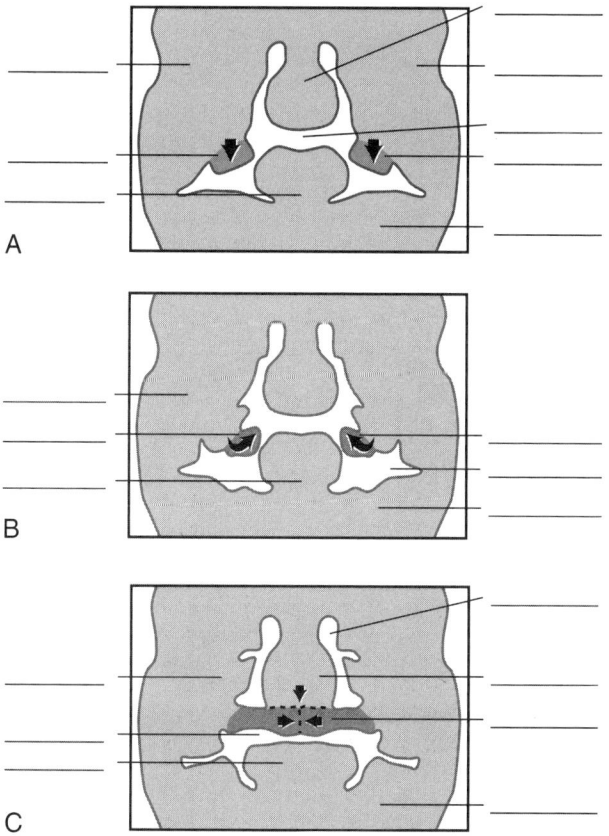

19. Figure 5.4, *B, C, D*

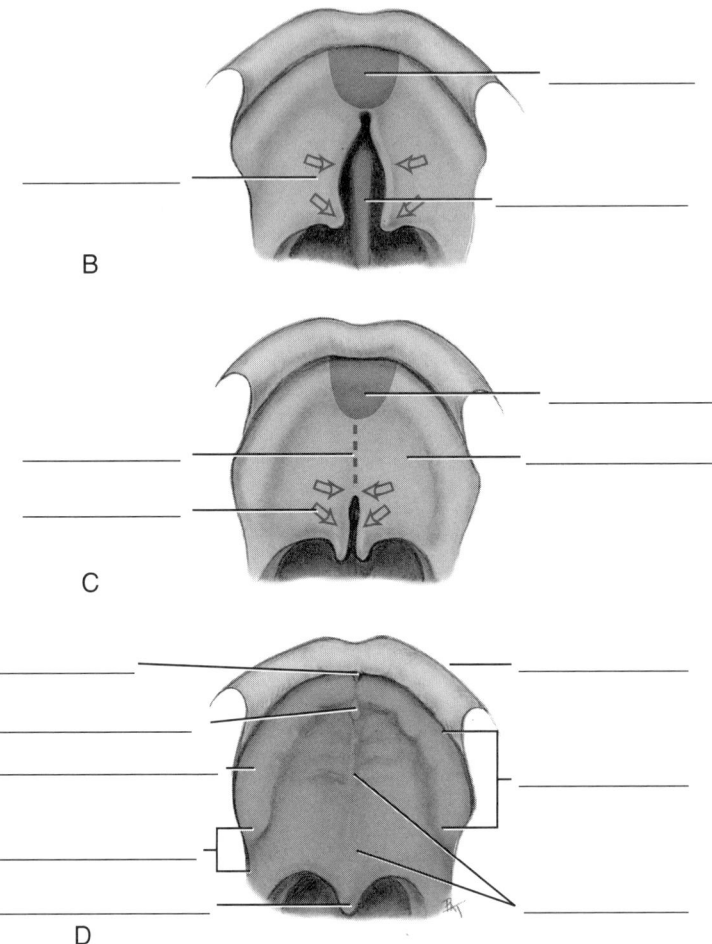

20. Figure 5.5, *A*

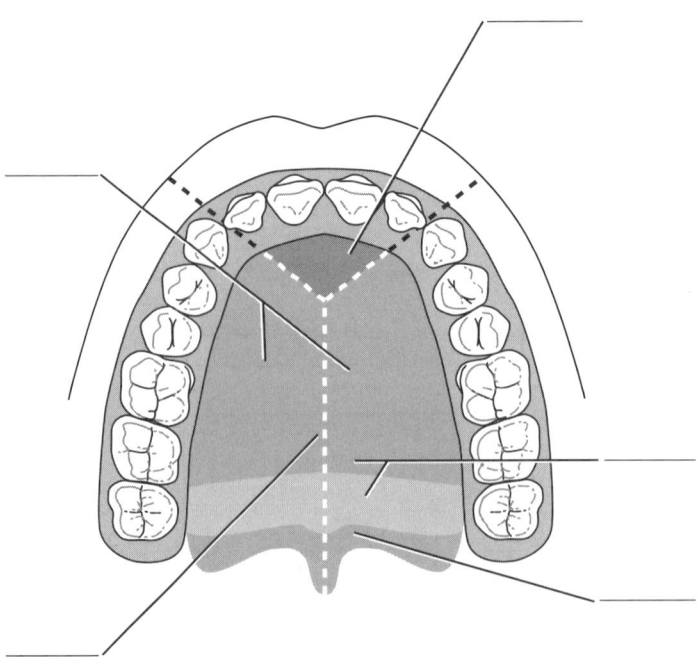

21. Figure 5.8, *A, B, C*

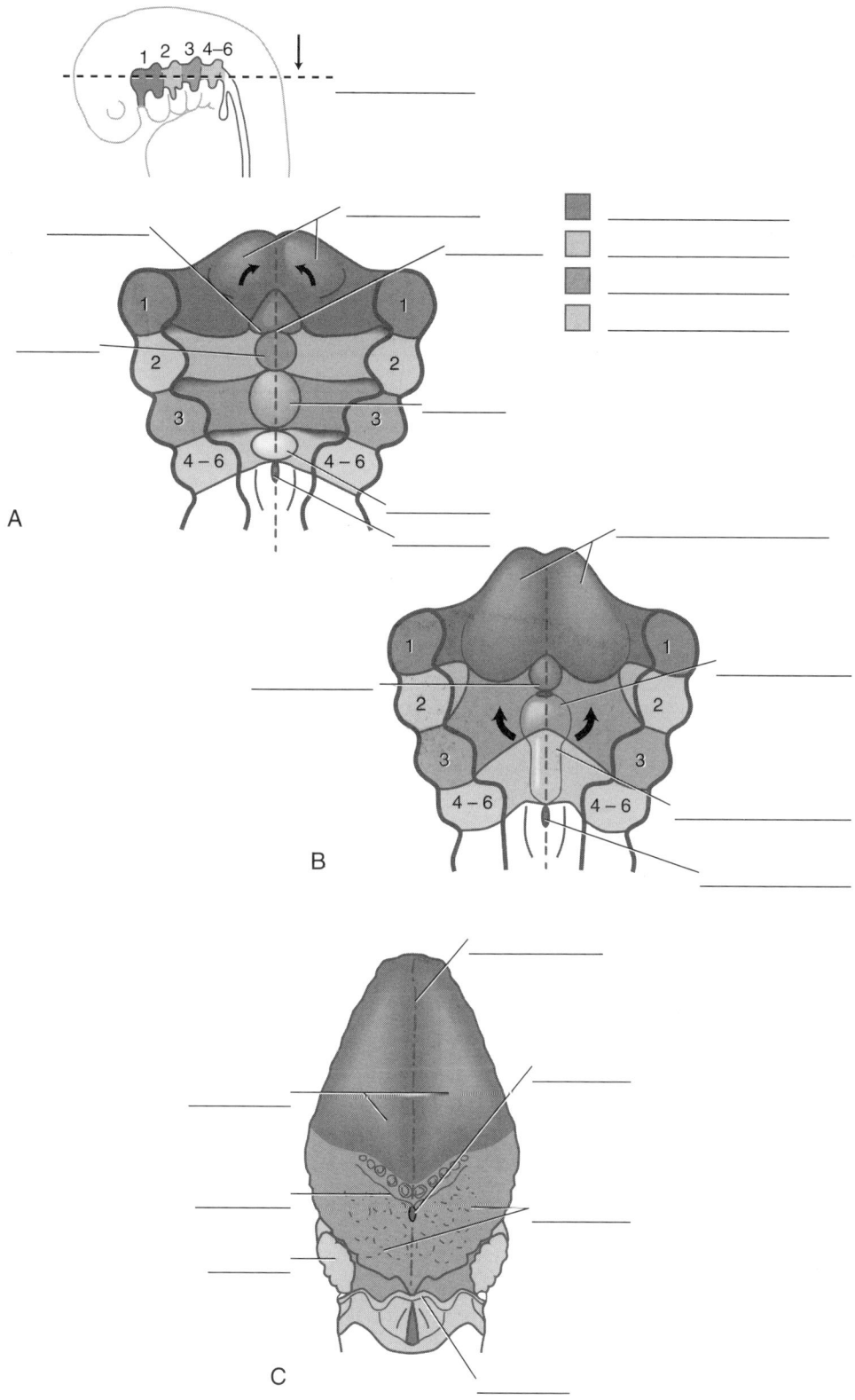

Chapter 6: Tooth Development and Eruption

22. Figure 6.1

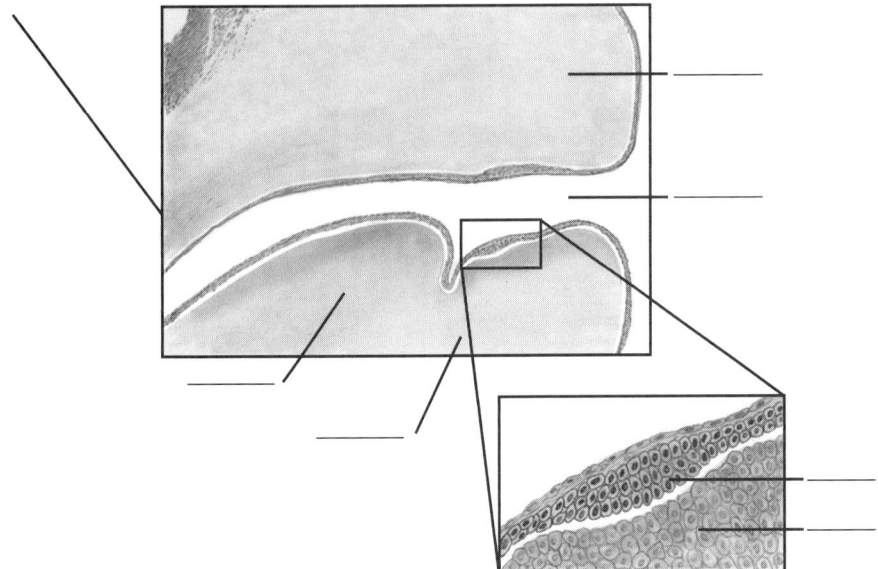

23. Figure 6.2

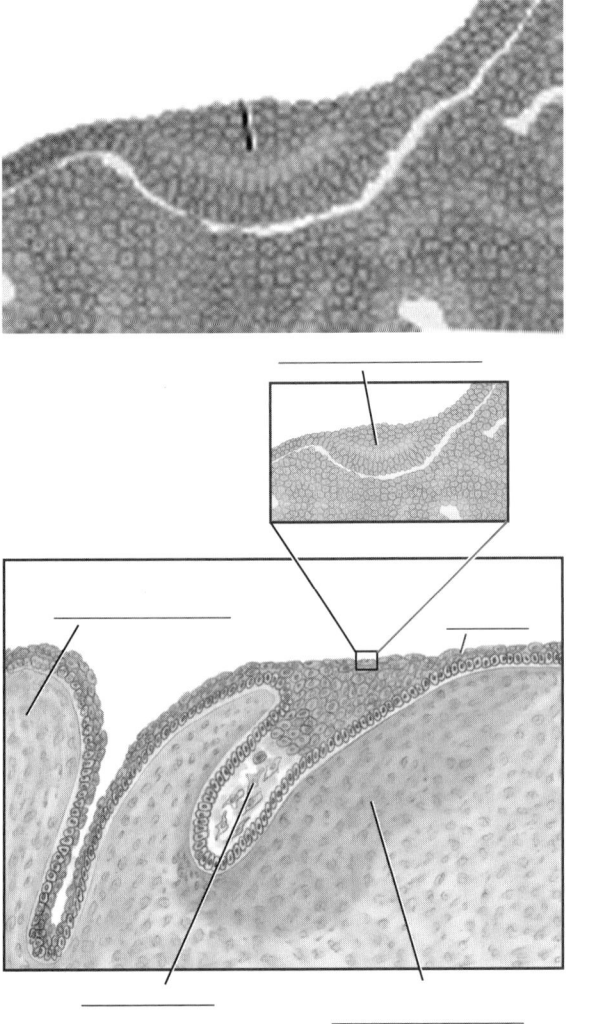

24. Figure 6.3

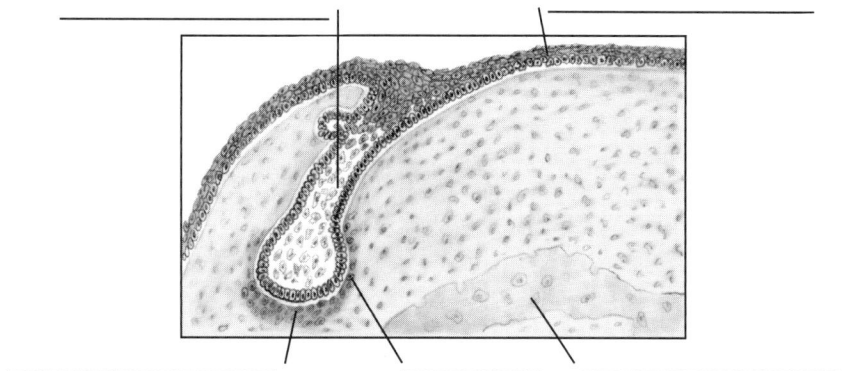

25. Figure 6.5

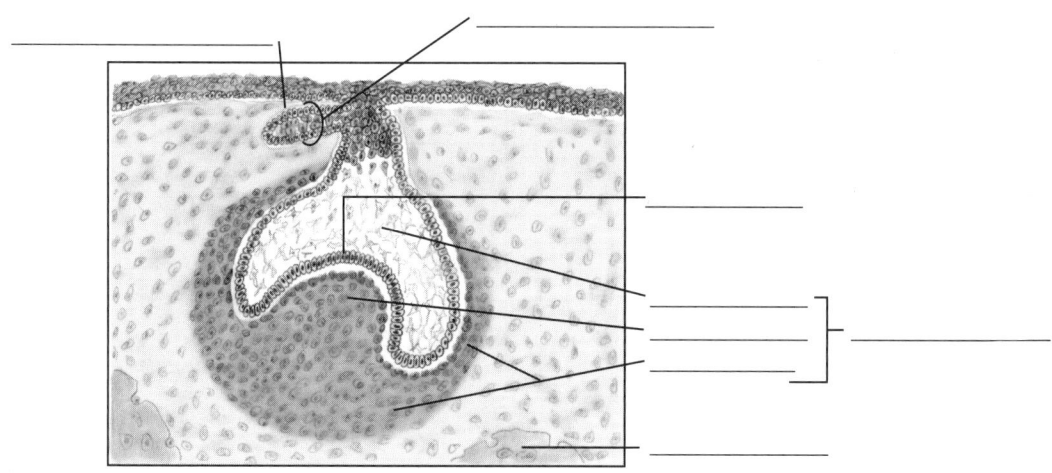

26. Figure 6.7

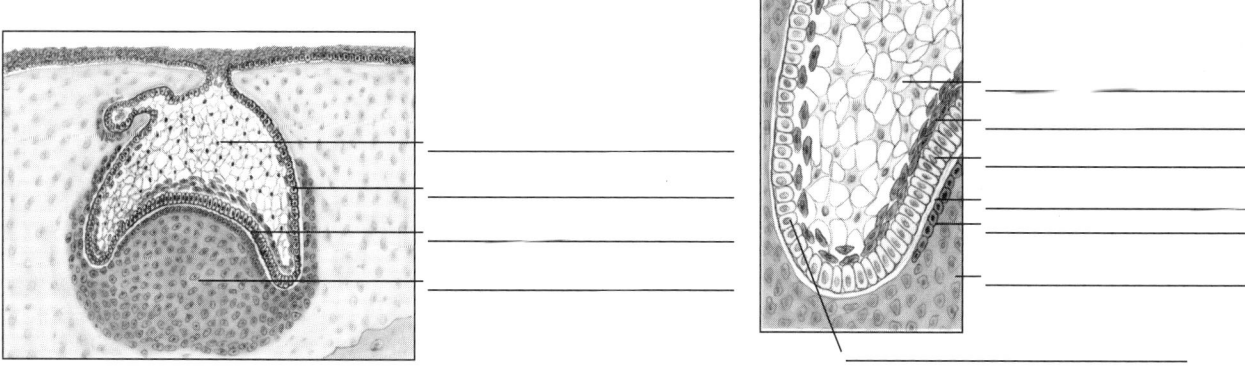

27. Figure 6.9, *A, B*

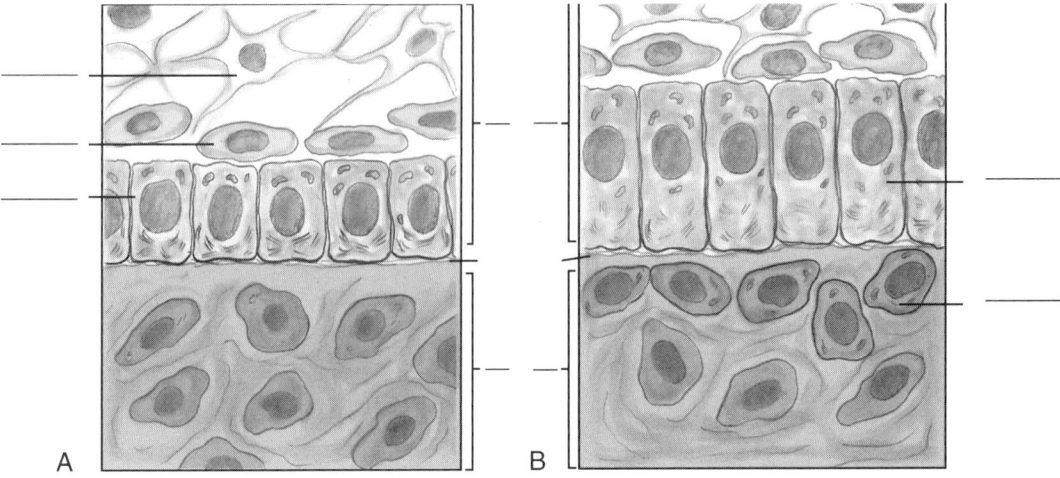

28. Figure 6.10, *A, B*

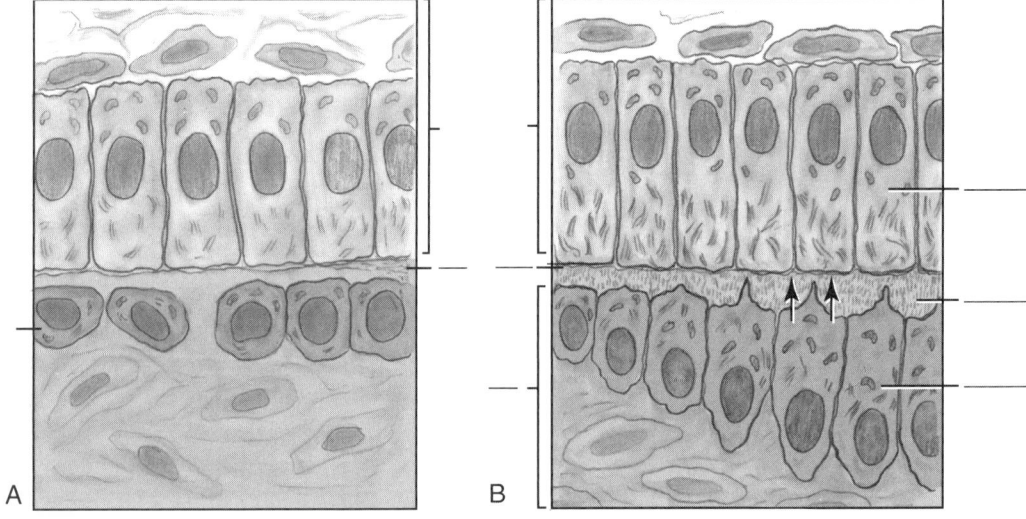

29. Figure 6.12

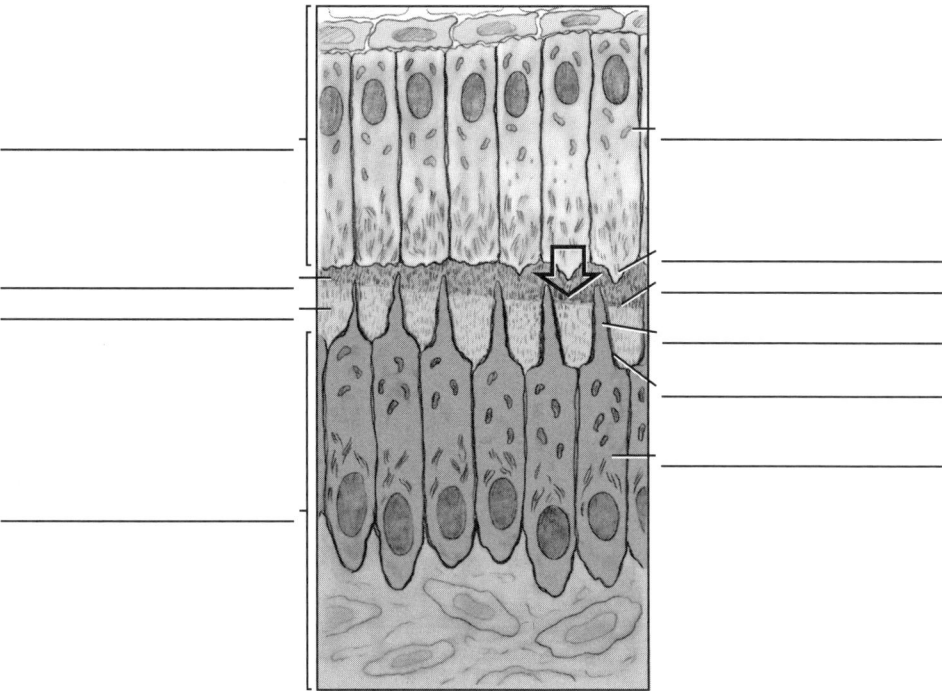

30. Figure 6.13

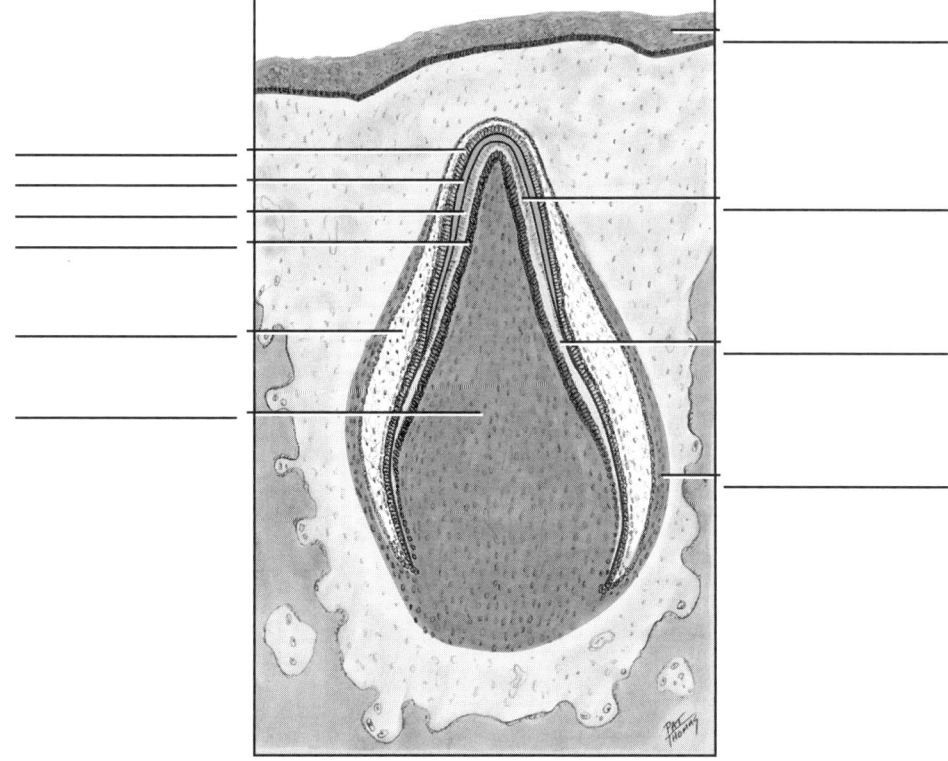

31. Figure 6.18, *A, B*

32. Figure 6.19

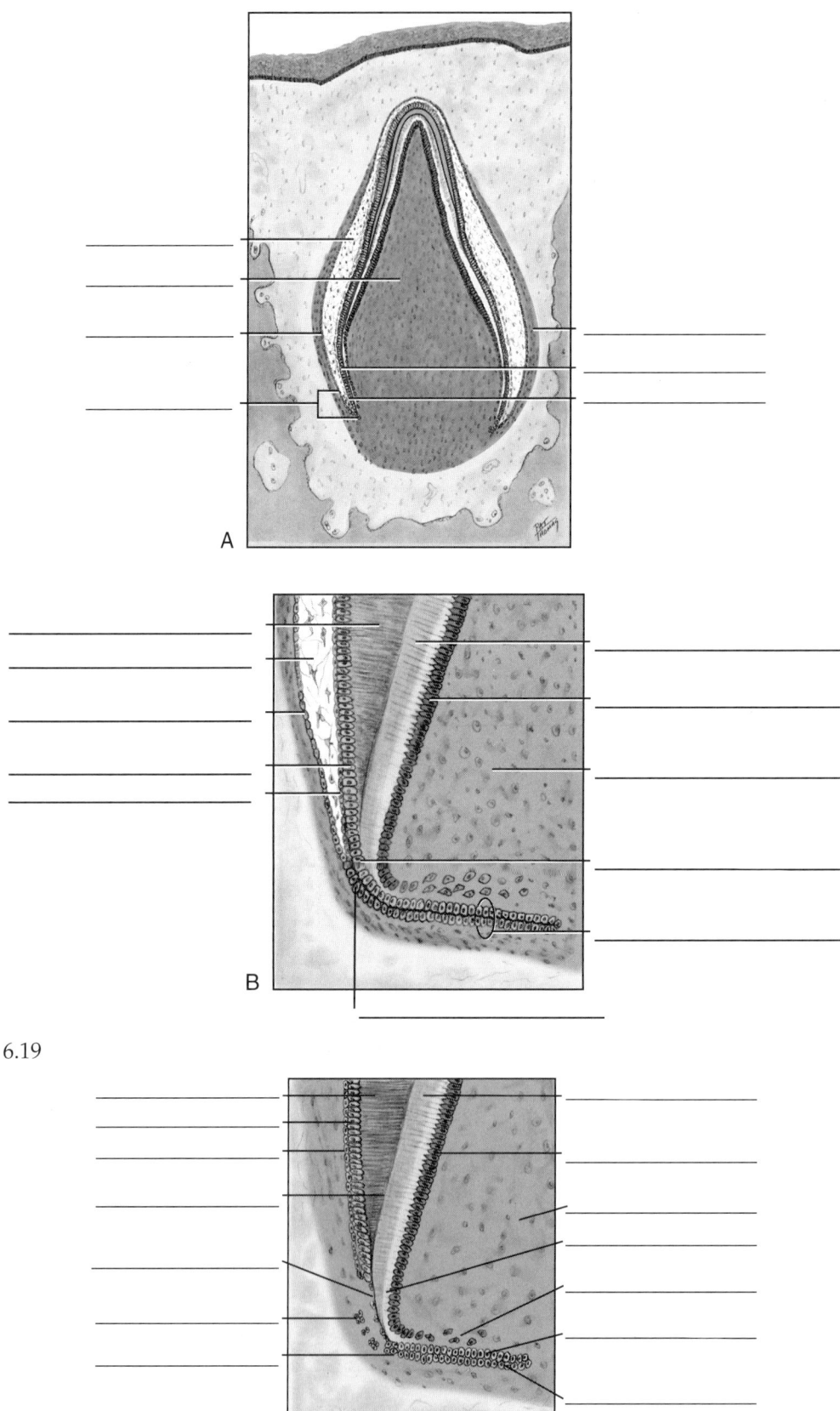

33. Figure 6.20

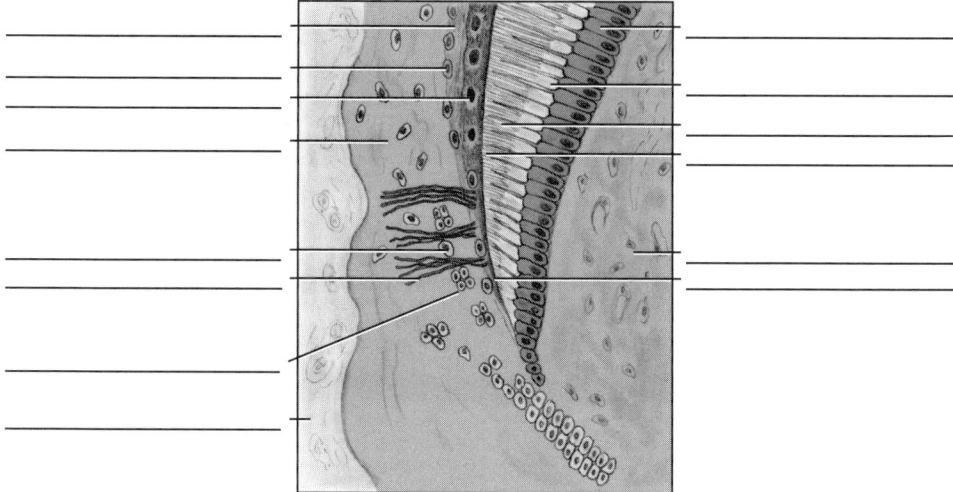

34. Figure 6.23

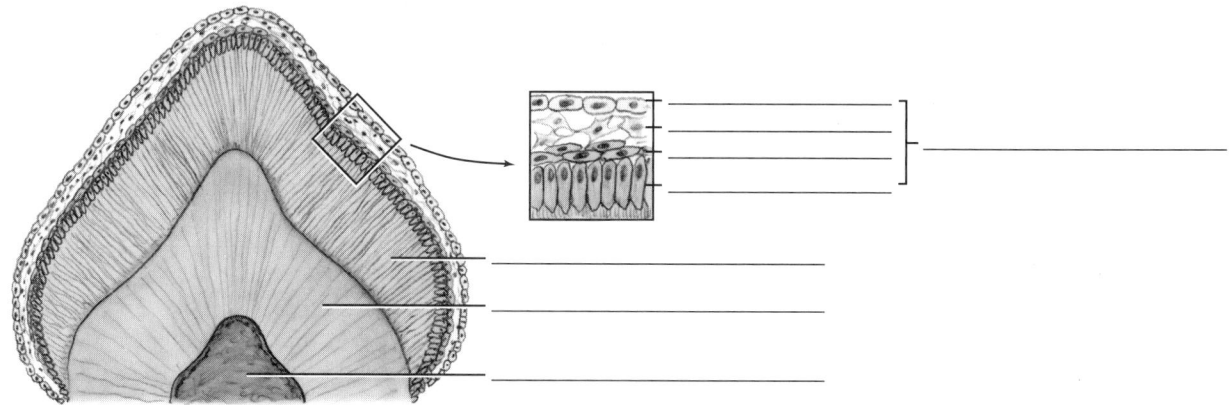

35. Figure 6.26

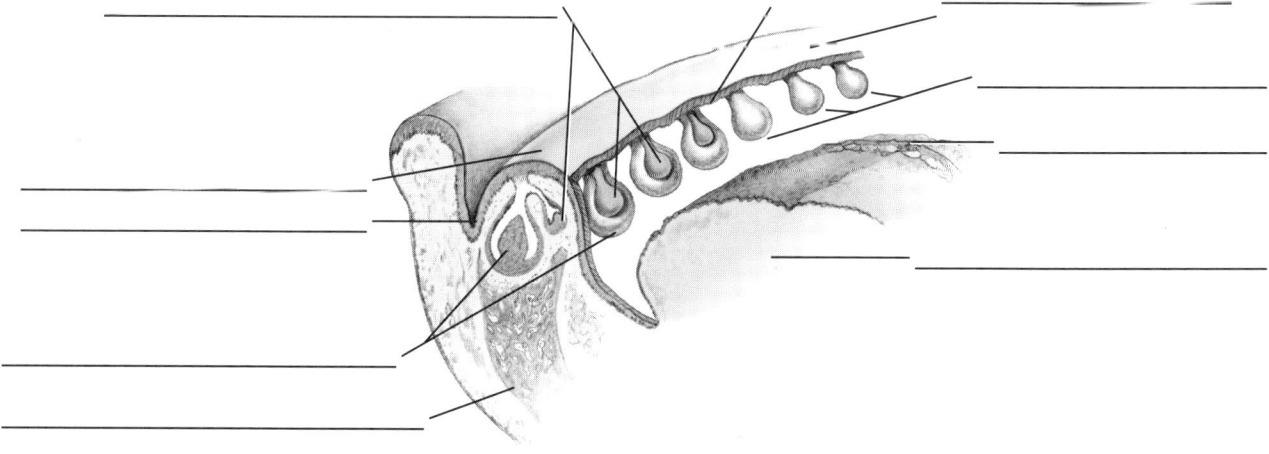

36. Figure 6.27, *B, C*

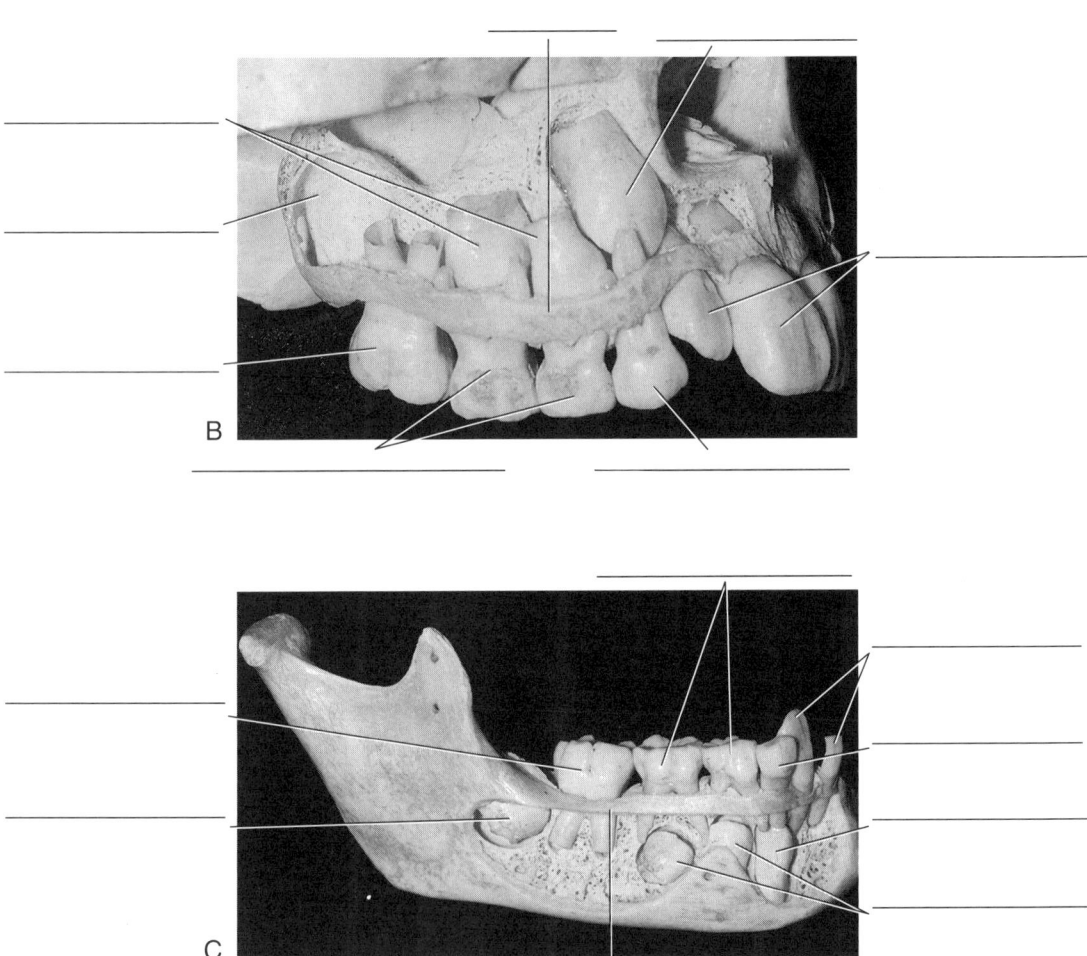

UNIT 3: DENTAL HISTOLOGY

Chapter 7: Basic Cell Properties and Processes

1. Figure 7.2

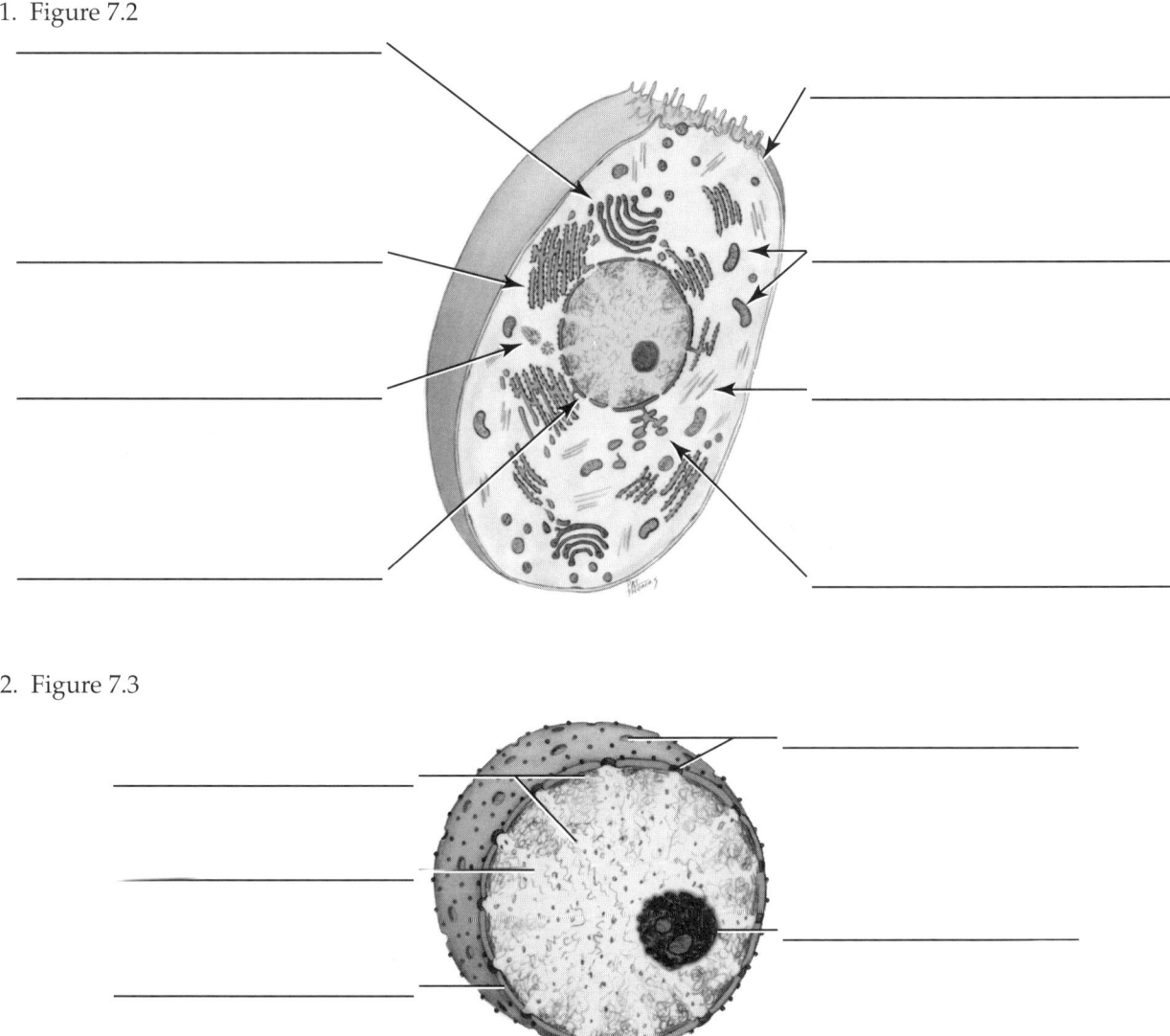

2. Figure 7.3

3. Figure 7.5, *A*

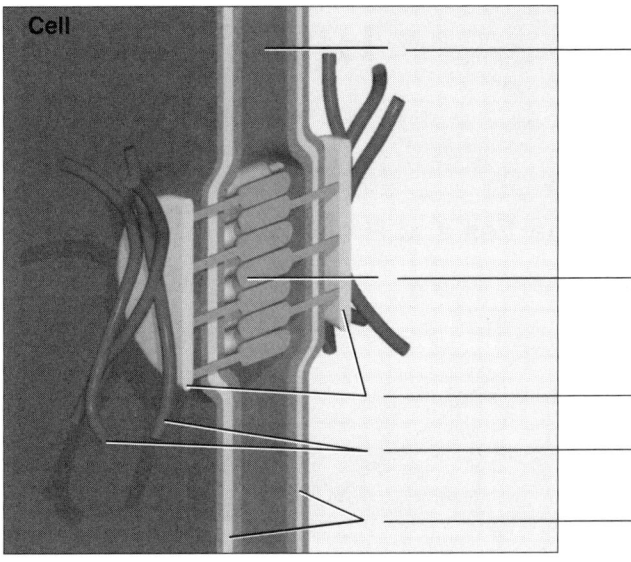

4. Figure 7.6, *A*

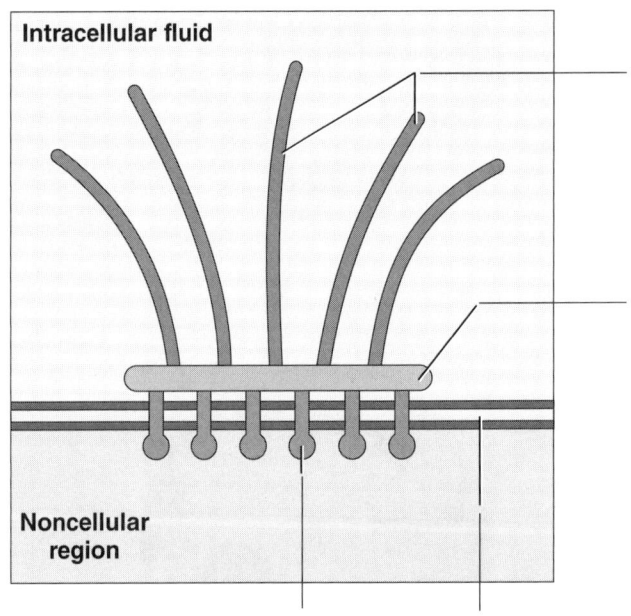

Chapter 8: Basic Tissue Properties and Processes

5. Figure 8.3

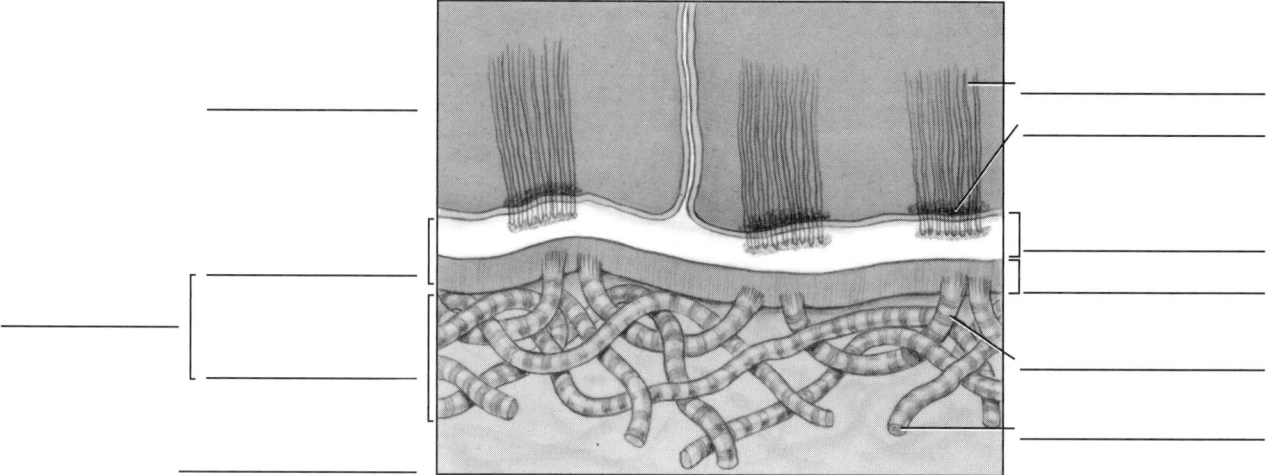

6. Figure 8.4, *A*

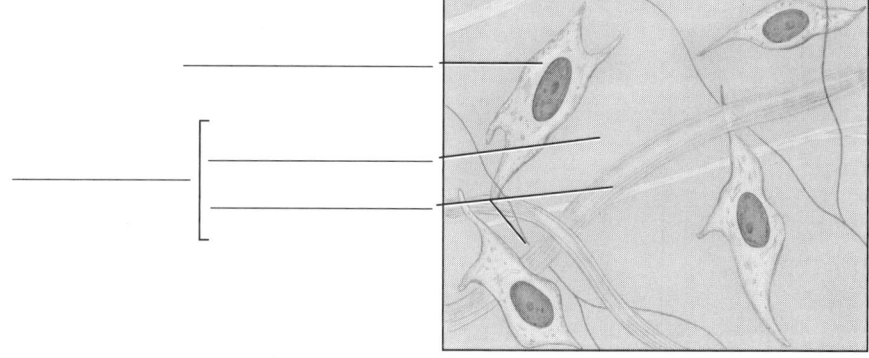

7. Figure 8.5

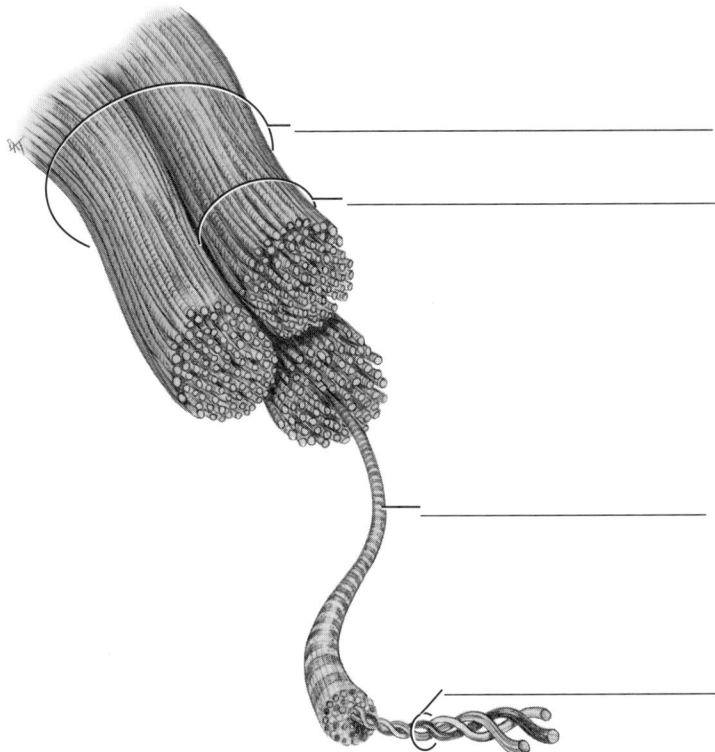

8. Figure 8.6

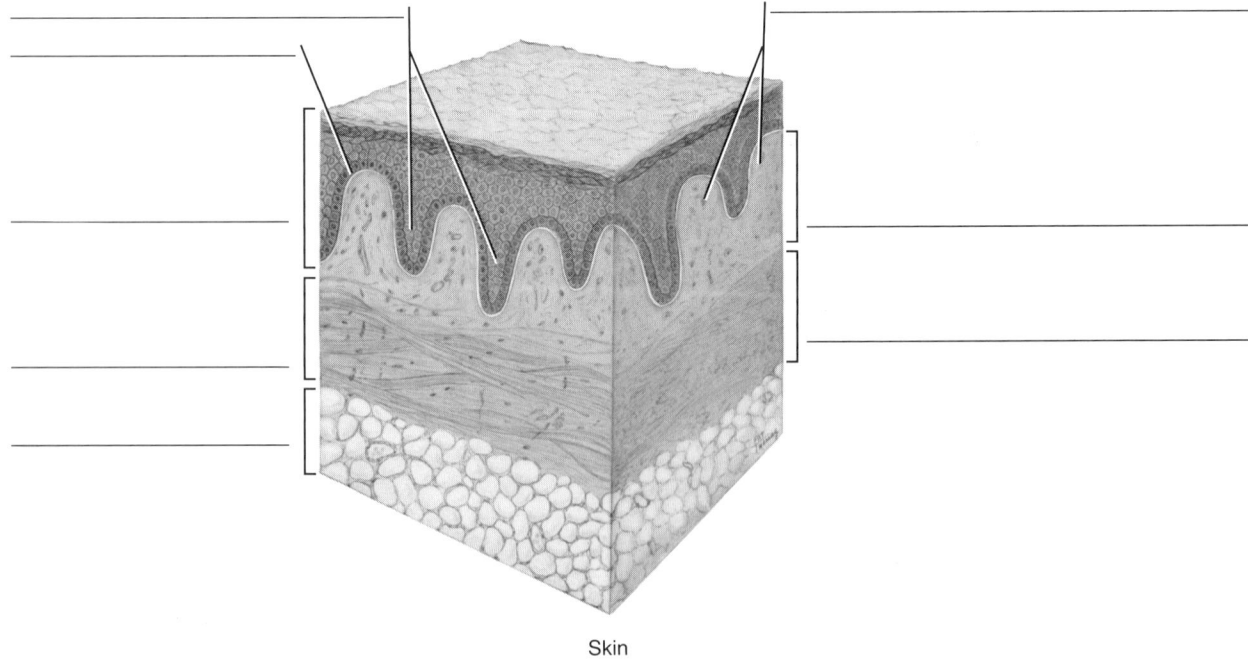

Skin

9. Figure 8.7

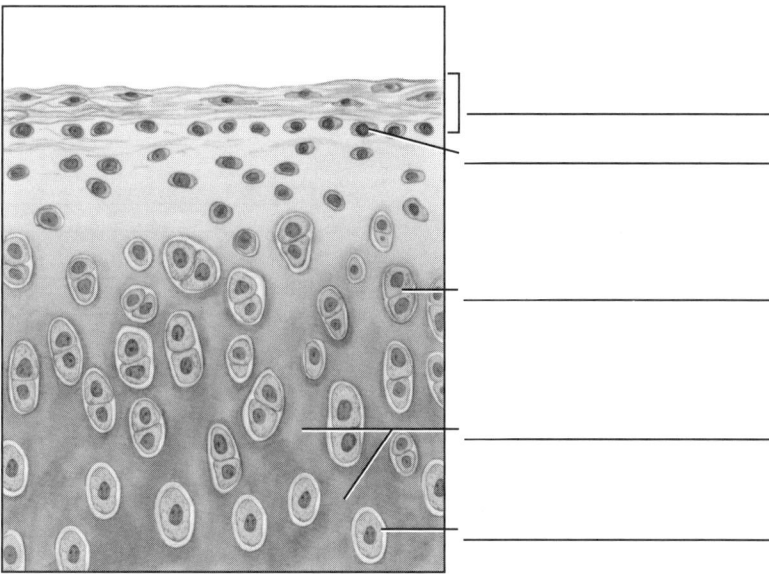

10. Figure 8.8

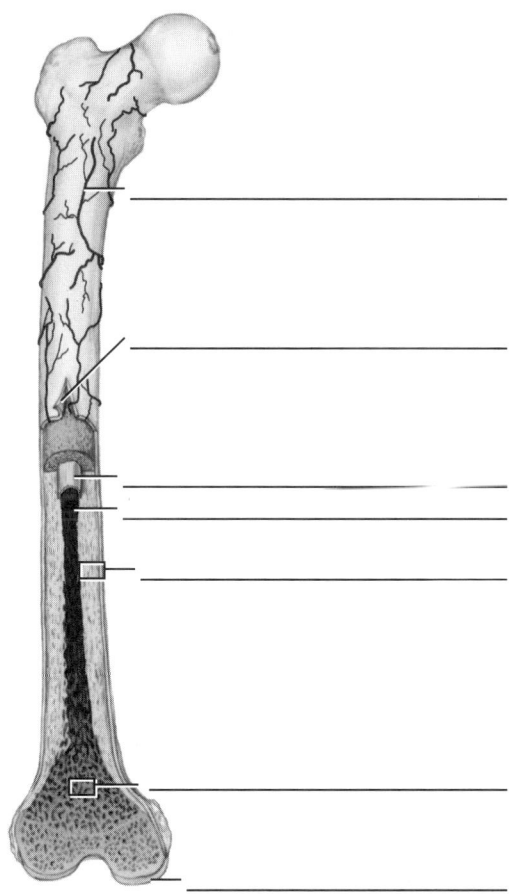

11. Figure 8.9

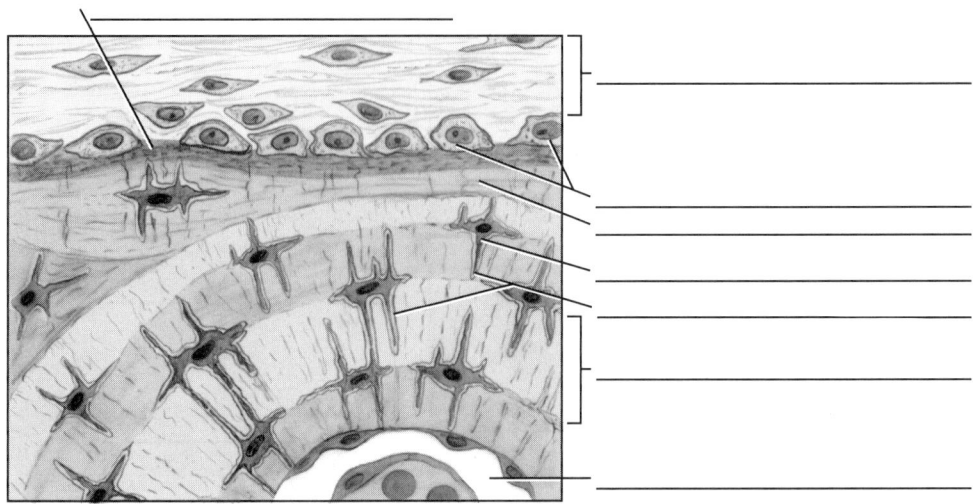

12. Figure 8.10, *A, B* (Courtesy M. J. Fehrenbach, RDH, MS.)

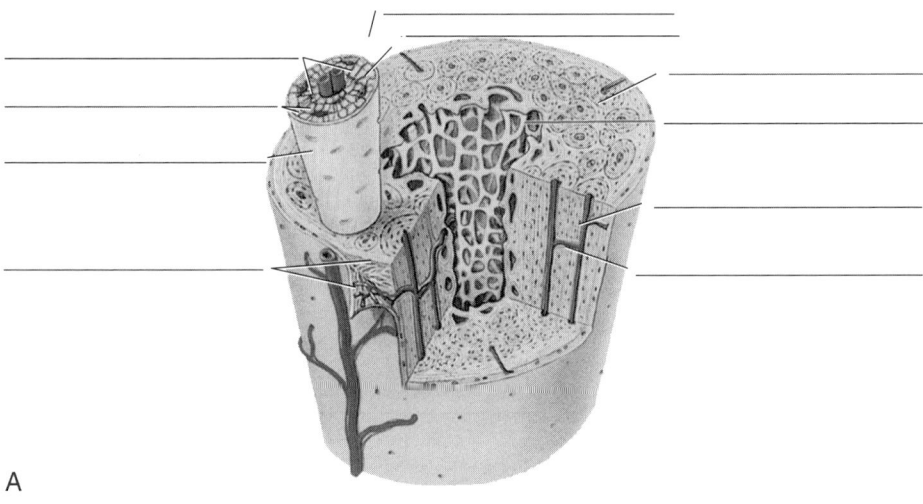

A

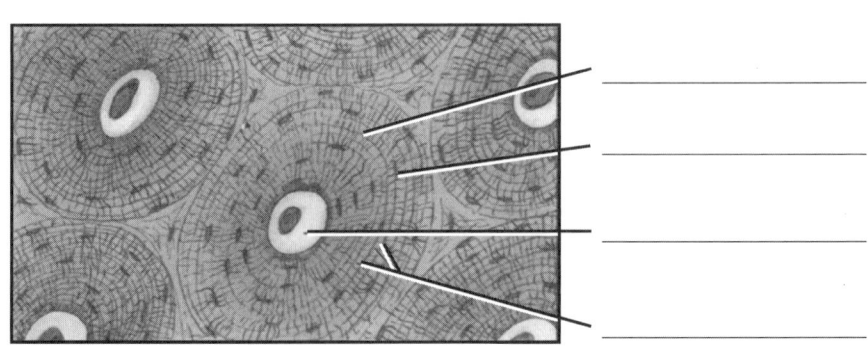

B

13. Figure 8.11

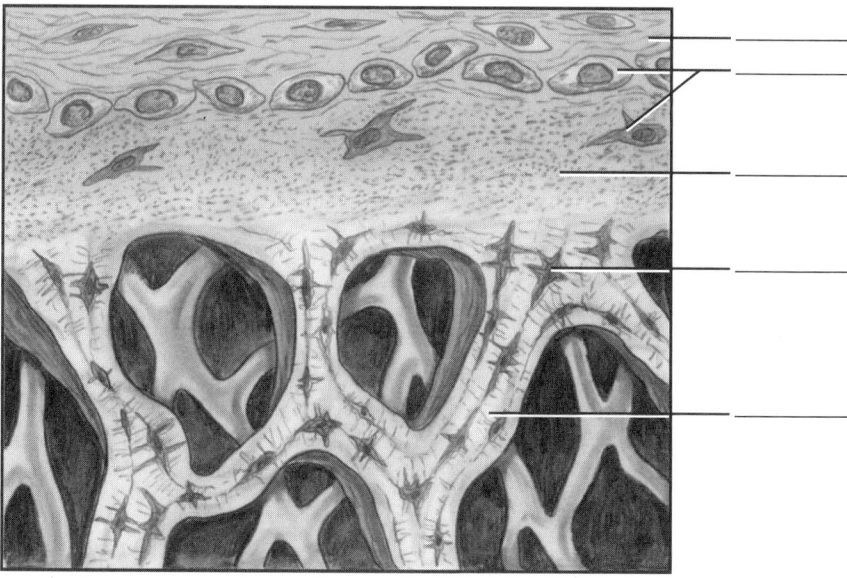

14. Figure 8.14, *A*

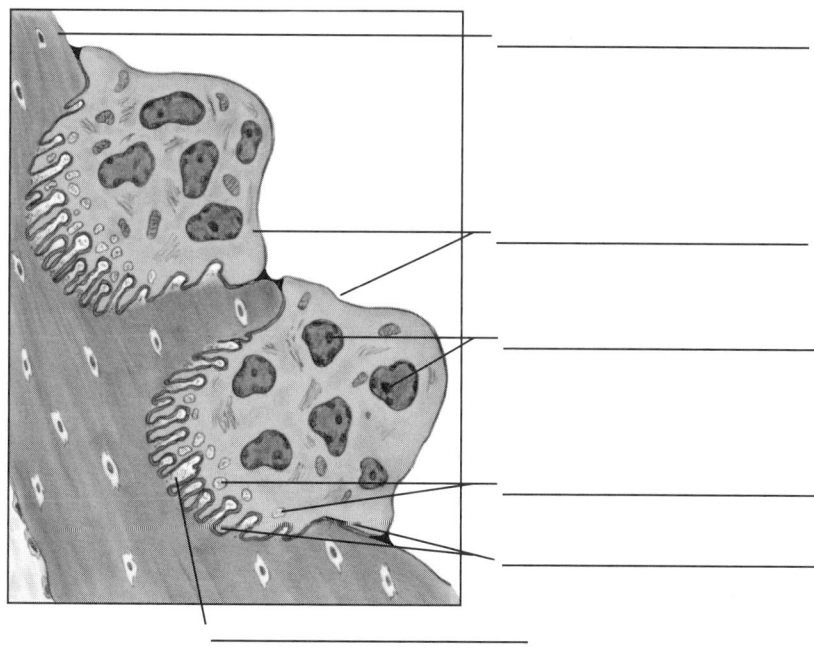

15. Figure 8.20

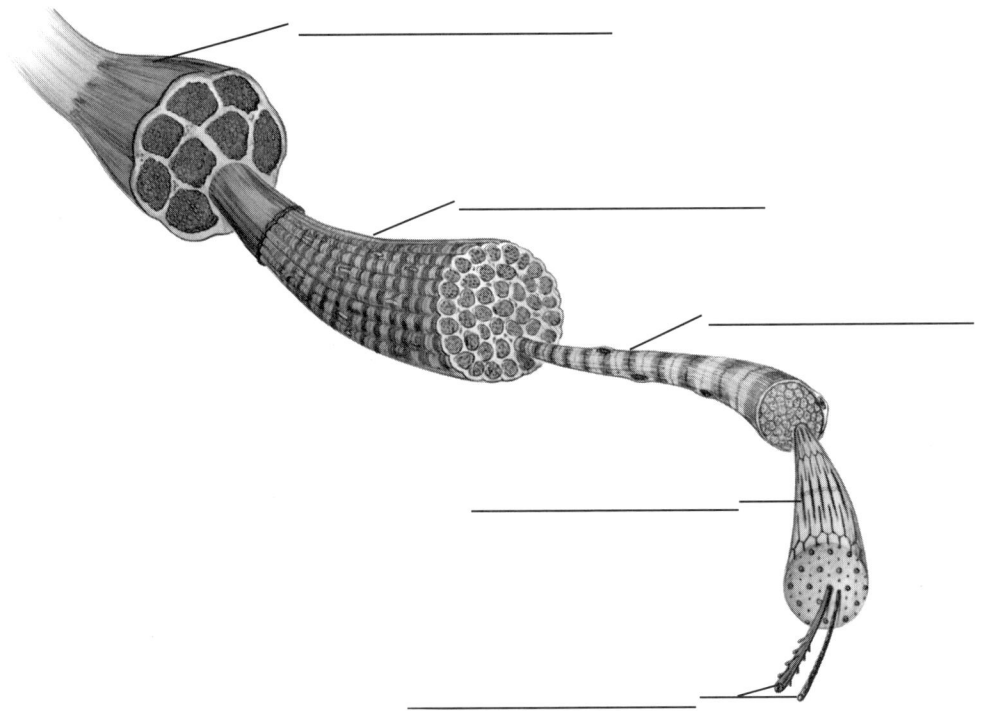

16. Figure 8.21

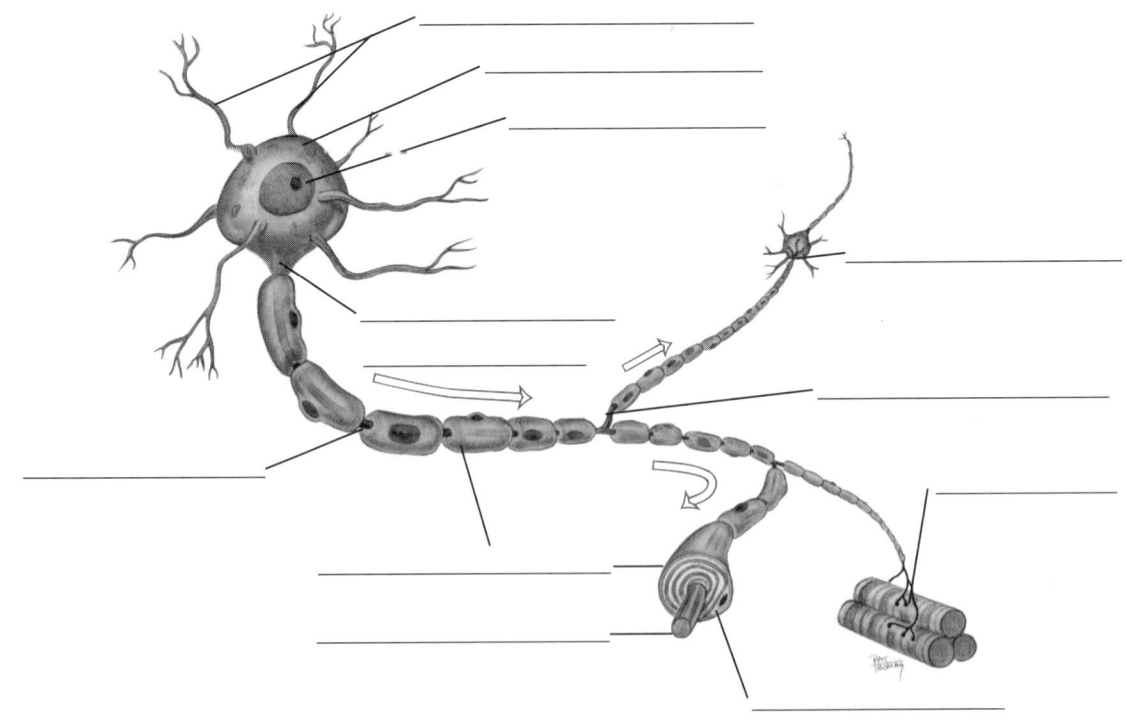

Chapter 9: Oral Mucosa

17. Figure 9.1

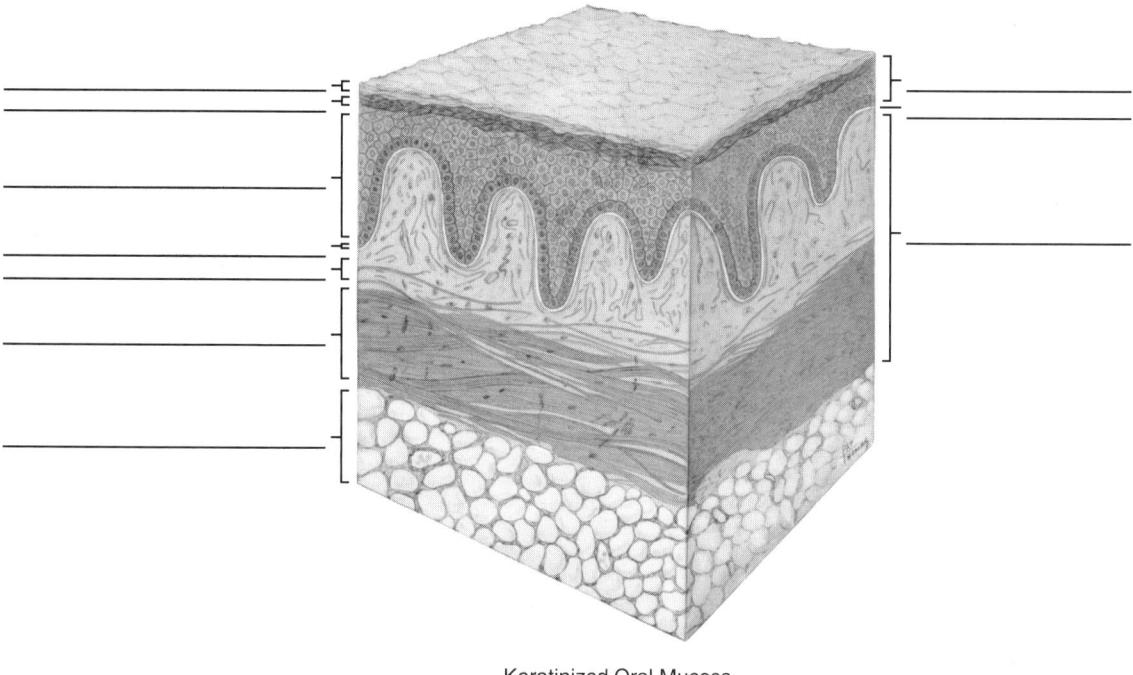

Keratinized Oral Mucosa
(and underlying tissue)

18. Figure 9.2

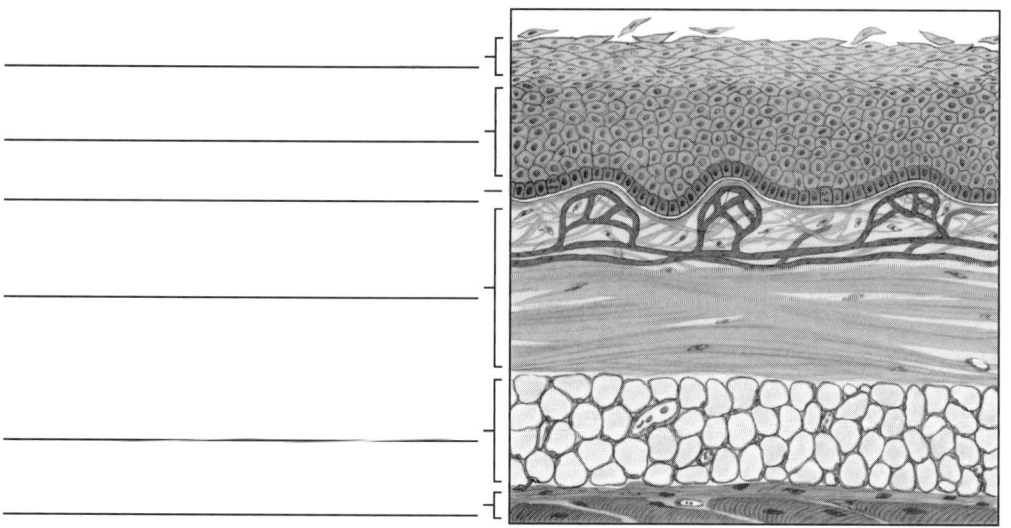

Nonkeratinized Stratified Squamous Epithelium
(and deeper tissue)

19. Figure 9.3

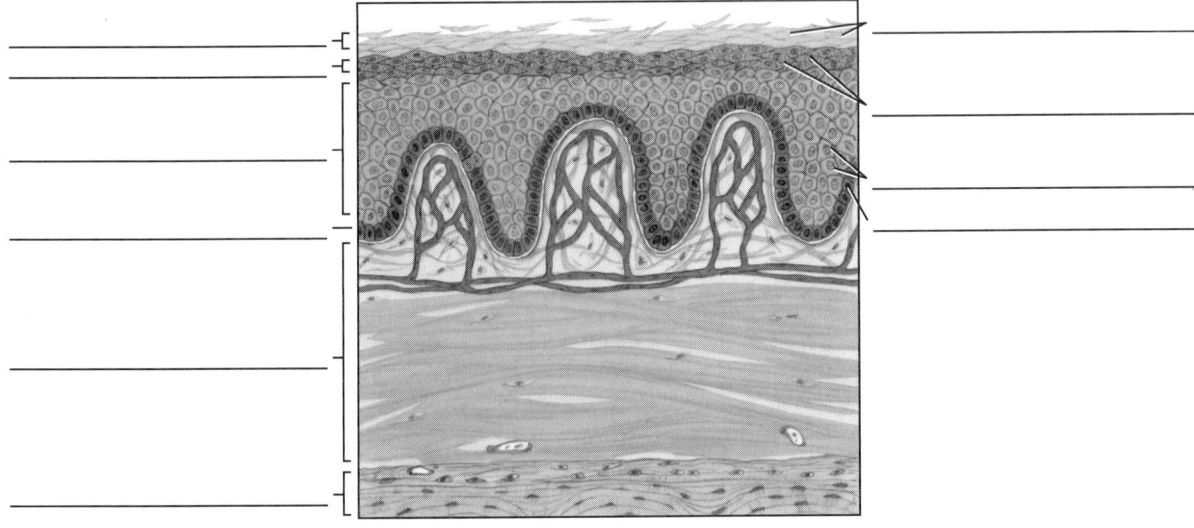

Orthokeratinized Stratified Squamous Epithelium
(and deeper tissue)

20. Figure 9.5

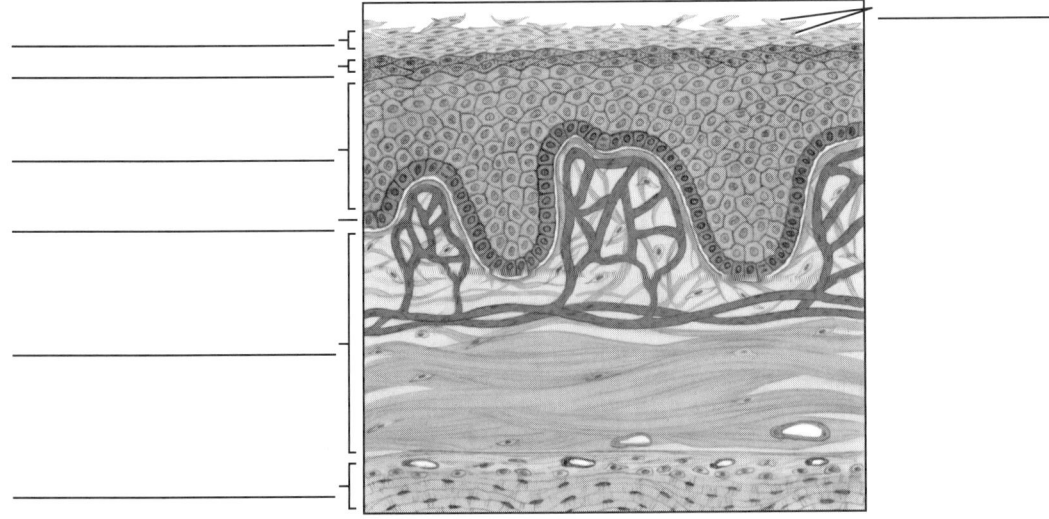

Parakeratinized Stratified Squamous Epithelium
(and deeper tissue)

21. Figure 9.6

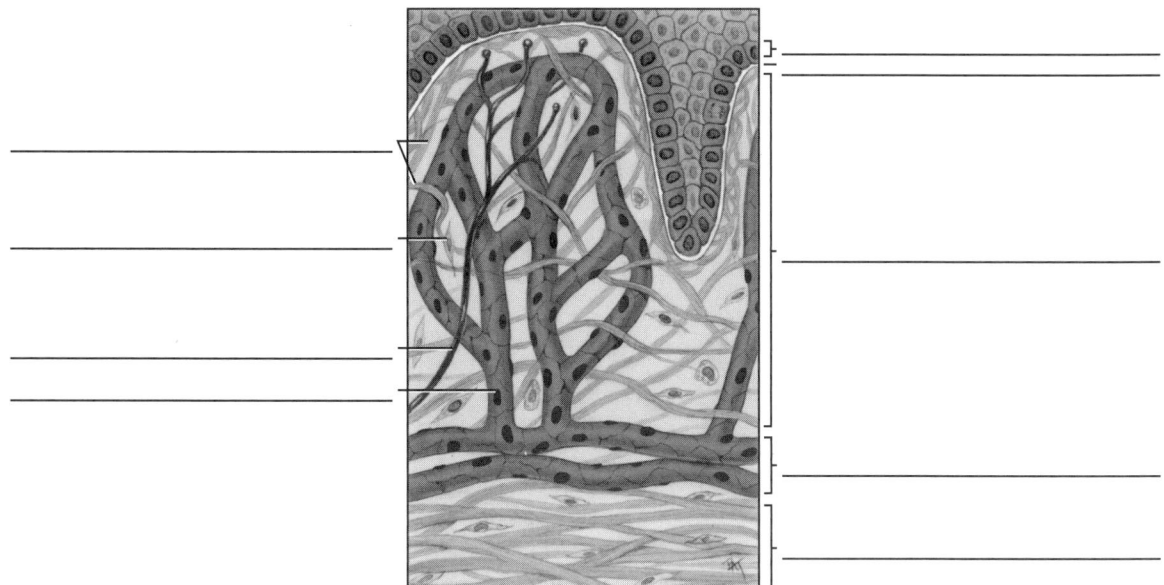

22. Figure 9.13

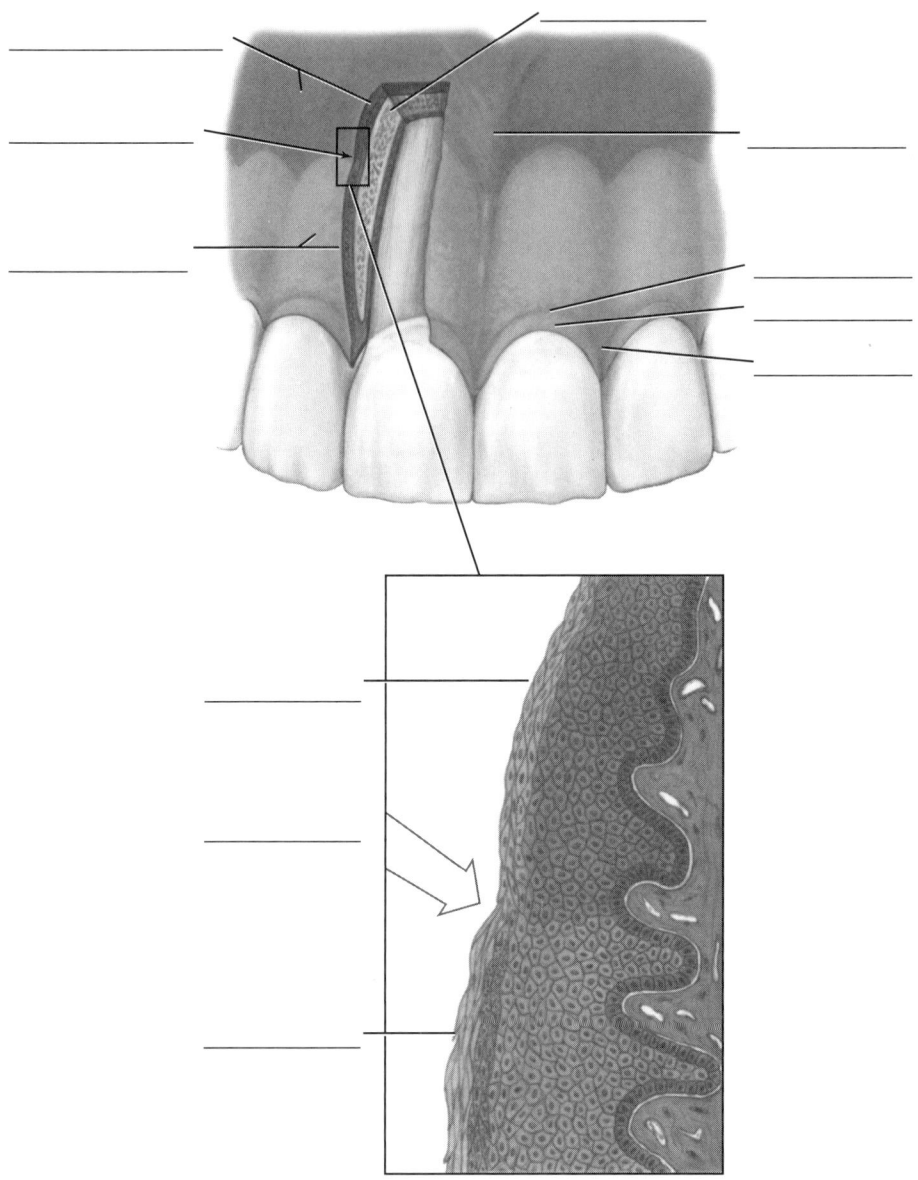

23. Figure 9.17

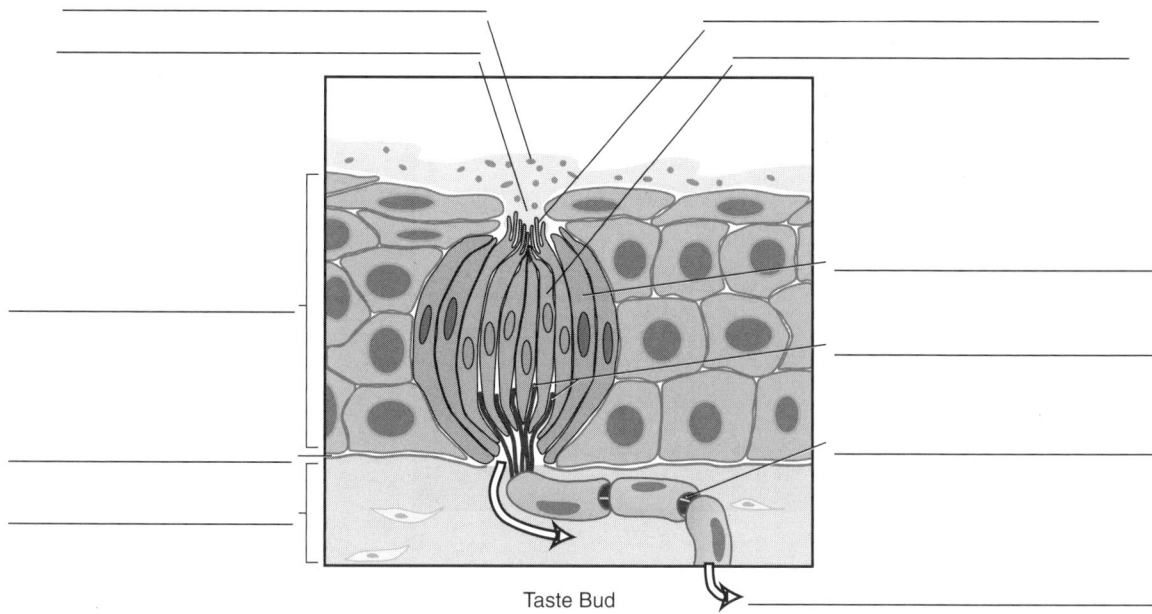

Taste Bud

Chapter 10: Gingival and Dentogingival Junctional Tissue

24. Figure 10.1

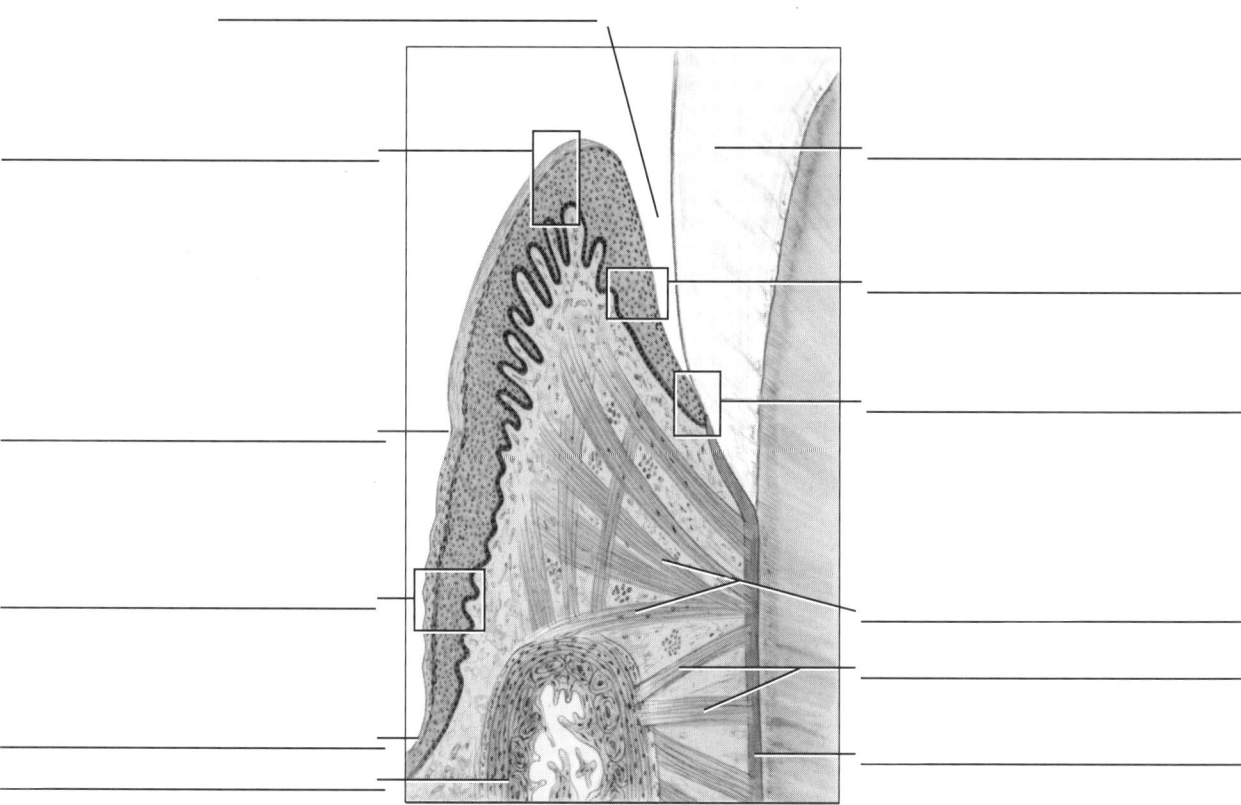

25. Figure 10.8

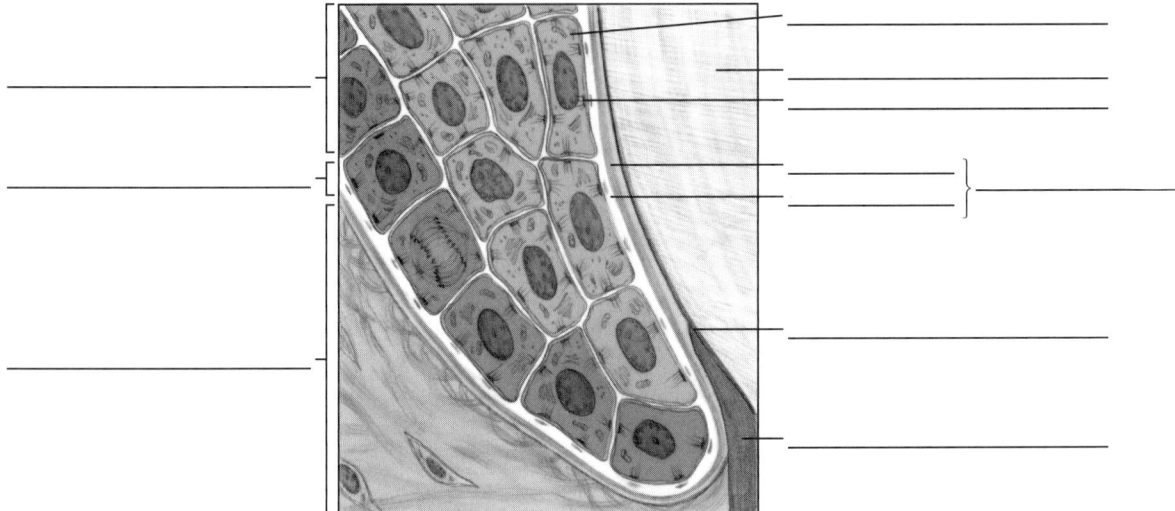

Chapter 11: Head and Neck Structures

26. Figure 11.1, *B*

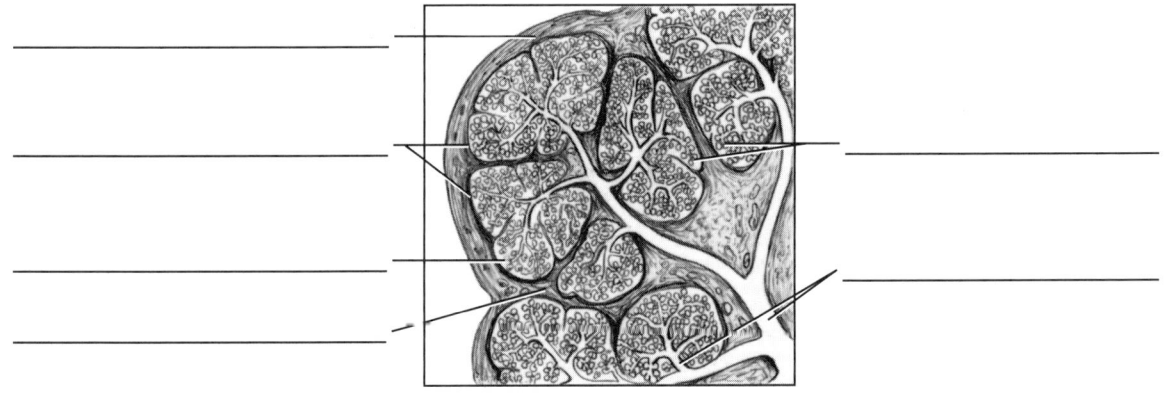

Salivary Gland

27. Figure 11.6

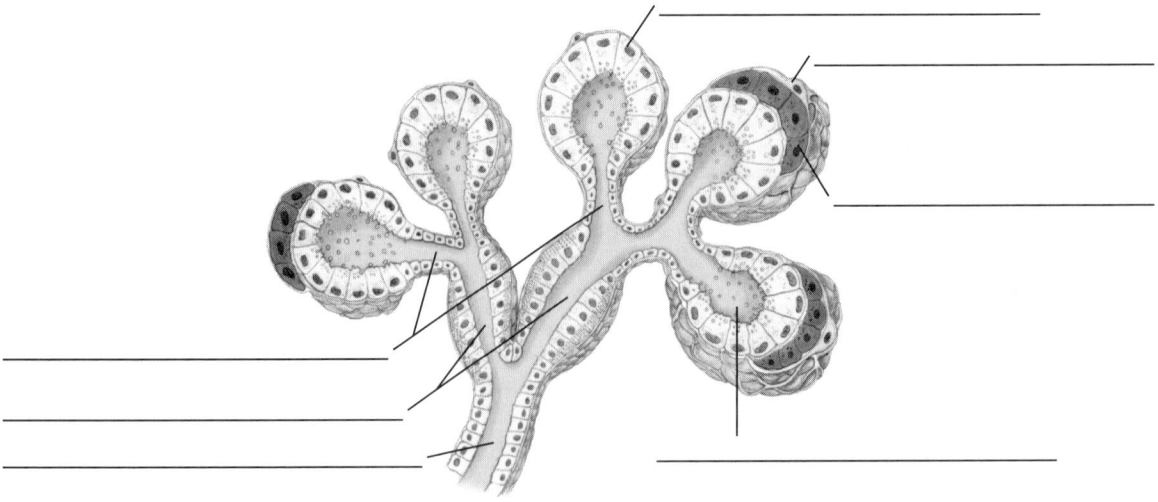

28. Figure 11.7, *A, B, C*

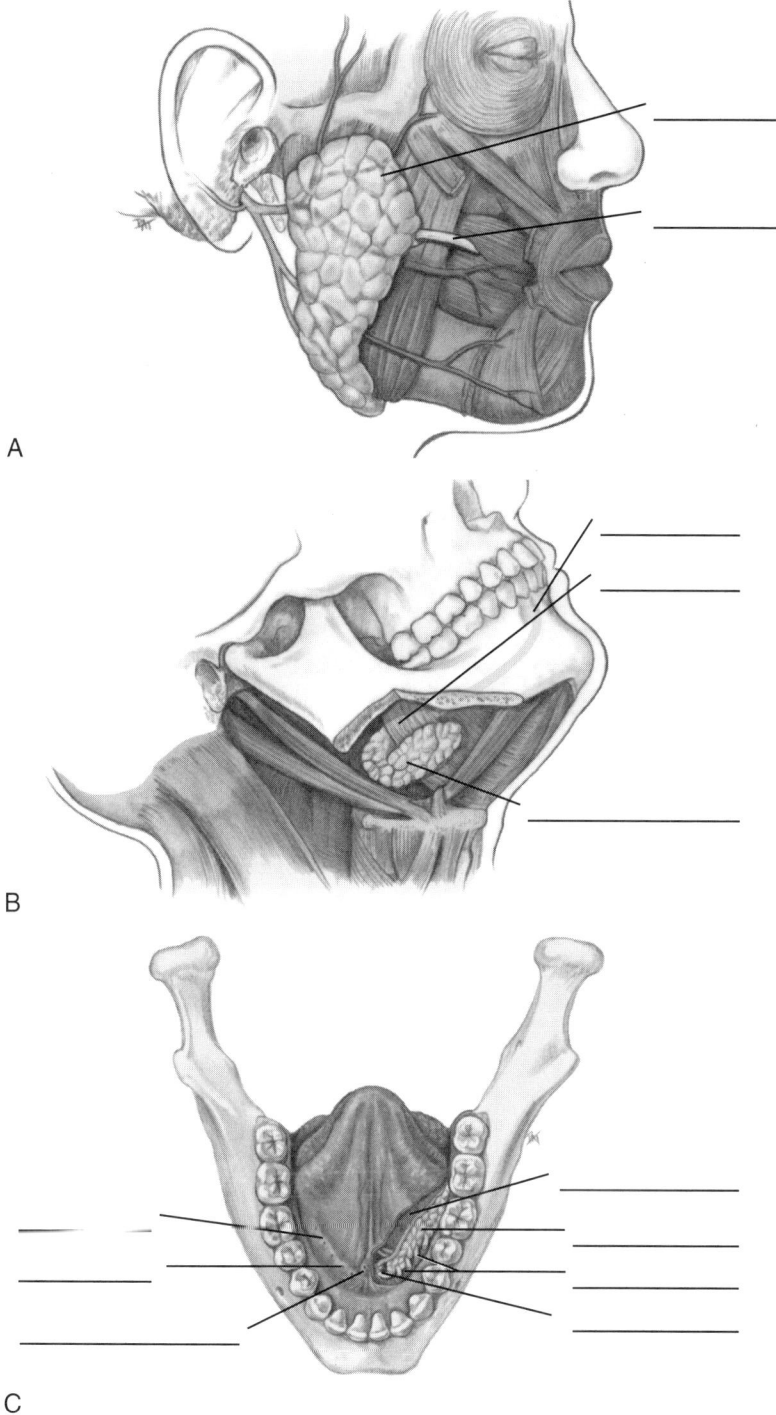

29. Figure 11.13, *B*

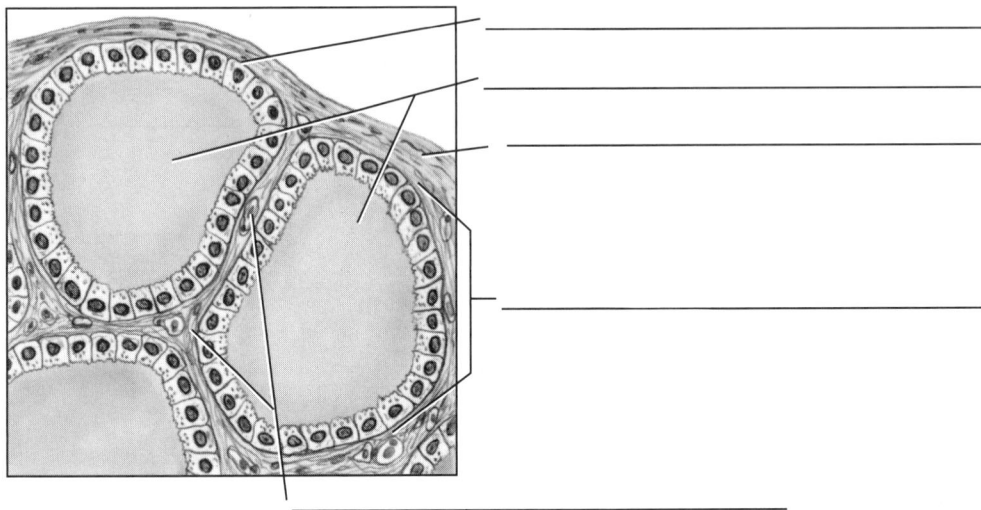

30. Figure 11.16, *A*

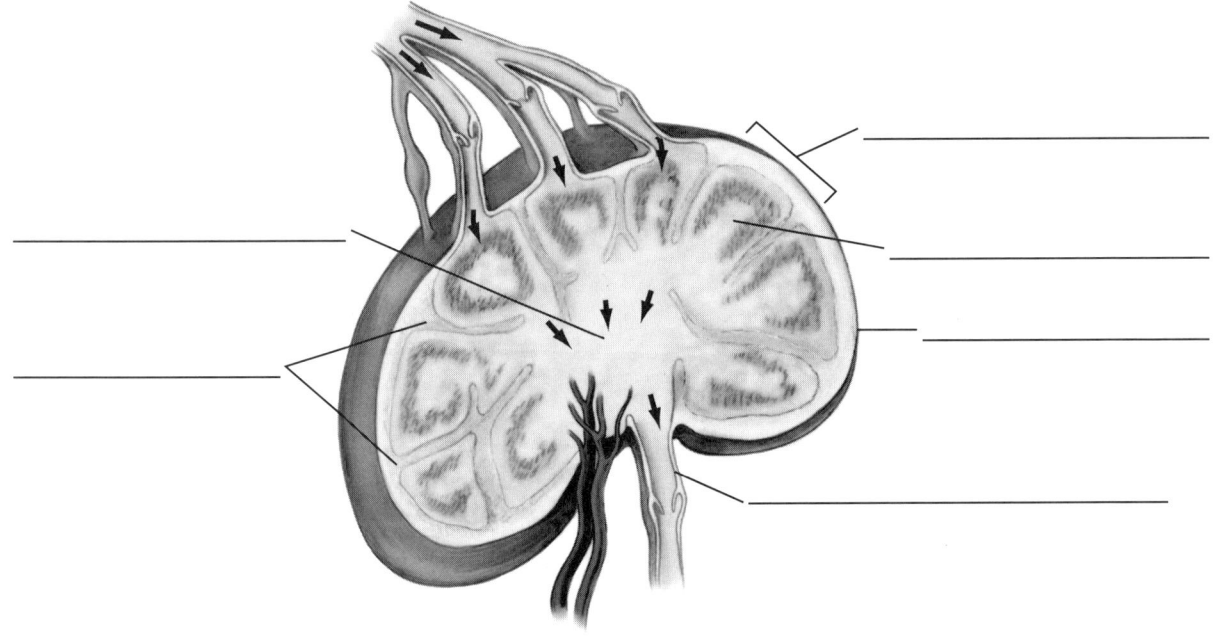

31. Figure 11.17, *A*

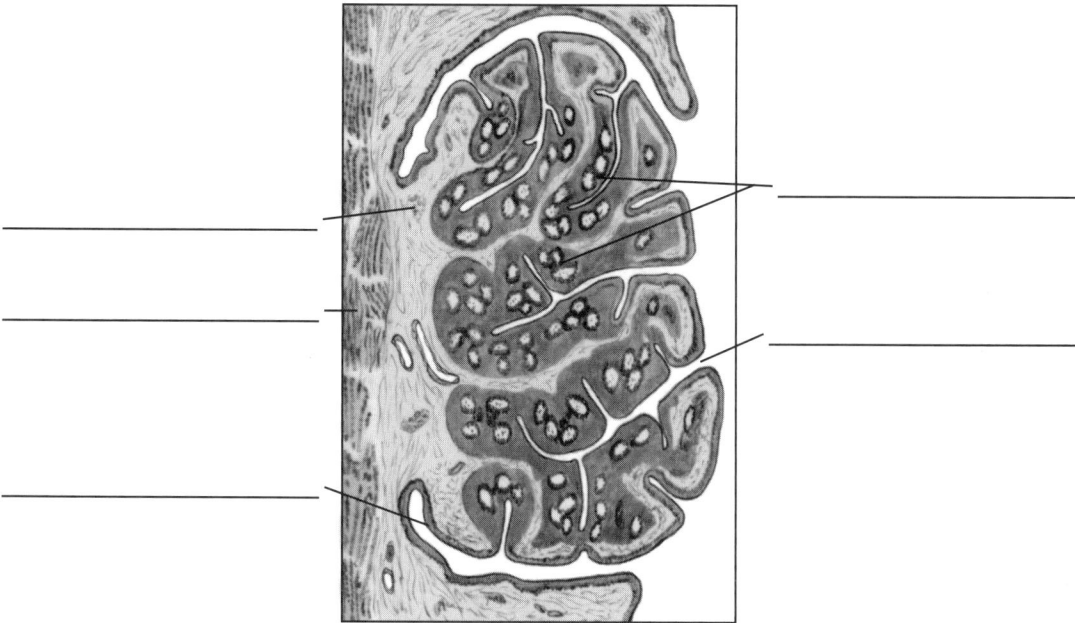

32. Figure 11.19

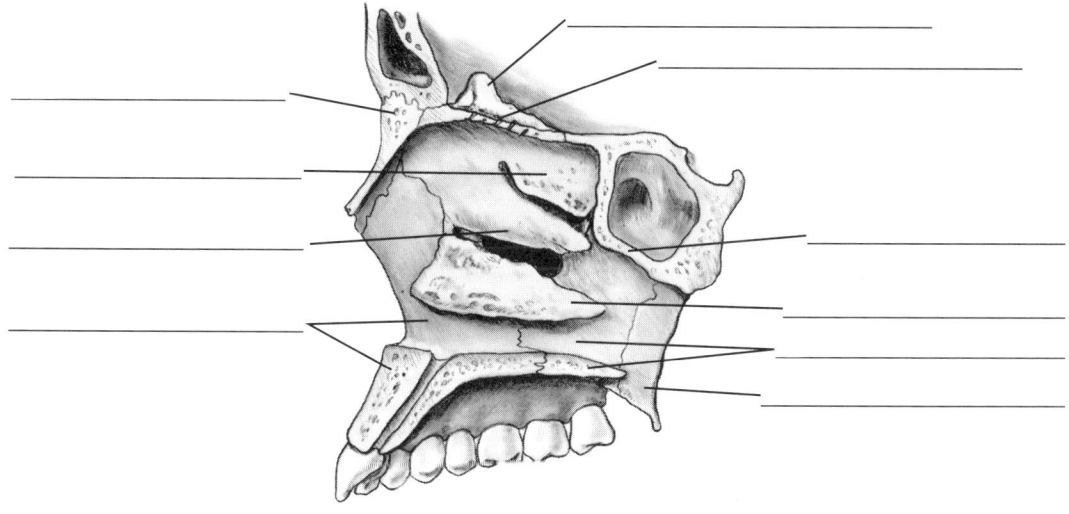

33. Figure 11.20

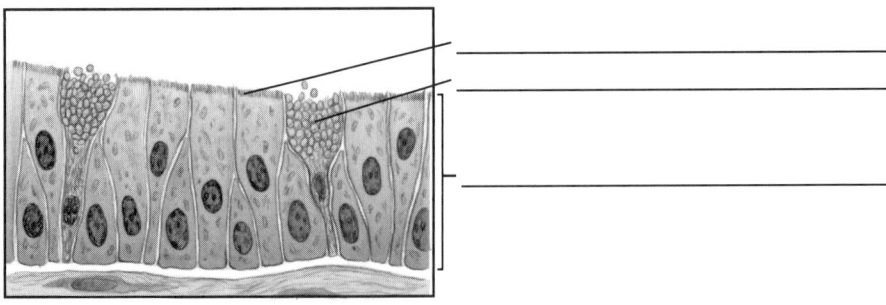

Nasal Cavity

34. Figure 11.21

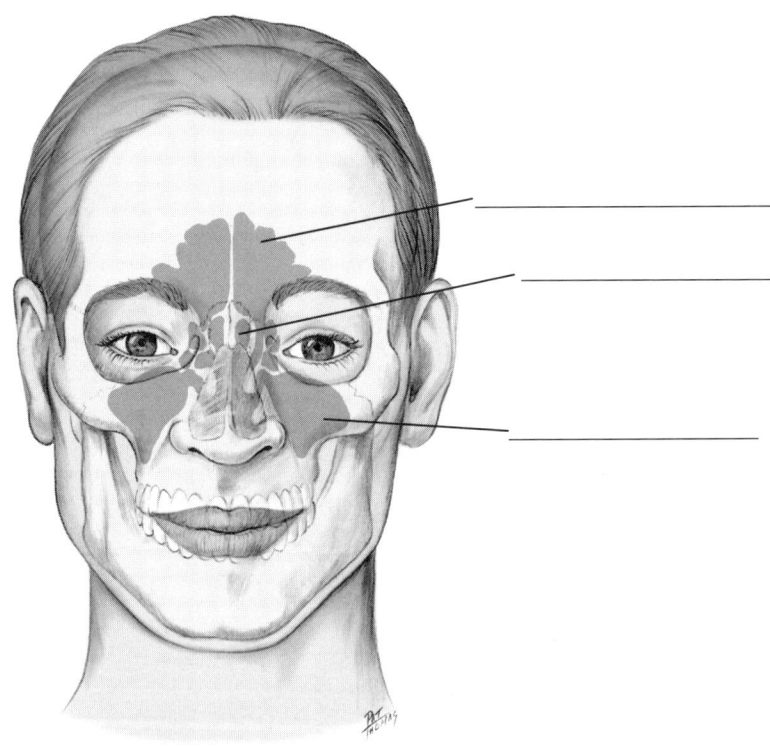

Chapter 12: Enamel

35. Figure 12.4, *A*

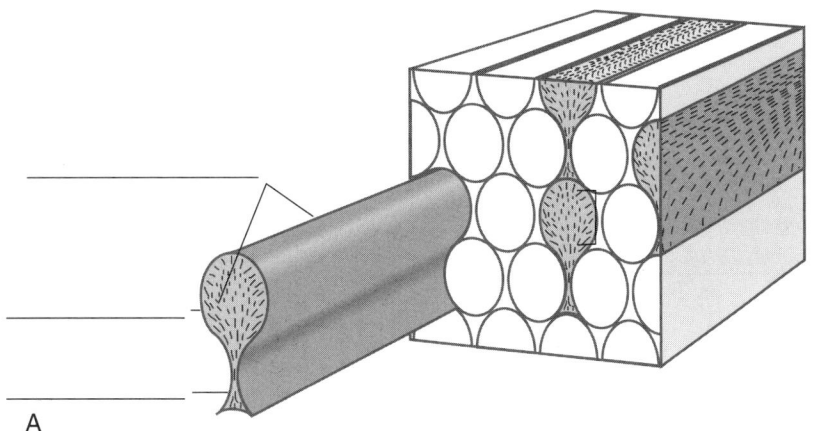

A

Chapter 13: Dentin and Pulp

36. Figure 13.8

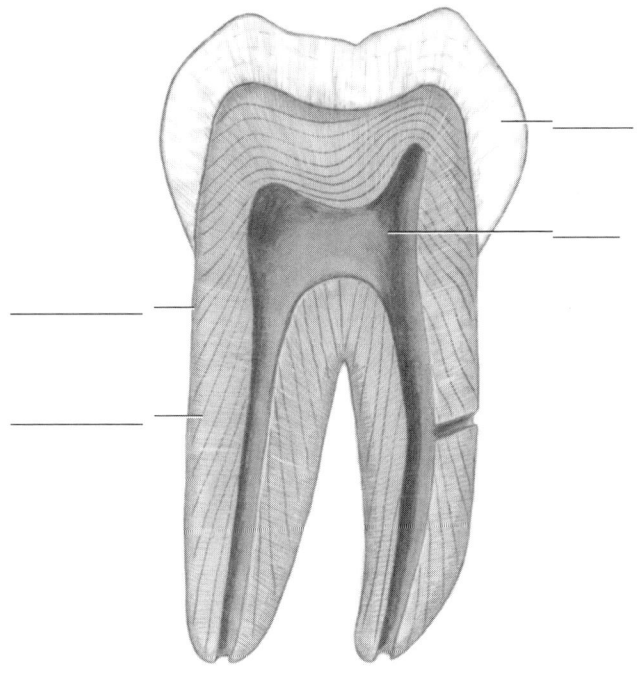

37. Figure 13.16, *B*

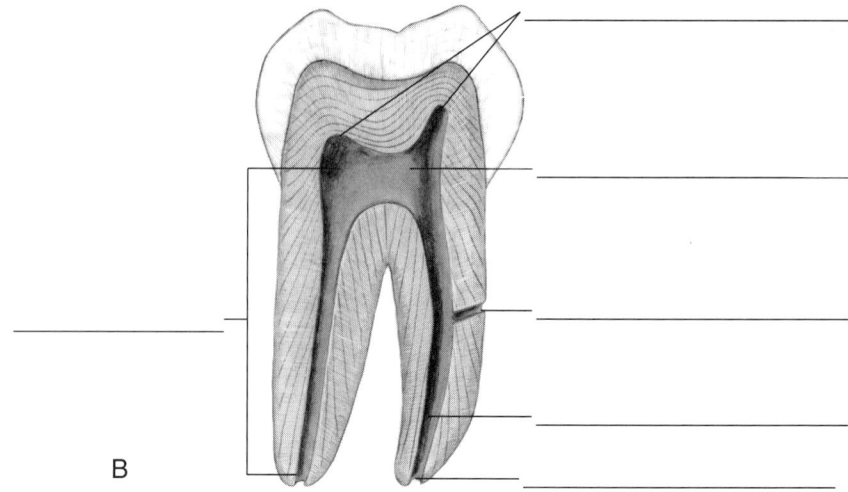

Chapter 14: Periodontium: Cementum, Alveolar Process, and Periodontal Ligament

38. Figure 14.1

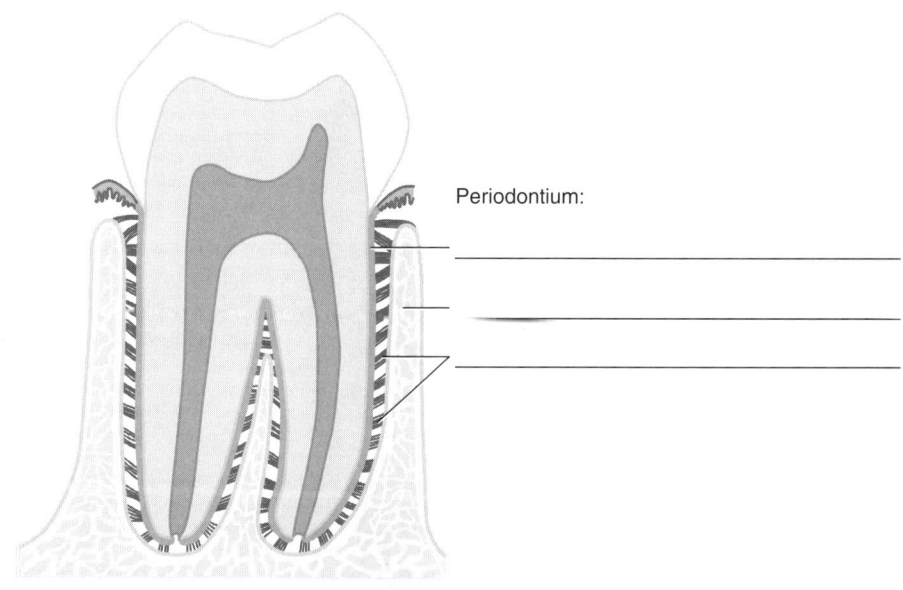

Periodontium:

39. Figure 14.2

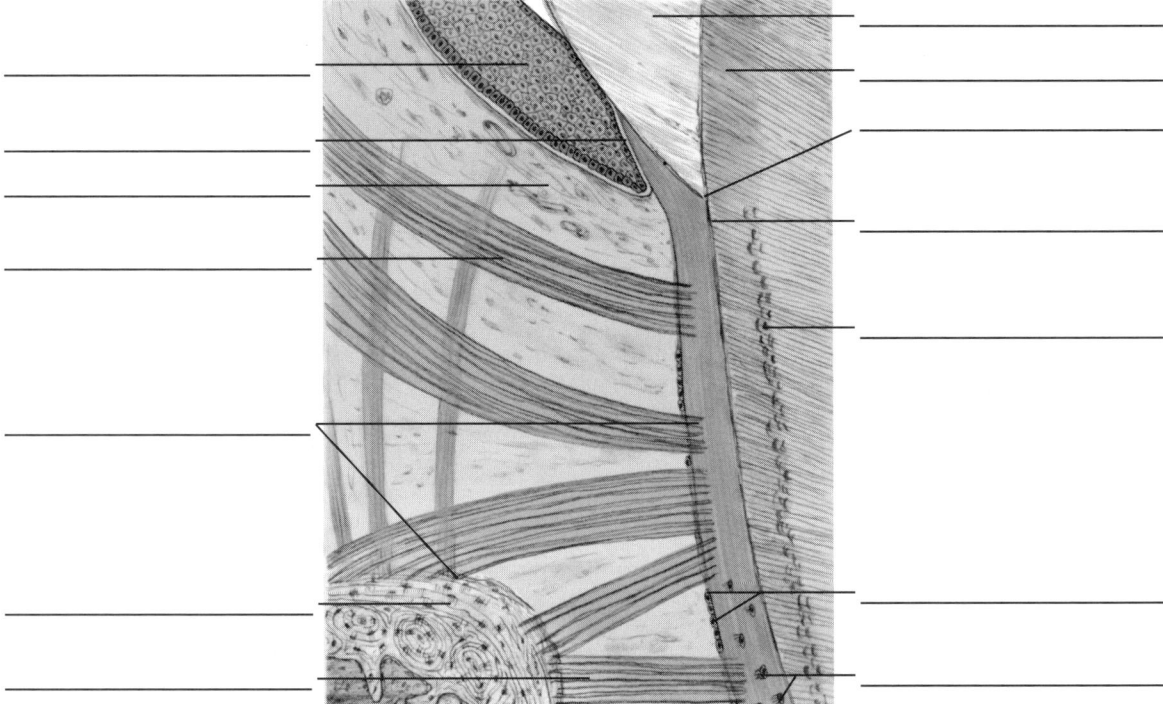

40. Figure 14.14, *A, B, C*

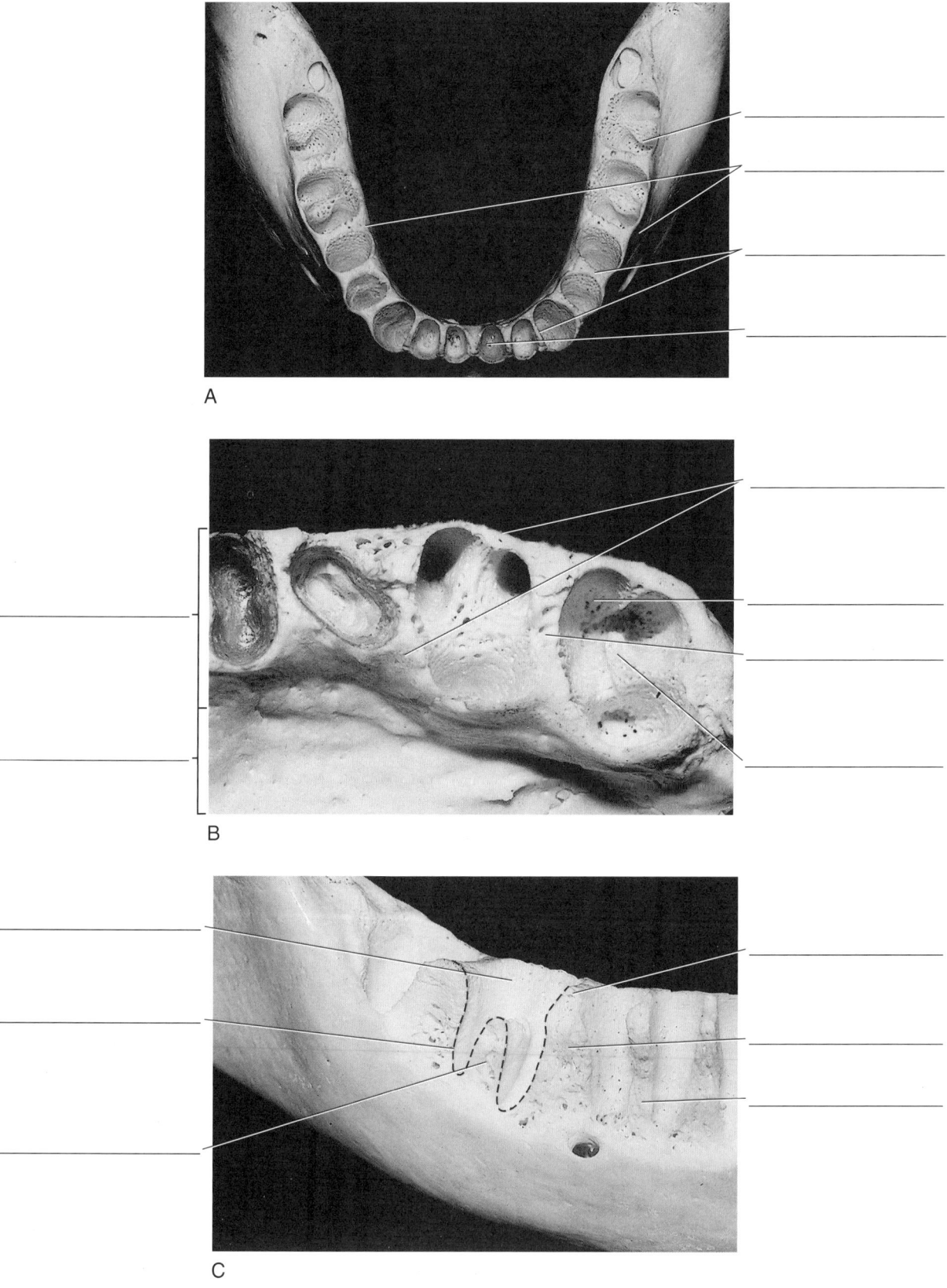

41. Figure 14.16, *A, B*

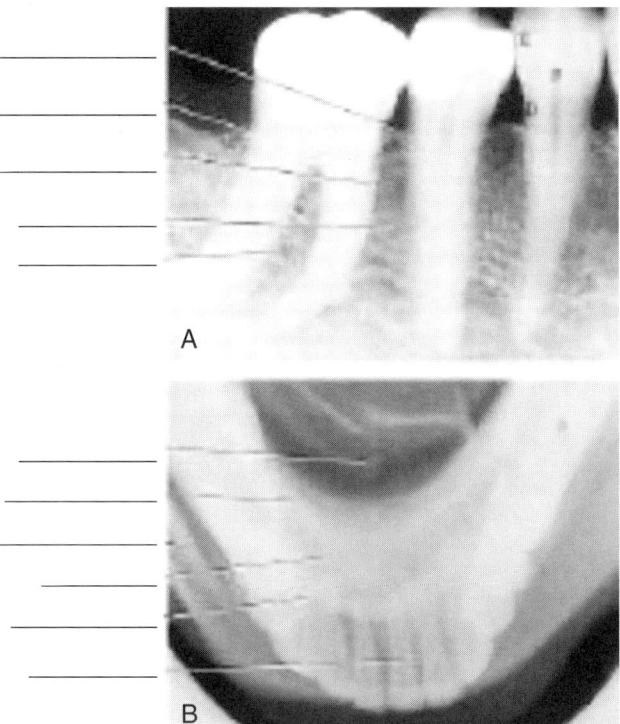

42. Figure 14.27

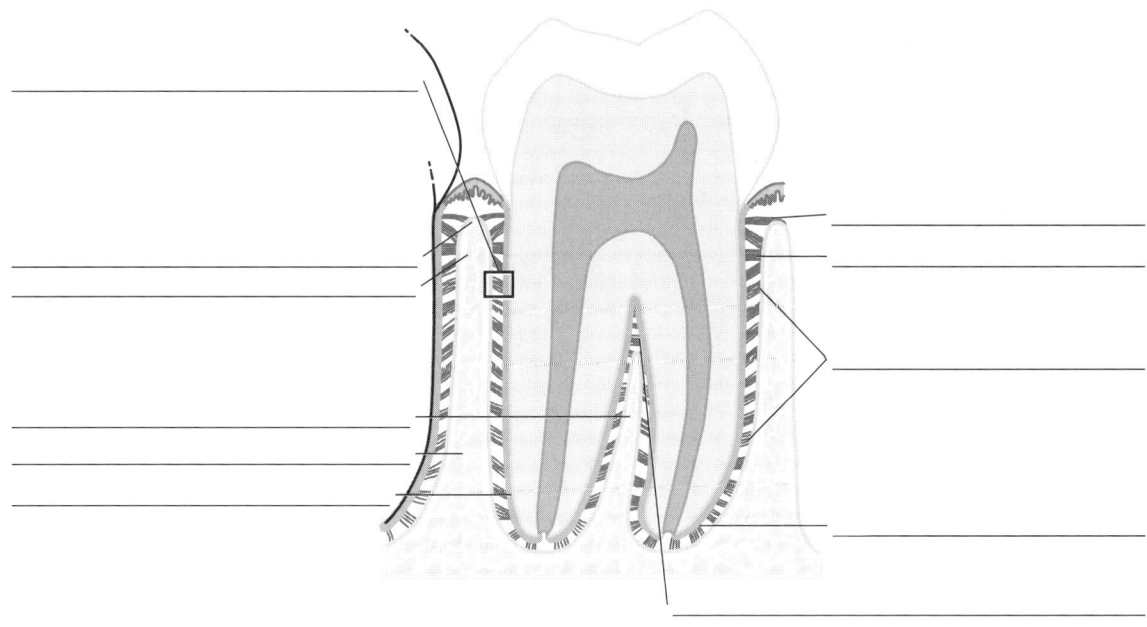

43. Figure 14.30

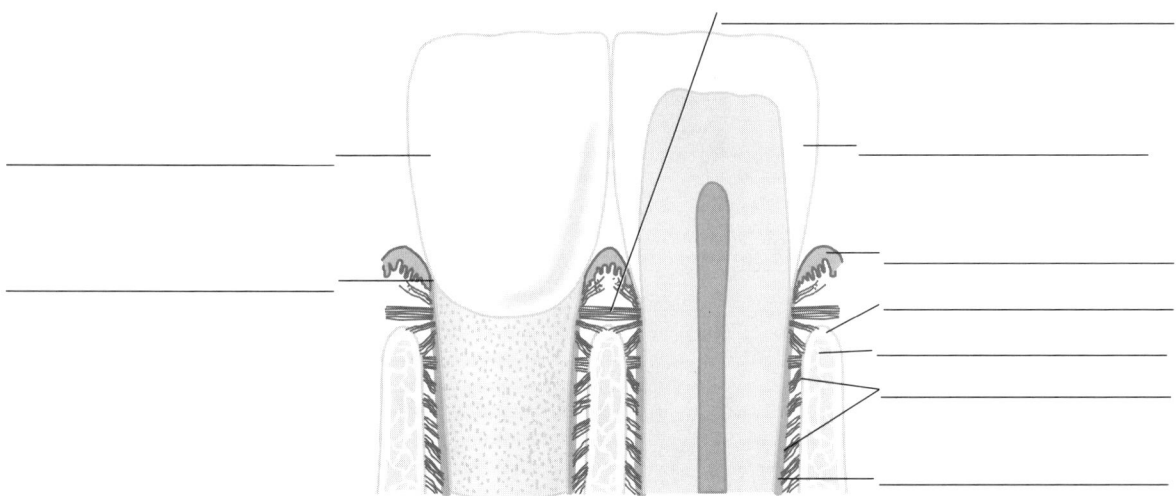

44. Figure 14.32

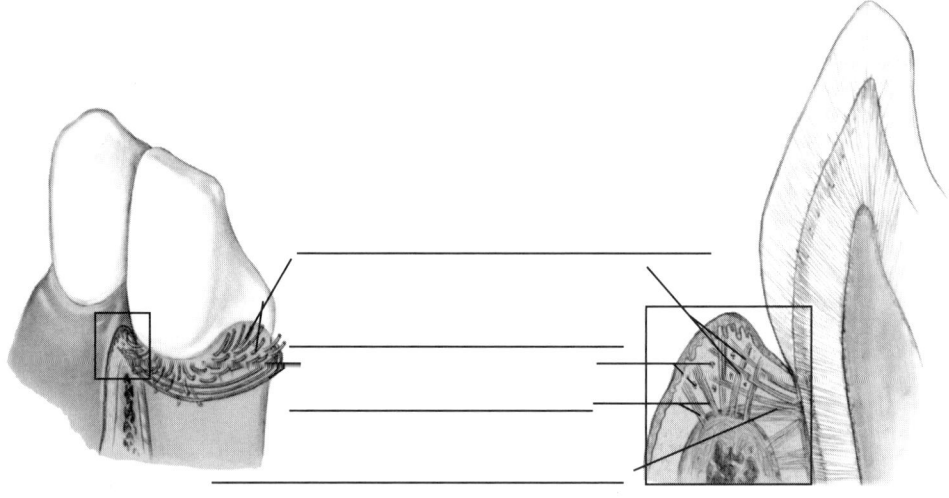

UNIT 4: DENTAL ANATOMY

Chapter 15: Overview of Dentitions

1. Figure 15.1

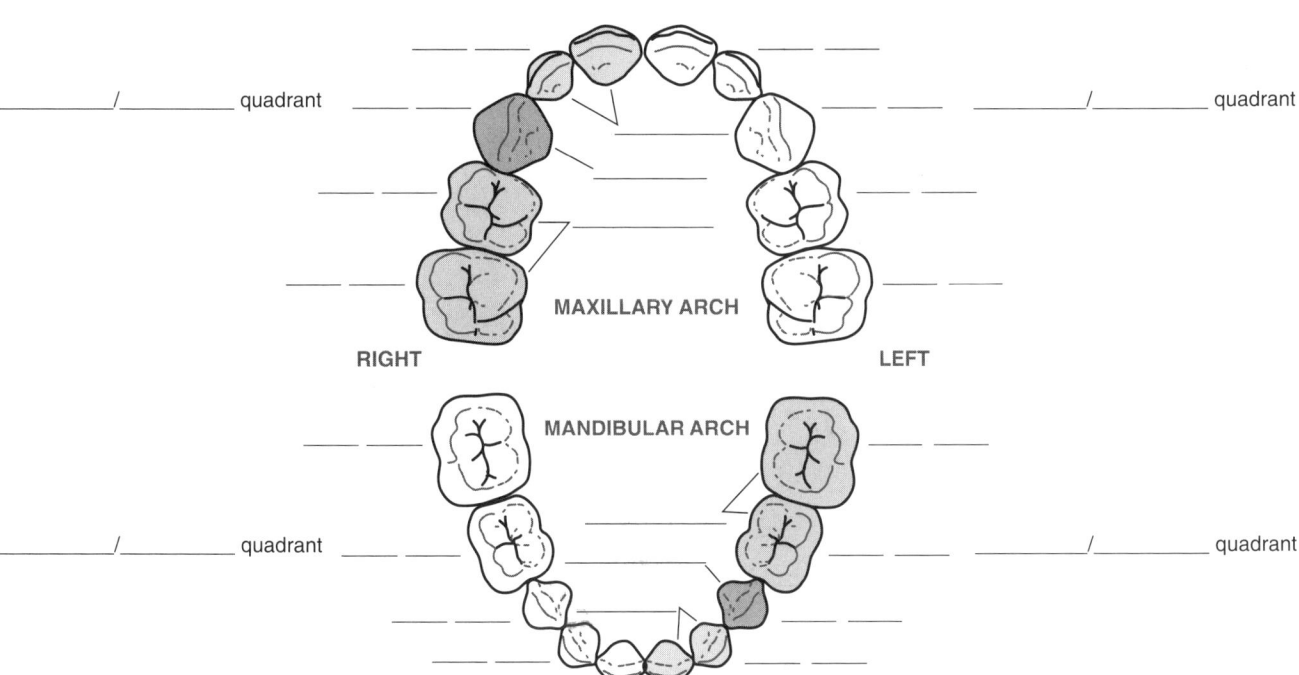

2. Figure 15.2

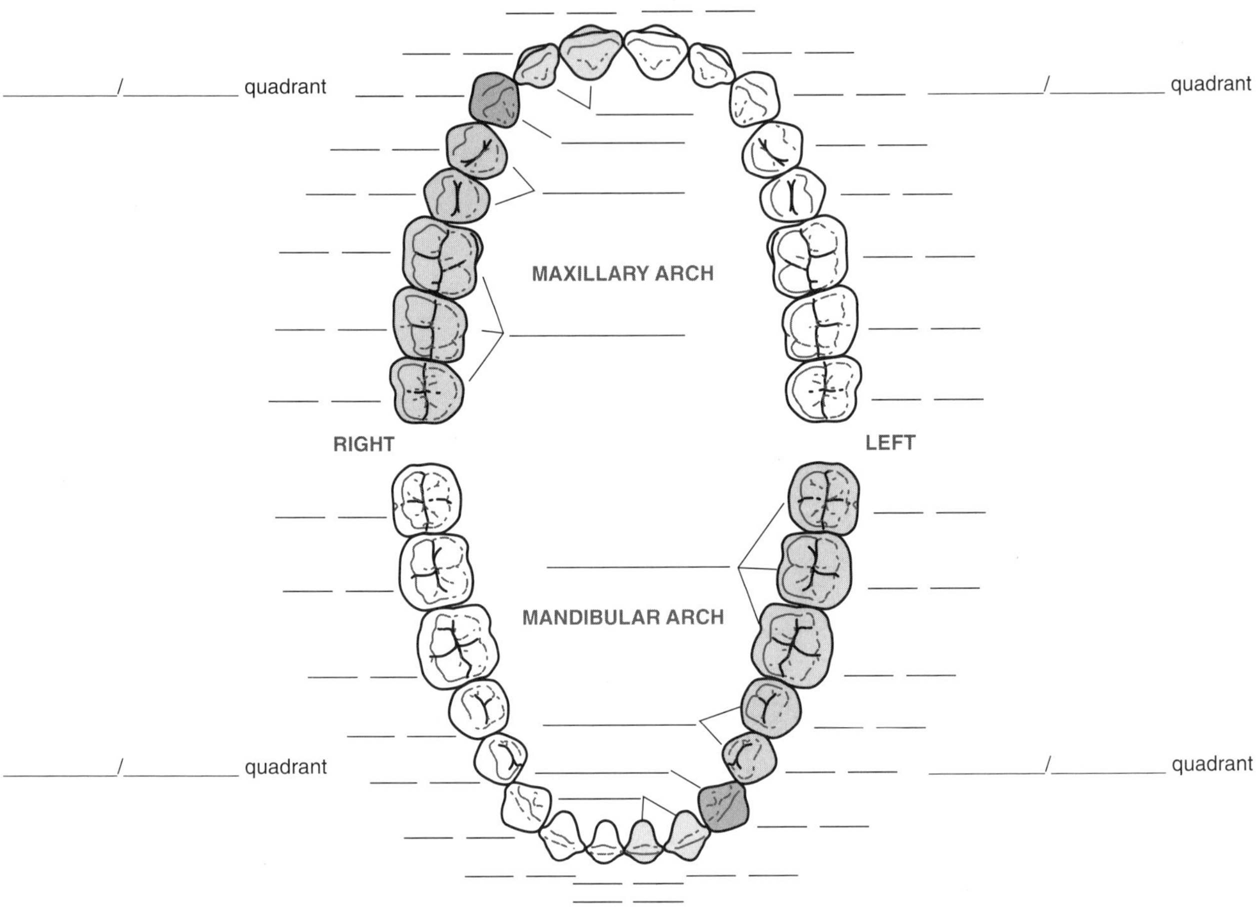

_____ / _____ quadrant   _____ / _____ quadrant

MAXILLARY ARCH

RIGHT   LEFT

MANDIBULAR ARCH

_____ / _____ quadrant   _____ / _____ quadrant

3. Figure 15.5

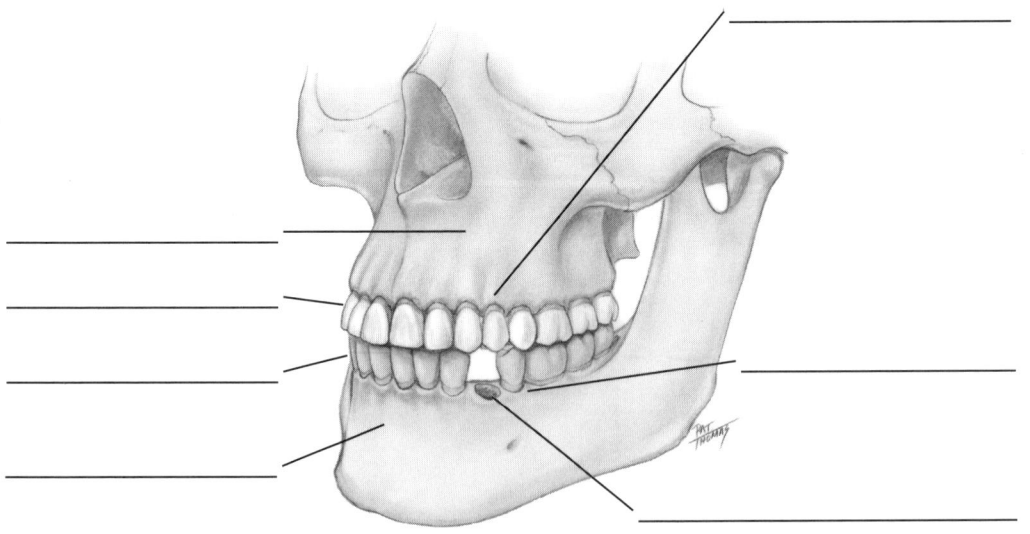

4. Figure 15.6

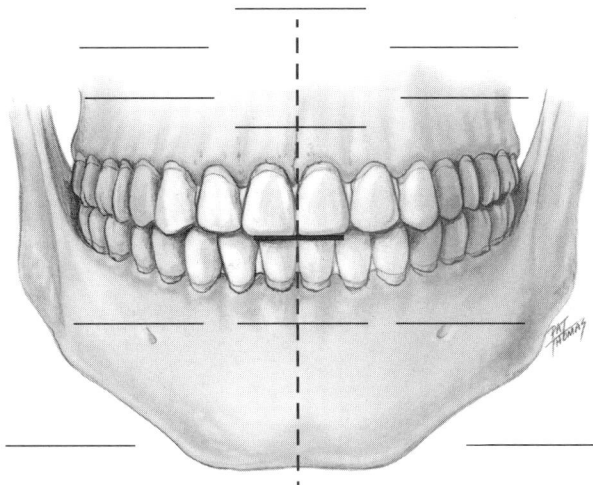

5. Figure 15.7

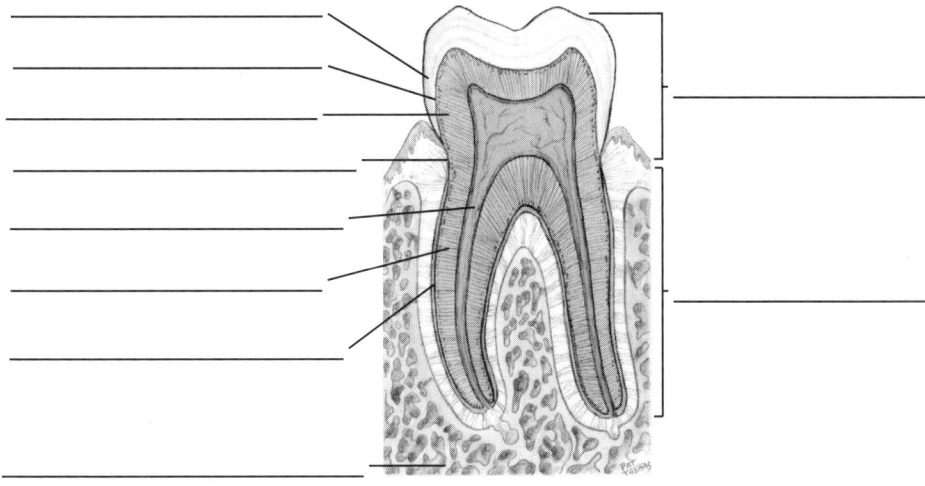

6. Figure 15.8, *A*

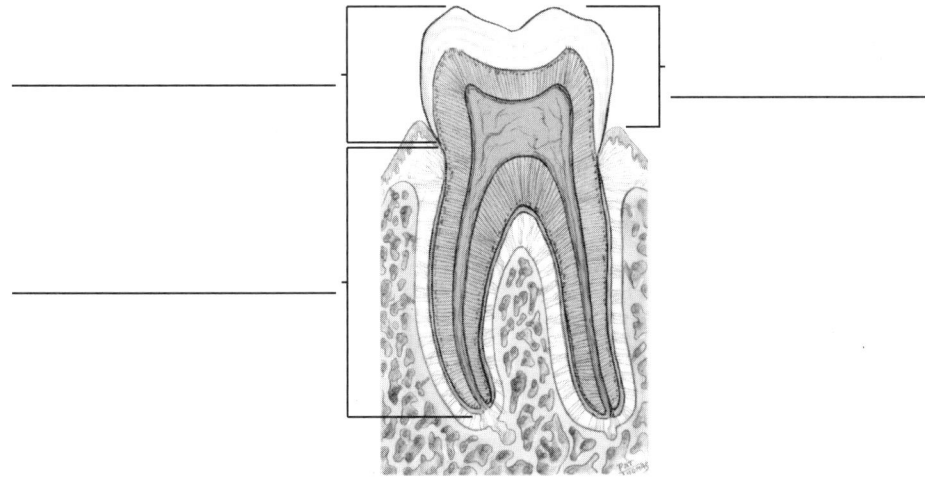

7. Figure 15.9

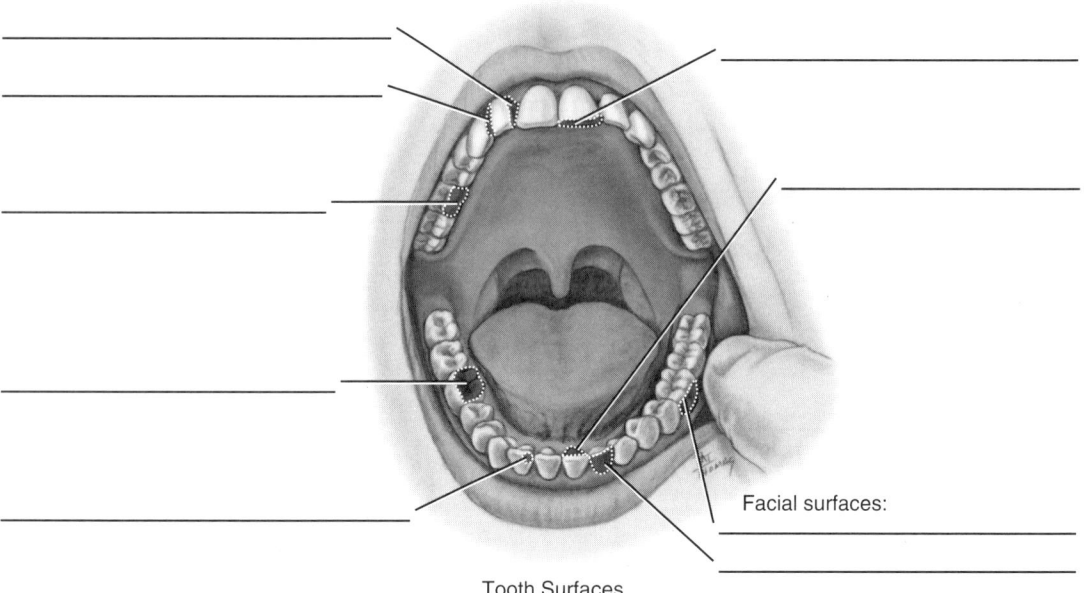

Facial surfaces:

Tooth Surfaces

8. Figure 15.11

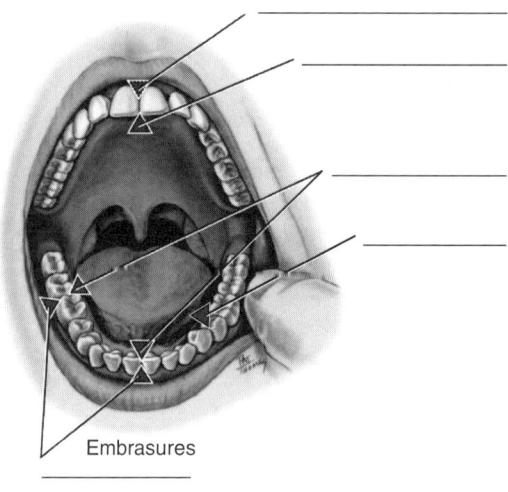

Embrasures

9. Figure 15.12

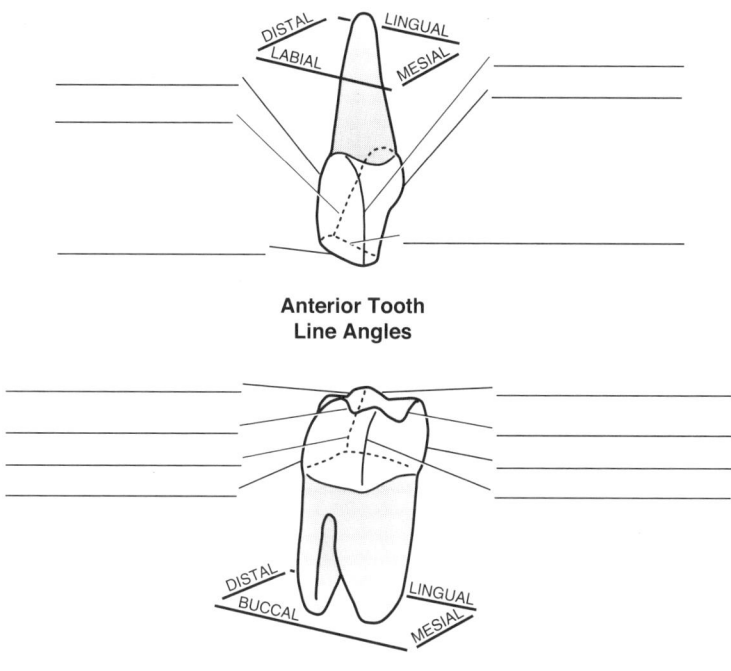

10. Figure 15.13

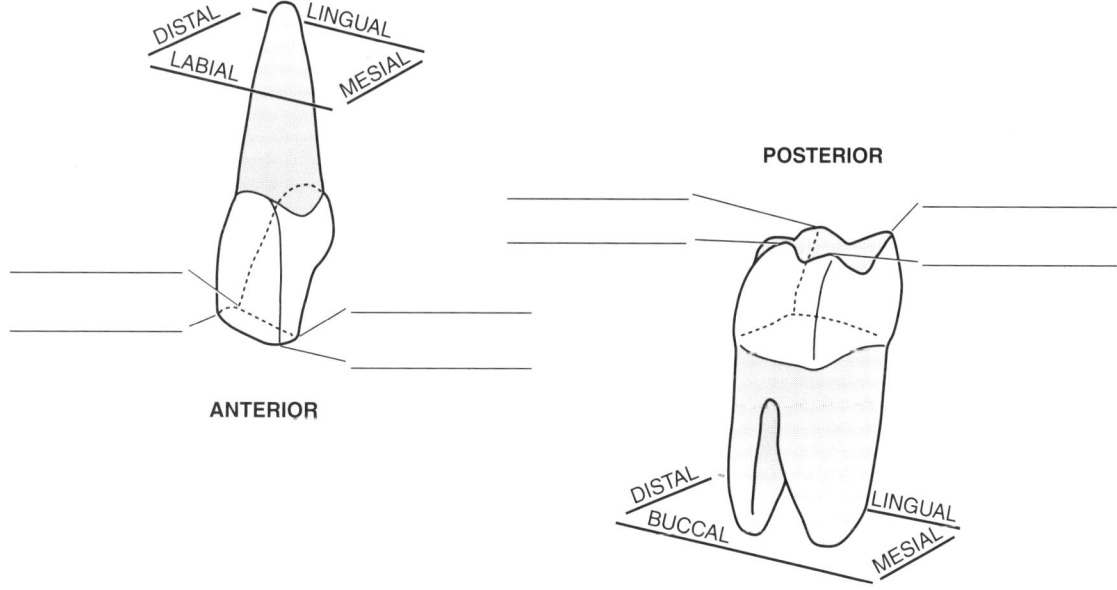

11. Figure 15.14

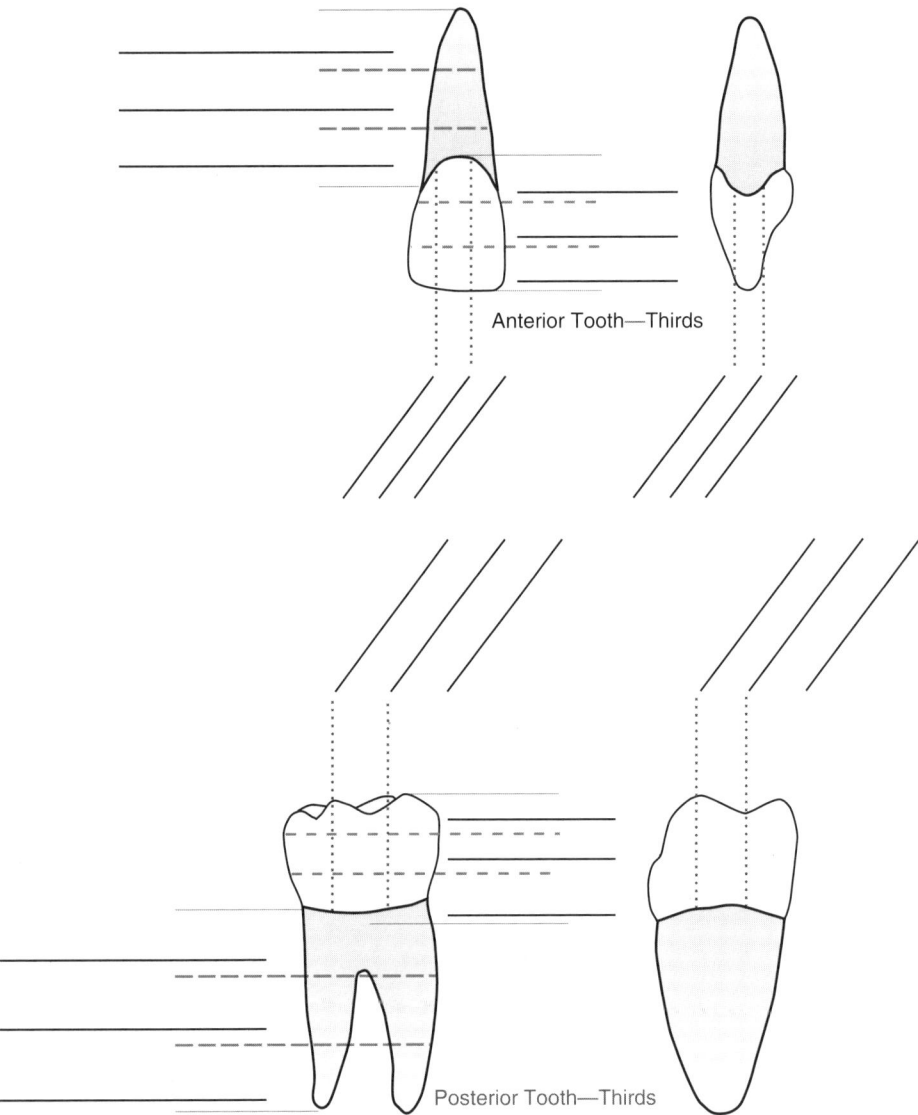

Chapter 16: Permanent Anterior Teeth

12. Figure 16.6

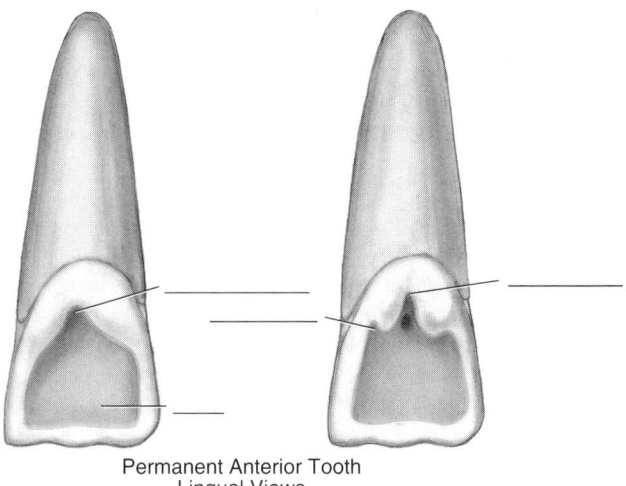

Permanent Anterior Tooth
Lingual Views

13. Figure 16.7

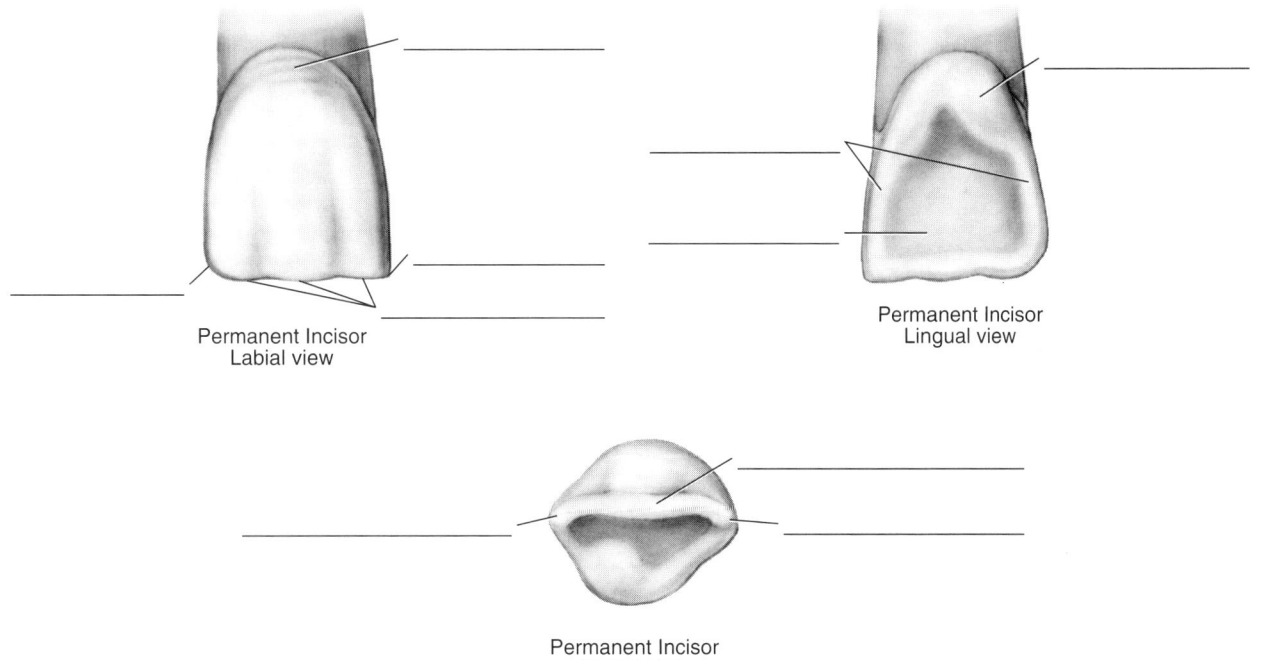

Permanent Incisor
Labial view

Permanent Incisor
Lingual view

Permanent Incisor
Incisal view

14. Figure 16.16

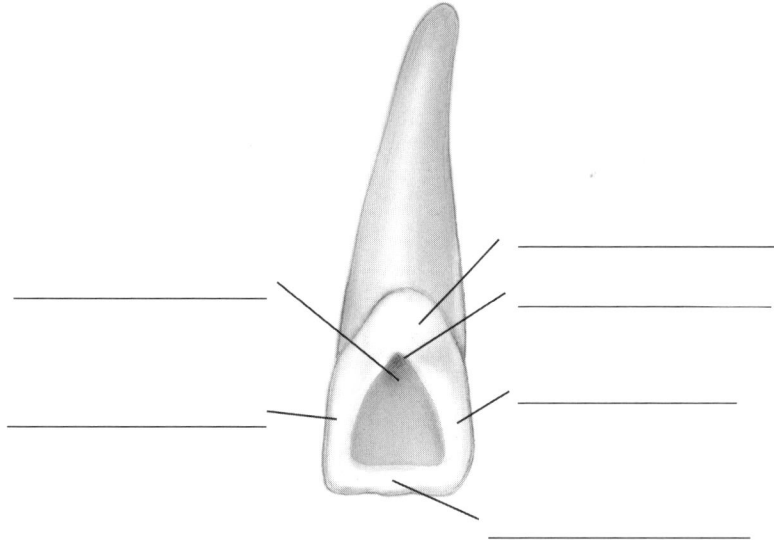

Permanent Maxillary Right Lateral Incisor
Lingual View

15. Figure 16.22

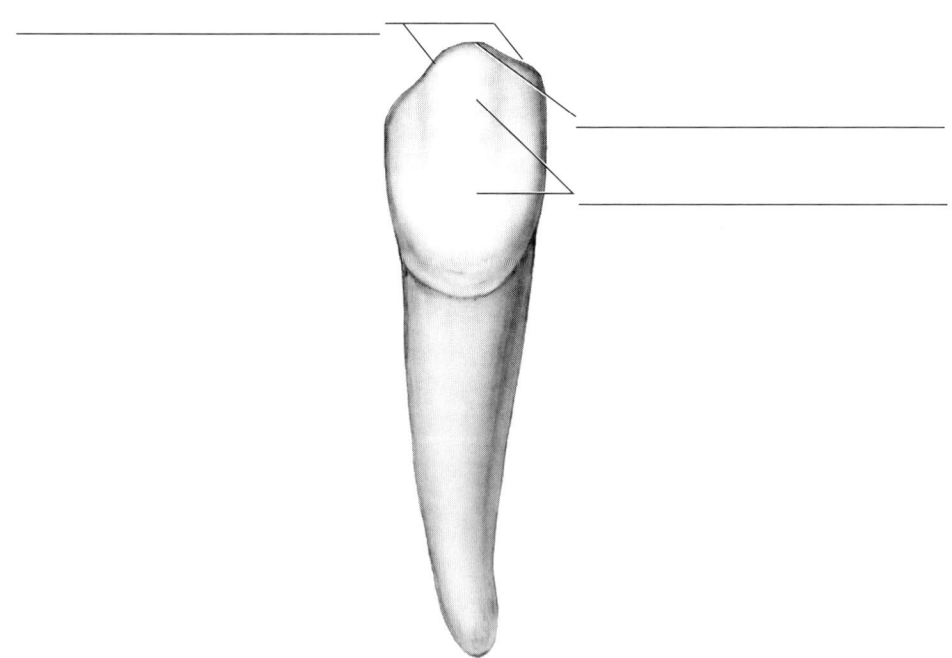

Permanent Mandibular Right Canine
Labial View

16. Figure 16.23

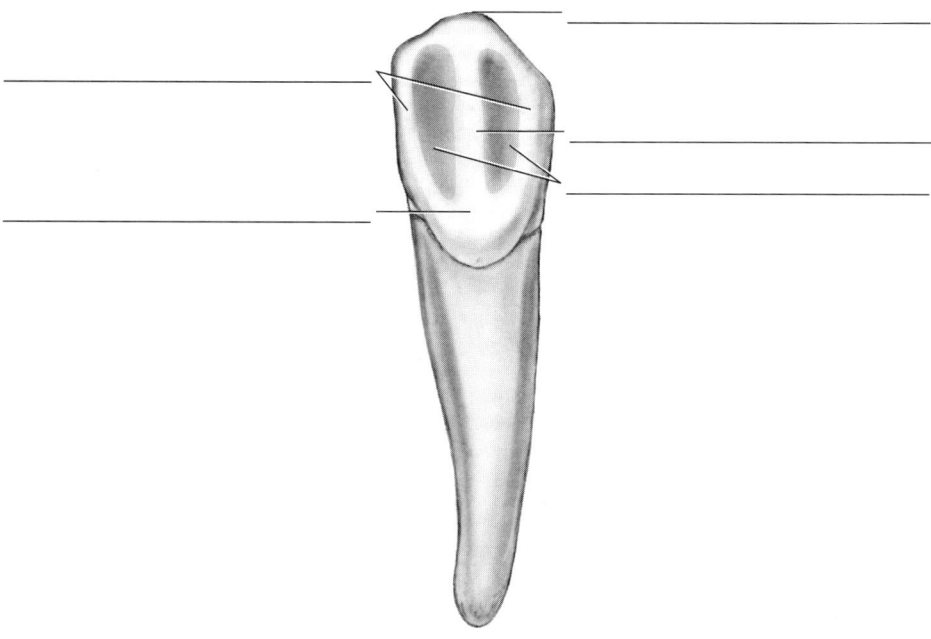

Permanent Mandibular Right Canine
Lingual View

17. Figure 16.27

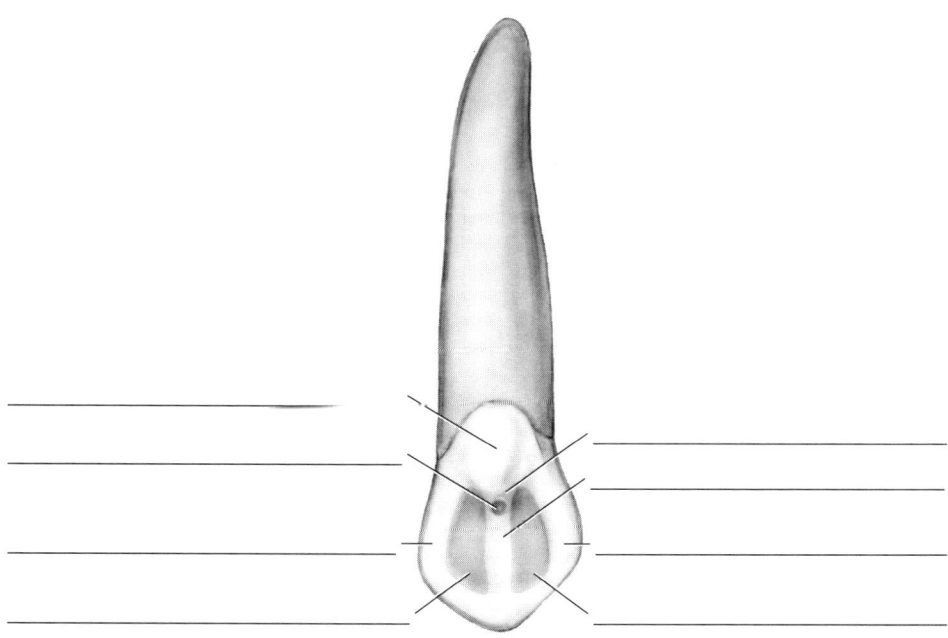

Permanent Maxillary Right Canine
Lingual View

Chapter 17: Permanent Posterior Teeth

18. Figure 17.2

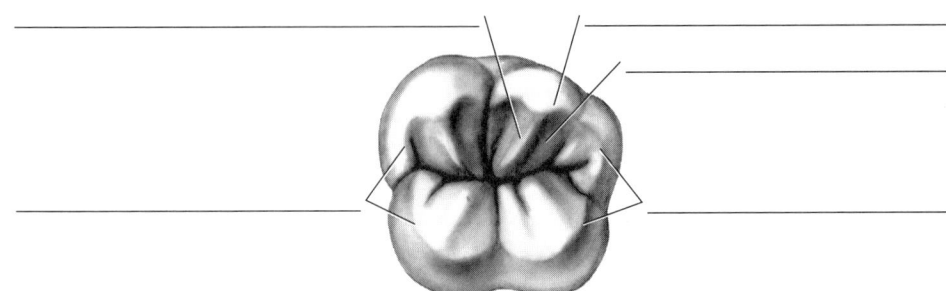

Permanent Posterior Tooth
Occlusal View

19. Figure 17.4

Developmental Grooves:

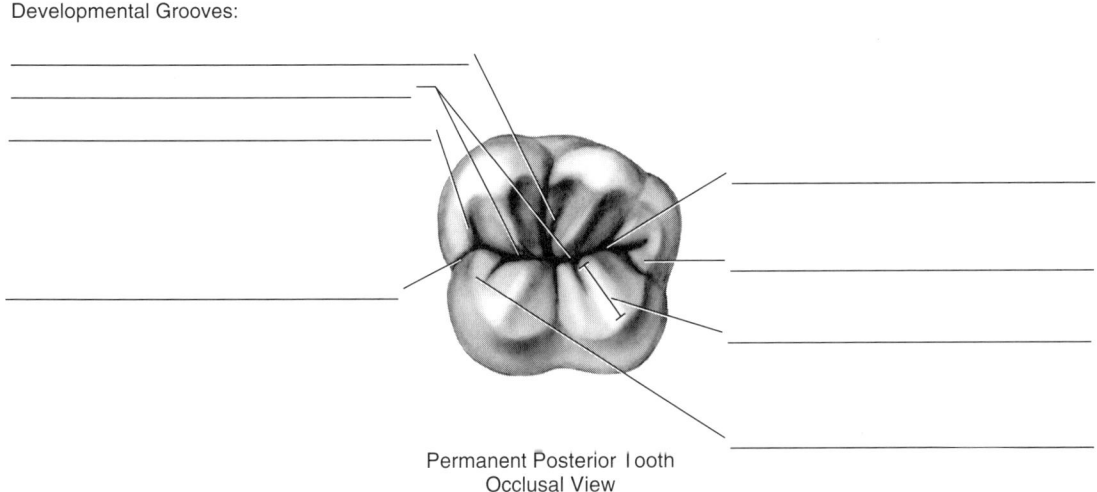

Permanent Posterior Tooth
Occlusal View

20. Figure 17.7

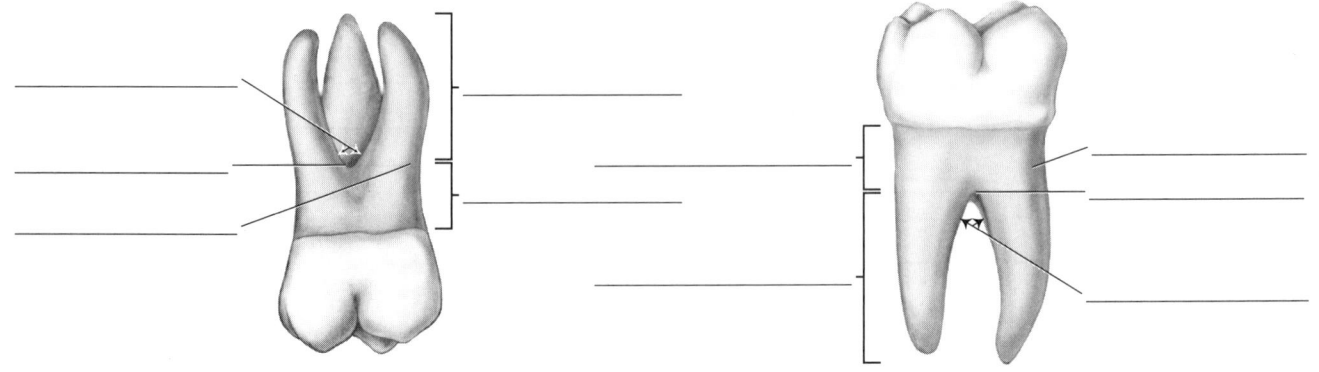

Permanent Posterior Molars: Maxillary and Mandibular
Buccal Views

21. Figure 17.10

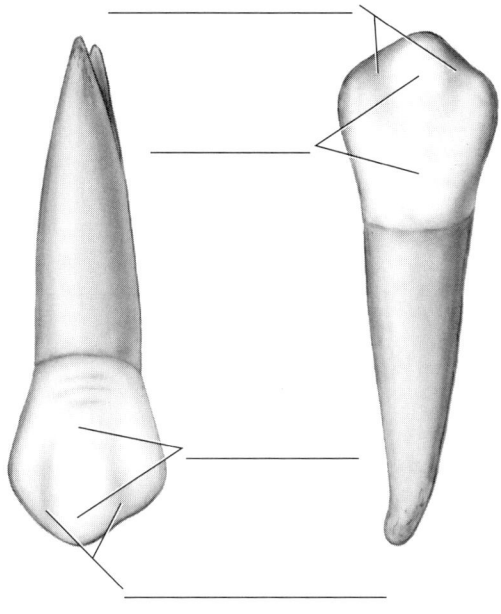

Permanent Premolars
Buccal Views

22. Figure 17.13

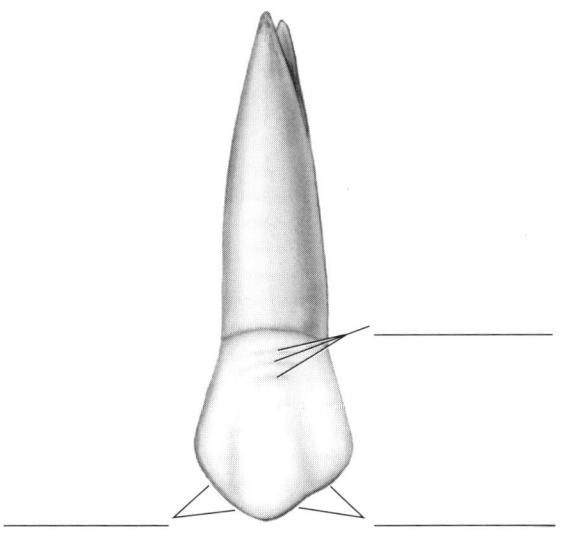

Permanent Maxillary Right First Premolar
Buccal View

23. Figure 17.14, *A*

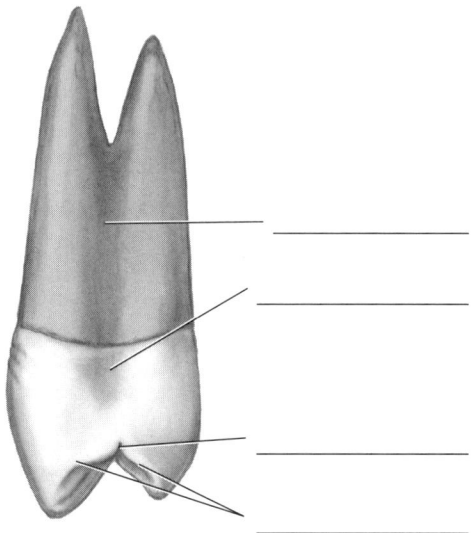

Permanent Maxillary Right First Premolar
Mesial view

24. Figure 17.15

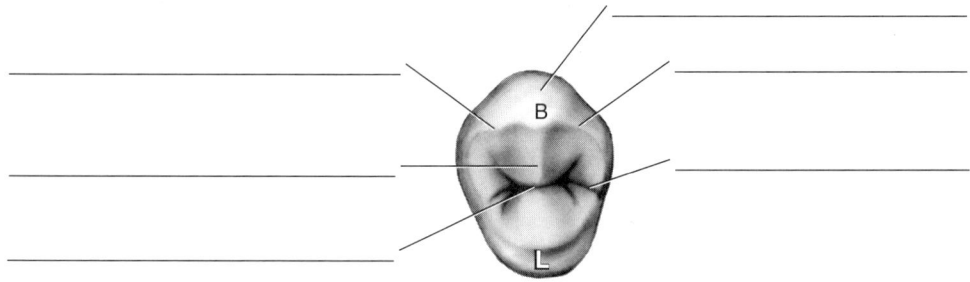

Permanent Maxillary Right First Premolar
Occlusal View

25. Figure 17.16

Transverse {
Ridge {

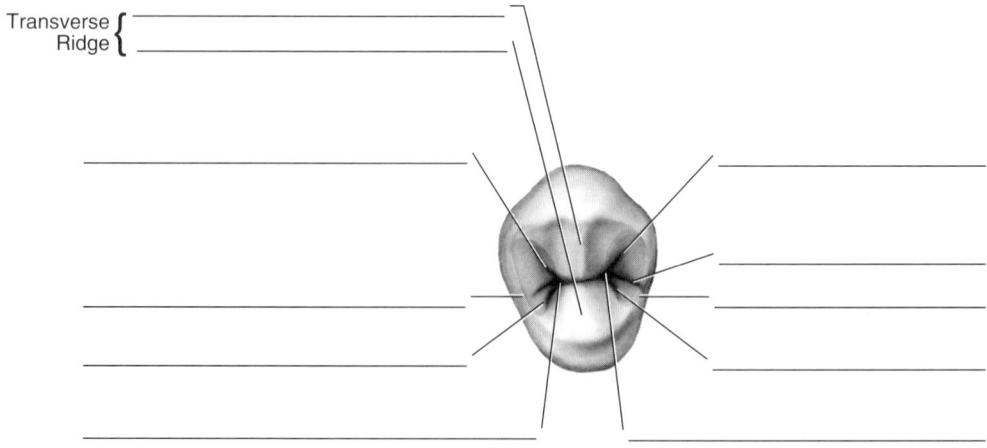

Permanent Maxillary Right First Premolar
Occlusal View

26. Figure 17.19

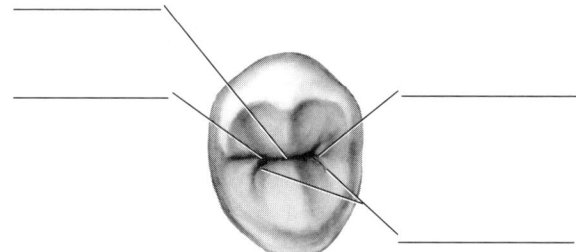

Permanent Maxillary Right Second Premolar
Occlusal View

27. Figure 17.22

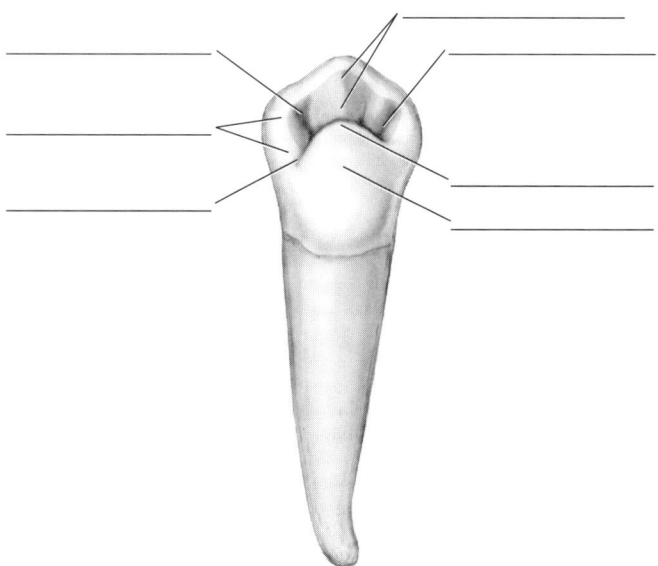

Permanent Mandibular Right First Premolar
Lingual View

28. Figure 17.23

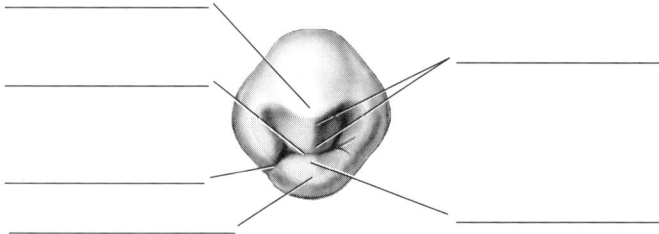

Permanent Mandibular Right First Premolar
Occlusal View

29. Figure 17.24

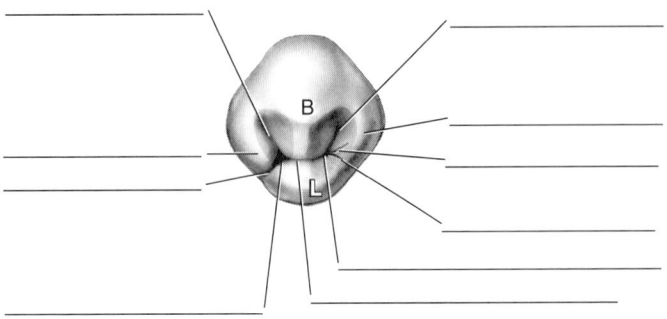

Permanent Mandibular Right First Premolar
Occlusal View

30. Figure 17.27

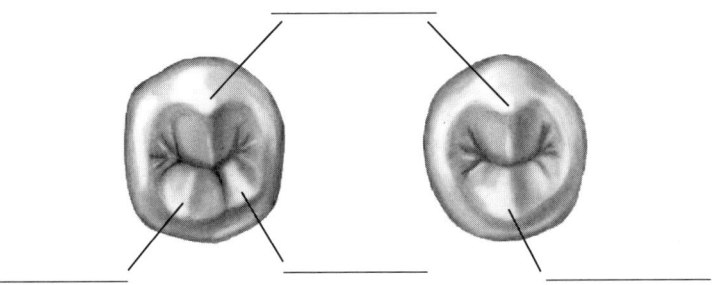

Three-Cusp type **Two-Cusp type**

Permanent Mandibular Second Premolars
Occlusal Views

31. Figure 17.29

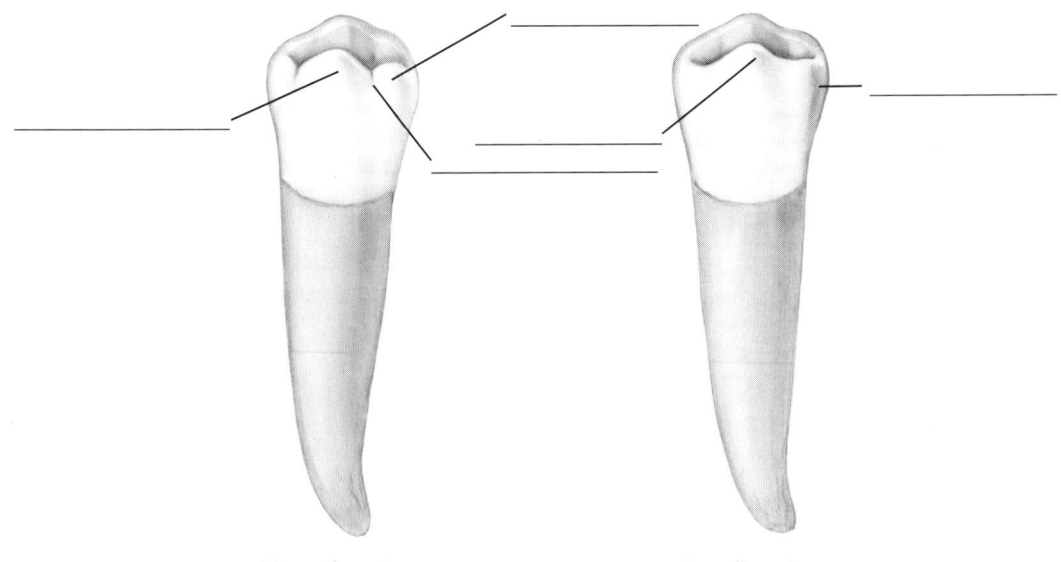

Three-Cusp type **Two-Cusp type**

Permanent Mandibular Right First Premolars
Lingual Views

32. Figure 17.30

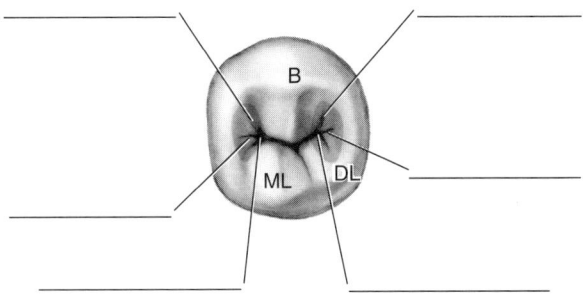

Permanent Mandibular Right Second Premolar: Three-Cusp Type
Occlusal View

33. Figure 17.31

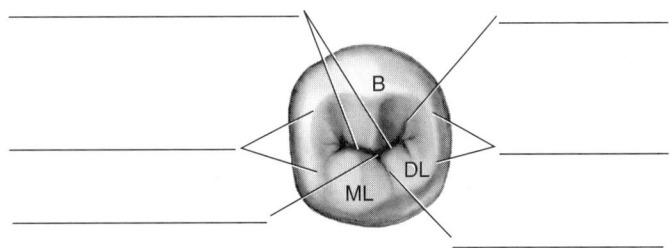

Permanent Mandibular Right Second Premolar: Three-Cusp Type, Y-Shaped Groove Pattern
Occlusal View

34. Figure 17.32

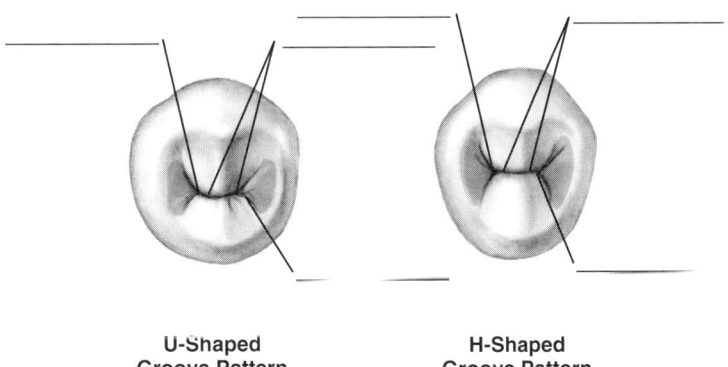

U-Shaped Groove Pattern **H-Shaped Groove Pattern**

Permanent Mandibular Right Second Premolars: Two-Cusp Type
Occlusal View

35. Figure 17.34

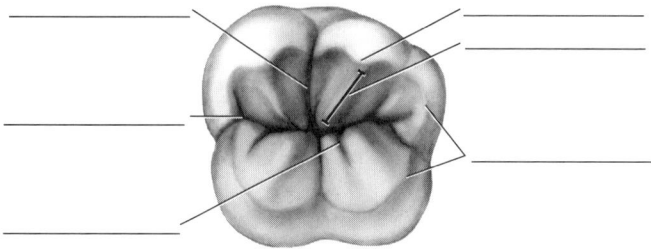

Permanent Molar
Occlusal View

36. Figure 17.37

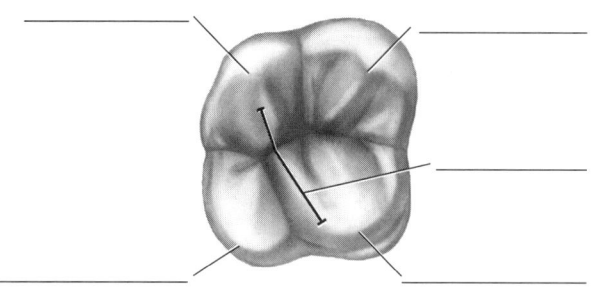

Permanent Maxillary Molar
Occlusal View

37. Figure 17.41

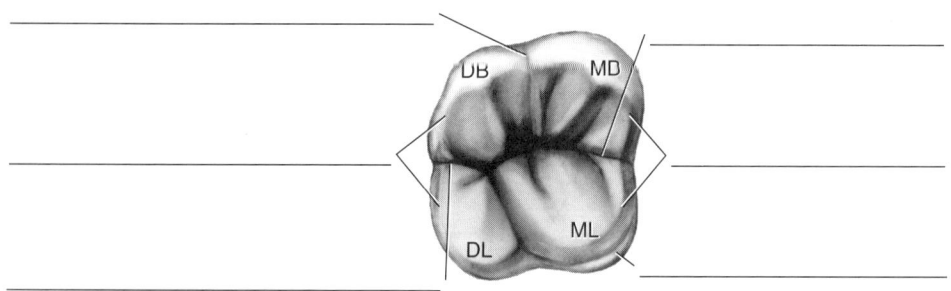

Permanent Maxillary Right First Molar
Occlusal View

38. Figure 17.42

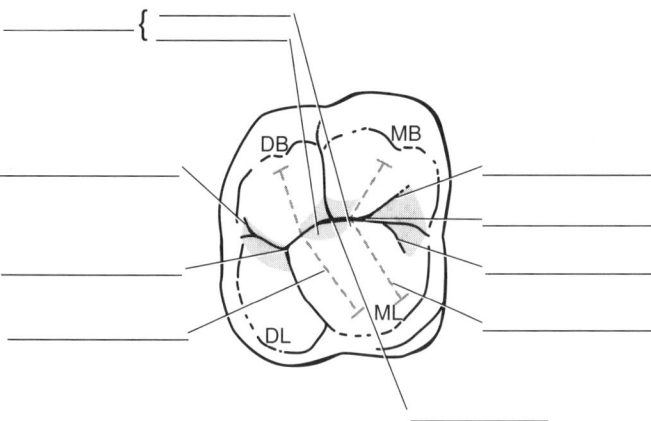

Permanent Maxillary Right First Molar
Occlusal View

39. Figure 17.46

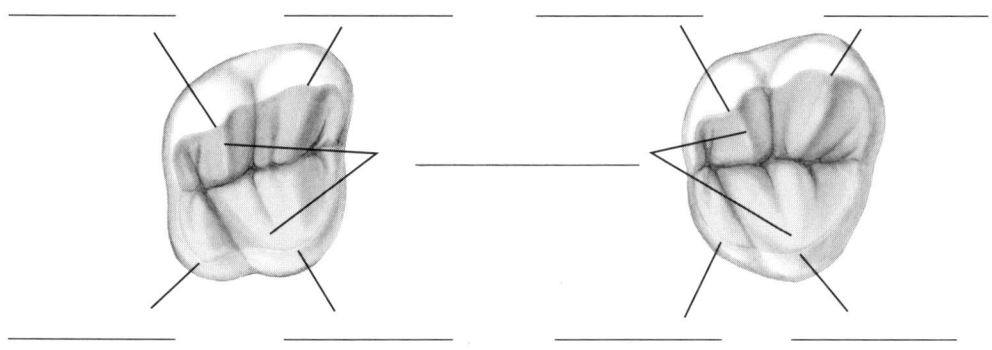

Rhomboidal Type   **Heart-Shaped Type**

Permanent Maxillary Right Second Molars
Occlusal Views

40. Figure 17.53

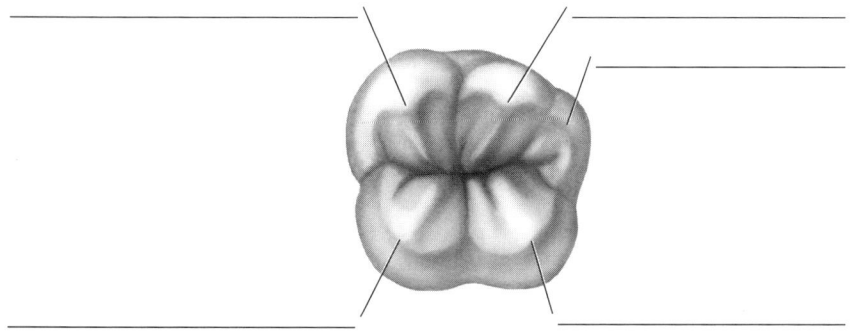

Permanent Mandibular Right First Molar
Occlusal View

41. Figure 17.54

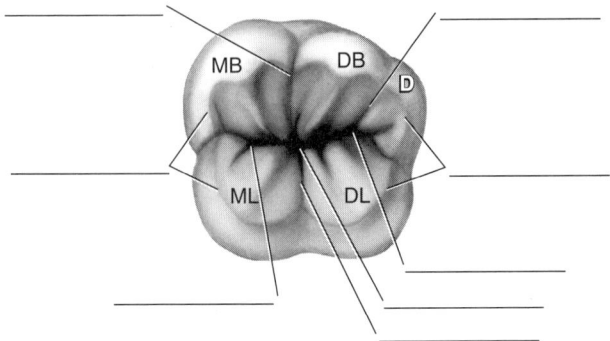

Permanent Maxillary Right First Molar
Occlusal View

42. Figure 17.59

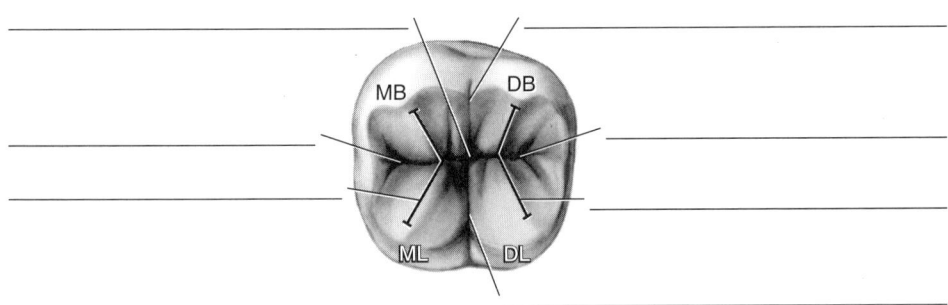

Permanent Mandibular Right Second Molar
Occlusal View

Chapter 18: Primary Dentition

43. Figure 18.2

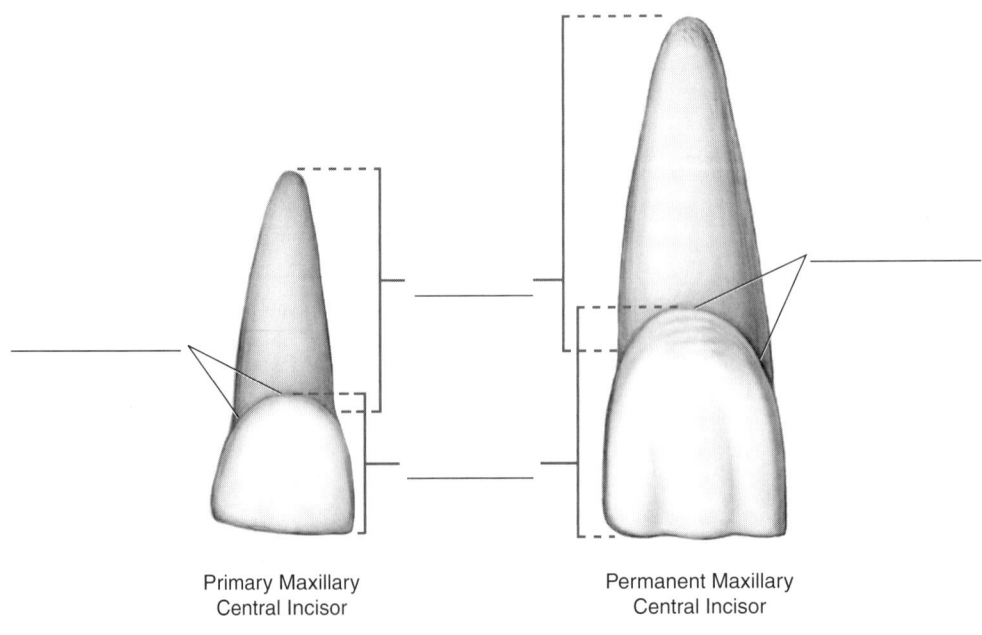

Primary Maxillary
Central Incisor

Permanent Maxillary
Central Incisor

Labial Views

44. Figure 18.3

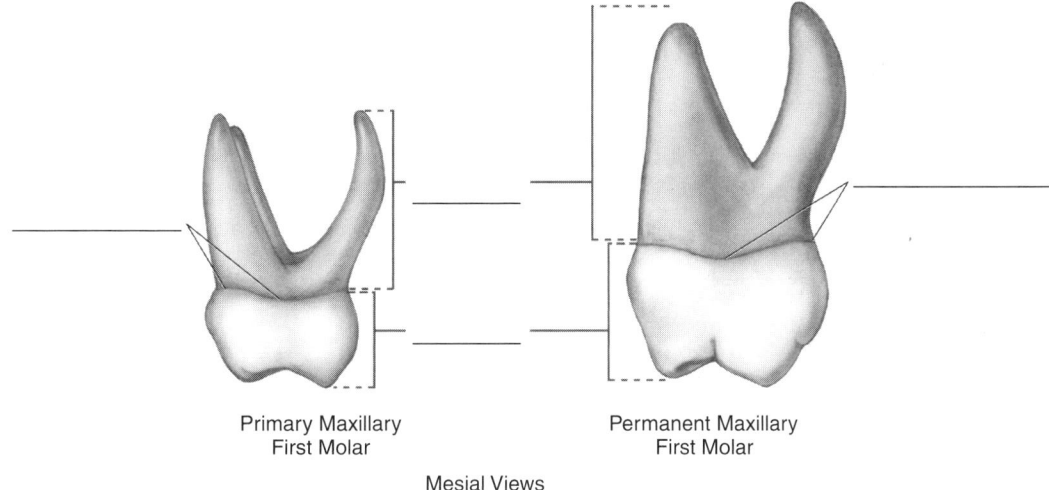

Primary Maxillary First Molar   Permanent Maxillary First Molar

Mesial Views

Chapter 19: Temporomandibular Joint

45. Figure 19.1

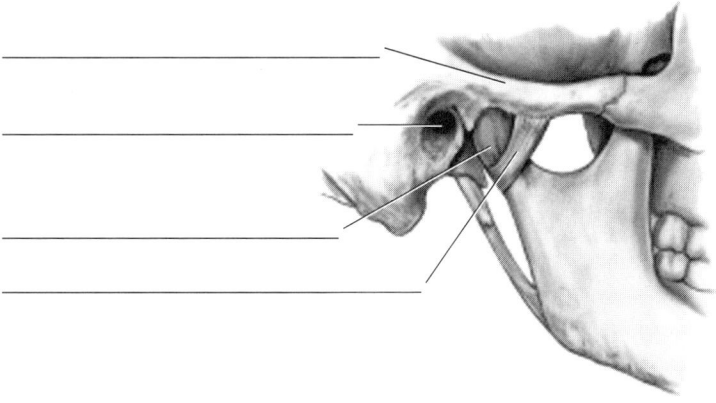

Temporomandibular Joint

46. Figure 19.5

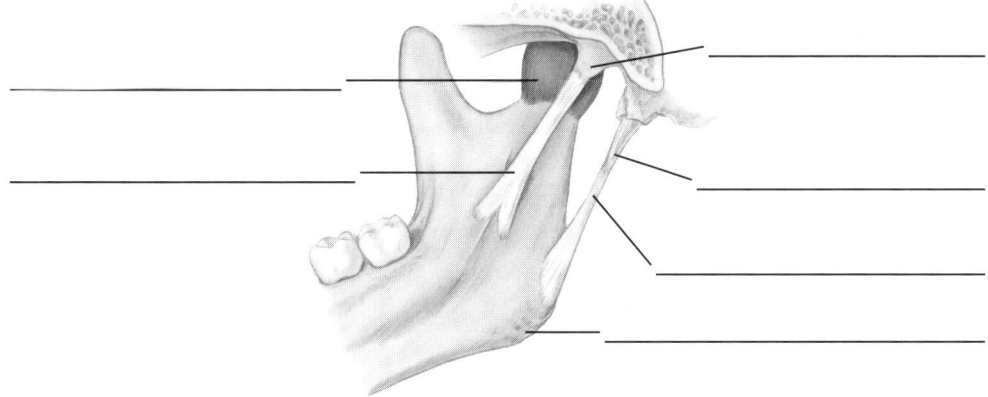

47. Figure 19.6

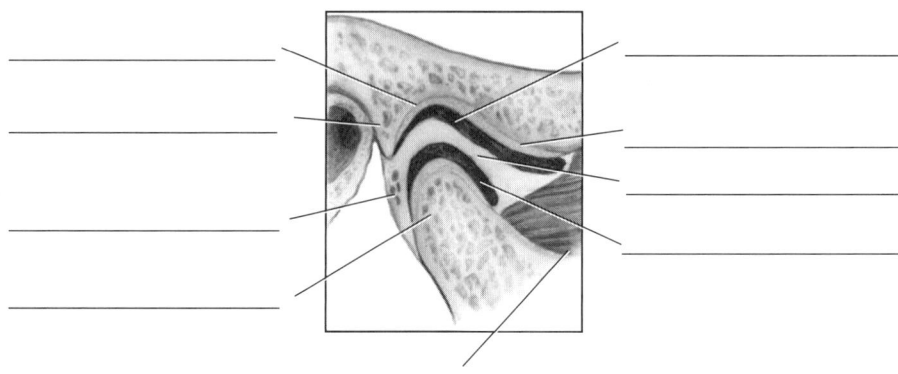

48. Figure 19.8, *A, B, C*

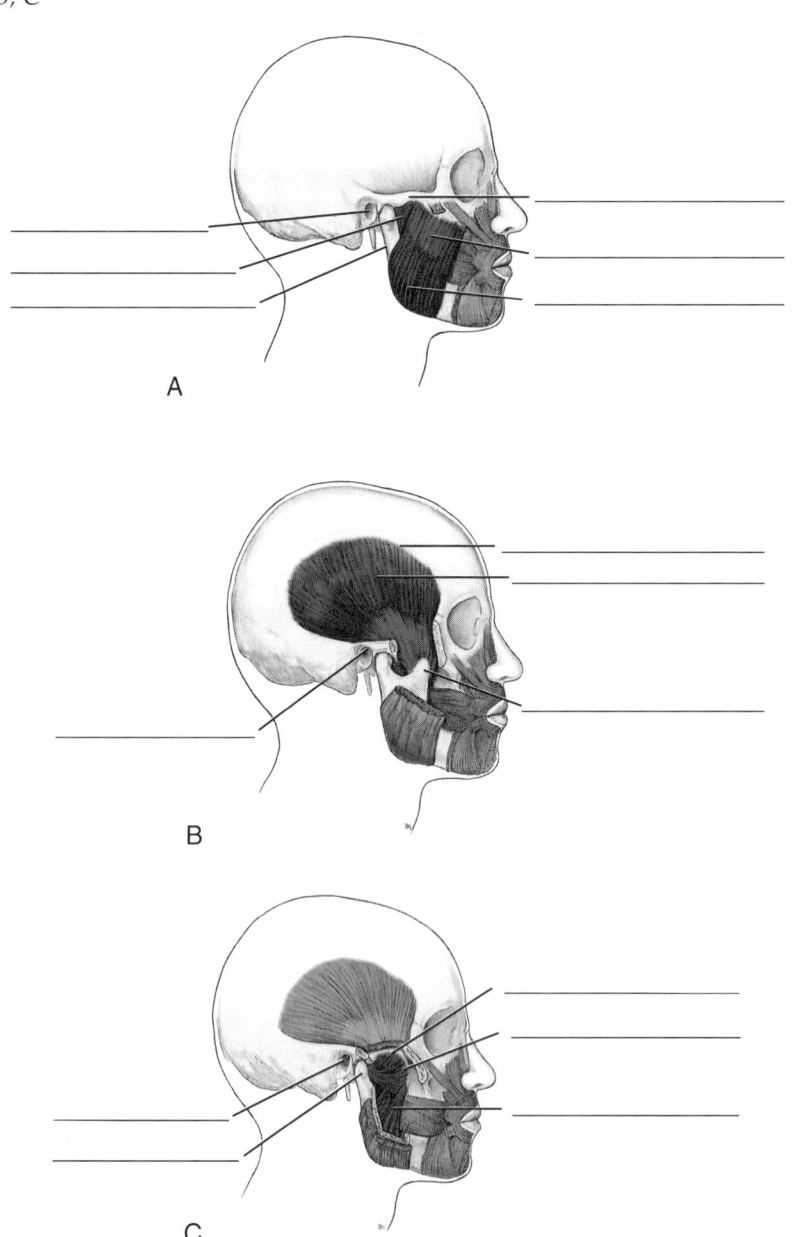

The following are exercises within the clinical setting for **identification through observation** as discussed and illustrated in the associated textbook. They include clinical observation of extraoral and intraoral structures, dentition, and occlusion. This student workbook and also a copy of associated textbook and any notes can be kept alongside oneself at the clinical setting as one goes through the exercises. These exercises will help the student dental professional tie in information about these clinical matters and then integrate them into future clinical situations. More in-depth examination can be done in the future by student dental professionals after additional coursework in oral pathology, periodontology, dental materials, dental imaging, and related clinical situations.

Directions for Parts 1 and 2: After completing the medical and dental history and/or review, the patient should be seated in a dental chair, either supine or upright as needed. Remove any pigmented lip products and apply nonpetroleum lubricant to dry lips; ask to take out any removable prostheses as needed. Good lighting and exposure of the region being observed are essential, e.g., collar and tie loosened, glasses removed. Follow your institution's current standard precautions for all patient care.

During this exercise in both extraoral and intraoral structure identification, check the items as noted. Make sure to also record any typical findings. Include specific location using nearby structures. Also record any atypical or abnormal findings; if found, take nonidentifiable clinical photographs as well as dental imaging, if possible, after being given permission to be shared with other students and instructors. Make appropriate referrals with assistance, if needed, through your institution. Also include any palpable lymph nodes of the face and neck.

The posterior part of the base of the tongue and its structures, such as the lingual tonsil, are usually not observable within the oral cavity; however, note the relationship of the nasopharynx and laryngopharynx to the oropharynx by indicating on the external neck the placement of these related internal regions. When observing oral mucosal surfaces, it is important to gently dry those surfaces with a gauze or air syringe if one can, so that color or texture changes will become more obvious. In addition, avoid contact with any structures near the soft palate or pharynx to prevent the gag reflex; use only observation in this region.

Explanations of the reasons for performing both extraoral and intraoral examinations for the patient and their relationship of these examinations to dental treatment, including the terminology used in these examinations, *are located* in the associated textbook in **Chapters 1 and 2**.

Basic Clinical Supplies Needed: The student dental professional will need the following basic supplies for the clinical identification exercises: dental chair and light, mirror instrument, hand mirror, and student workbook-included checklists.

CLINICAL IDENTIFICATION EXERCISE Part 1: Extraoral Structures

Extraoral Identification Checklist		
Frontal, Orbital, and Nasal Regions	**Typical Findings**	**Atypical or Abnormal Findings**
Forehead		
Orbits		
External Nose: Root of Nose, Apex of Nose, Nares, Nasal Septum, Nasal Alae		
Infraorbital and Zygomatic Regions	**Typical Findings**	**Atypical or Abnormal Findings**
Zygomatic Arches		
Temporomandibular Joints		
Buccal Regions	**Typical Findings**	**Atypical or Abnormal Findings**
Cheeks and Masseter Muscles		
Angles of the Mandible		
Parotid Salivary Glands		
Oral Region	**Typical Findings**	**Atypical or Abnormal Findings**
Lips: Vermilion Zones/Borders, Mucocutaneous Junctions, Labial Commissures		
Maxillae, Philtrum, Tubercle of Upper Lip		

Extraoral Identification Checklist		
Mental Region	Typical Findings	Atypical or Abnormal Findings
Mandible: Mandibular Symphysis, Rami, Coronoid Processes, Coronoid Notches, Mandibular Condyles, Mandibular Notches		
Regions of the Neck	Typical Findings	Atypical or Abnormal Findings
Sternocleidomastoid Muscles		
Hyoid Bone		
Thyroid Cartilage		
Thyroid Gland		
Submandibular Salivary Glands		
Sublingual Salivary Glands		

CLINICAL IDENTIFICATION EXERCISE Part 2: Intraoral Structures

Intraoral Identification Checklist		
Oral Vestibules	Typical Findings	Atypical or Abnormal Findings
Labial Mucosa		
Buccal Mucosa, Buccal Fat Pads		
Parotid Salivary Glands, Parotid Papillae		
Vestibular Fornices		
Alveolar Mucosa, Mucobuccal Folds		
Labial Frena: Maxillary and Mandibular		
Jaws, Alveolar Processes, Teeth, Arches	Typical Findings	Atypical or Abnormal Findings
Maxillae: Body, Maxillary Sinuses, Alveolar Process, Alveoli, Maxillary Teeth, Maxillary Tuberosities		
Mandible: Body, Alveolar Process, Alveoli, Mandibular Teeth, Retromolar Pads		
Permanent Teeth within Maxillary and Mandibular Arches: Crowns, Enamel, Anterior Teeth (Incisors, Canines), Posterior Teeth (Premolars, Molars)		
Gingival Tissue	Typical Findings	Atypical or Abnormal Findings
Attached Gingiva		
Mucogingival Junctions		
Marginal Gingiva: Free Gingival Crests and Grooves		
Gingival Sulci (location only)		
Interdental Gingiva: Interdental Papillae		
Oral Cavity Proper	Typical Findings	Atypical or Abnormal Findings
Fauces: Anterior and Posterior Pillars		
Palatine Tonsils		

Intraoral Identification Checklist		
Palate	Typical Findings	Atypical or Abnormal Findings
Hard Palate: Median Palatine Raphe, Incisive Papilla, Palatine Rugae		
Soft Palate, Uvula		
Pterygomandibular Folds		
Tongue	Typical Findings	Atypical or Abnormal Findings
Base of Tongue (anterior part only)		
Body of Tongue		
Dorsal Surface: Median Lingual Sulcus, Sulcus Terminalis, Foramen Cecum (if possible)		
Filiform Lingual Papillae		
Circumvallate Lingual Papillae		
Lateral Surfaces		
Foliate Lingual Papillae		
Ventral Surface		
Plicae Fimbriatae		
Floor of the Mouth	Typical Findings	Atypical or Abnormal Findings
Lingual Frenum		
Sublingual Folds		
Sublingual Caruncles		
Sublingual Salivary Glands		
Submandibular Salivary Glands		
Pharynx	Typical Findings	Atypical Findings
Oropharynx		

Directions for Parts 2 and 3: Follow basic preparations as noted for previous clinical exercises. Explanations of the reasons for performing patient examination of both the dentition and occlusion and their relationship of these examinations to dental treatment, including the terminology used in these examinations, *are located* in the associated textbook in **Chapters 15 and 20**. Both Universal and International Numbering Systems are included in the checklists.

CLINICAL IDENTIFICATION EXERCISE Part 3: Dentition

During this exercise in observing the patient's dentition (permanent), circle the items as noted on the crowns of the tooth types listed. Place NA (aka Not Applicable) if trauma, restoration, or extraction has occurred so that it is impossible to tell what is present; third molars will not be specifically examined, but take notes on crown anatomy, if present.

Compare both quadrants of each arch; the sequence is the same as used in the associated textbook. Use the instrument mirror during observation. Also record any atypical or abnormal findings; if found, take nonidentifiable clinical photographs as well as dental imaging, if possible, after being given permission to be shared with other students and instructors. Make appropriate referrals with assistance, if needed, through your institution.

INCISORS CHECKLIST

TOOTH NUMBER	INCISAL SURFACE	CINGULUM/MARGINAL RIDGES	LINGUAL FOSSA	NOTES
8, 9 (11, 21)	Ridge/Edge	Well-developed/ Less developed	Deep/Shallow	
7, 10 (12, 22)	Ridge/Edge	Well-developed/ Less developed	Deep/Shallow	
24, 25 (31, 41)	Ridge/Edge	Well-developed/ Less developed	Deep/Shallow	
23, 26 (32, 42)	Ridge/Edge	Well-developed/ Less developed	Deep/Shallow	

CANINE CHECKLIST

TOOTH NUMBER	CUSP TIP	CINGULUM/LINGUAL RIDGE/MARGINAL RIDGES	LINGUAL FOSSA	NOTES
6, 11 (13, 23)	Centered/Offset	Well-developed/Less developed	Deep/Shallow	
22, 27 (33, 43)	Centered/Offset	Well-developed/Less developed	Deep/Shallow	

PREMOLAR CHECKLIST

TOOTH NUMBER	OCCLUSAL SHAPE	CUSPS	RIDGES	PROXIMAL SHAPE	NOTES
5, 12 (14, 24)	Hexagonal/Diamond-Shaped/Square	2 or 3	Transverse/ Not Transverse	Trapezoidal/ Rhomboidal	
4, 13 (15, 25)	Hexagonal/Diamond-Shaped/Square	2 or 3	Transverse/ Not Transverse	Trapezoidal/ Rhomboidal	
21, 28 (34, 44)	Hexagonal/Diamond-Shaped/Square	2 or 3	Transverse/ Not Transverse	Trapezoidal/ Rhomboidal	
20, 29 (35, 45)	Hexagonal/Diamond-Shaped/Square	2 or 3	Transverse/ Not Transverse	Trapezoidal/ Rhomboidal	

MOLAR CHECKLIST

TOOTH NUMBER	OCCLUSAL SHAPE	CUSPS	RIDGES	PROXIMAL SHAPE	PITS	NOTES
3, 14 (16, 26)	Rhomboidal/ Heart-Shaped	4 or 5	Oblique/ Transverse	Trapezoidal/ Rhomboidal	Lingual/ Buccal	
2, 15 (17, 27)	Rhomboidal/ Heart-Shaped	4 or 5	Oblique/ Transverse	Trapezoidal/ Rhomboidal	Lingual/ Buccal	
19, 30 (36, 46)	Rectangular/ Pentagonal	4 or 5	Oblique/ Transverse	Trapezoidal/ Rhomboidal	Lingual/ Buccal	
18, 31 (37, 47)	Rectangular/ Pentagonal	4 or 5	Oblique/ Transverse	Trapezoidal/ Rhomboidal	Lingual/ Buccal	
1, 16 (18, 28)						

MOLAR CHECKLIST

TOOTH NUMBER	OCCLUSAL SHAPE	CUSPS	RIDGES	PROXIMAL SHAPE	PITS	NOTES
17, 32 (38, 48)						

CLINICAL IDENTIFICATION EXERCISE Part 4: Occlusion

Additional Supplies Needed: Will also need periodontal probe instrument, articulating paper, and floss. Because many steps are involved in this procedure, the sequence used can be modified as needed; the following sequence is the same used in the associated textbook. Also record any atypical or abnormal findings; if found, take nonidentifiable clinical photographs as well as dental imaging, if possible, after being given permission to be shared with other students and instructors. Make appropriate referrals with assistance, if needed, through your institution.

Step 1. Occlusal History: Extraoral and Intraoral Findings

Before performing the clinical identification of an occlusion, include the **occlusal history** of the patient. Note in the chart section any removable prostheses (flippers, retainers, night and sports mouthguards, and partial or complete dentures as well as overdentures); however, have the patient keep them in their oral cavity during the procedure if worn regularly to complete the masticatory function of the dentition. Note any occlusal complaints, habits, and applicable physical or psychological findings from the patient's or dental and medical history that may be pertinent to the patient's occlusal history. Record all of these in that chart section labeled as "Occlusal History."

Additionally, include any additional findings noted during the extraoral observation that may be pertinent to the patient's occlusion (see earlier observation exercises) and record in that chart section labeled as "Extraoral Findings." This includes facial profile and asymmetries, vertical dimension loss, mandibular deviation upon opening, lip seal loss, and temporomandibular disorder signs. Also include any additional findings noted during the intraoral observation that may be pertinent to the patient's occlusion such as cheek chewing and biting with large areas of mucosal hyperkeratosis from habits or abnormal tongue placement with improper swallowing and record in that chart section labeled as "Intraoral Findings."

Record the general amount of tooth loss in that chart section labeled as "Attrition" and "Abfraction" as well as circling the involved teeth in red with **attrition** or **abfraction** in that part of the chart. Also record the location of associated **wear facets** by circling the involved teeth in red in that part of the chart. Finally, record any **mobility** by circling the involved teeth in red in that part of the chart.

Record any **sensitivity** to thermal changes using ice or cold spray and percussion by using gentle tapping in that chart section labeled as "Sensitivity". Note any changes in the **intra-arch form or alignment** such as loss of interdental contact with pathologic migration, plunging cusps, open bite, crossbites, and any arch collapse. Note also any missing, rotated, drifted, supererupted, or fractured teeth. Include any major changes in restorations since occlusal trauma is the main reason for early restoration failure. Changes in the midline of the dentition for each of the two dental arches should also be noted. Record all these in that chart section labeled as "Intra-arch Form/Alignment."

Finally, note any pertinent information from **dental imaging** if available such as loss of the lamina dura support, alterations of the periodontal ligament space, root resorption or excess cementum, and nonvital and fixed prosthetic teeth, including veneers, crowns, and implants. Record these findings in that chart section labeled as "Dental Imaging."

Step 2. Centric Relation

To allow the student dental professional to identify the occlusion of a patient, the patient must be placed in **centric relation (CR)**. The position of CR is the end point of closure of the mandible in the most retruded position, which will serve as a baseline.

To achieve CR, first put the patient in an upright position, sitting or standing in front and to the side of the patient. The patient should be relaxed, looking straight ahead with lips parted. Using the operating hand, place a thumb against the outside of the patient's chin, with the fingers placed under the inferior border of the mandible to alternately lift and loosen the mandible. Then second, establish the hinge movement of the mandible by gently arcing the mandible with the fingers several times in a closing and opening manner. Then third, guide the loosened mandible into closure, with the mandible placed in its most retruded position.

Step 3. Angle Classification of Malocclusion

Once the patient is in CR, determine the **Angle classification of malocclusion** of the patient's dentition. Most cases can be placed into one of three main classes on the basis of the position of the permanent maxillary first molar relative to the permanent mandibular first molar (see associated text). The use of the canines in each arch instead must also be recorded if the first molars cannot be used for classification by entering tooth used for determination in that chart section. A tendency to any type of malocclusion, which is considered less than the width of a premolar, can be recorded using either the molar or canine relationship by entering any tendencies in that chart section. Additionally, any subgroups within the classification must be recorded as well if the right or left side is not symmetrical within Angle classification by entering two notations in that chart section. The classification and any additional notes as discussed are recorded in that chart section labeled as "Angle Classification."

Step 4. Overjet

With the patient maintained in CR, **overjet** or horizontal overlap between the two arches is determined by measuring it in millimeters with the tip of the periodontal probe. Place the probe at a right angle to the labial surface of a mandibular incisor at the base of the incisal ridge of a maxillary incisor. The measurement is taken from the labial surface of the mandibular incisor to the lingual surface of the maxillary incisor. Note that the labiolingual width of the maxillary incisor is not included in the measurement. Ideally at 1 to 3 mm for comparison. The overjet measurement is recorded in that chart section labeled as "Overjet."

Step 5. Overbite

With the patient maintained in CR, **overbite** or vertical overlap between the two arches is determined also by measuring it in millimeters with the tip of the periodontal probe. Place the probe on the incisal ridge of the maxillary incisor at a right angle to the mandibular incisor. As the patient opens the mouth or depresses the jaws, then place the probe vertically against the mandibular incisor to measure the distance to the incisal ridge of the mandibular incisor. Ideally at 2 to 5 mm for comparison. The overbite measurement is recorded in that chart section labeled as "Overbite."

Step 6. Interocclusal Clearance and Range of Motion

Now allow the patient to relax the mandible while observing **interocclusal clearance**, the space when the mandible is at rest. In this rest position, ideally 2 to 3 mm can be noted between the masticatory surfaces of the maxillary and mandibular teeth for comparison. Thus failure of a patient to assume this position when the jaws are not at work may mean the patient is habitually tense or has an **orofacial parafunctional habit** such as clenching or grinding (bruxism). Interocclusal clearance is measured in millimeters and recorded in that chart section labeled as "Interocclusal Clearance." If there is no interocclusal clearance noted during mandibular rest, follow-up questions may be necessary to ascertain any habitual tension or any orofacial parafunctional habit.

Additionally, the **range of motion** of the mandible can determined by measuring it in millimeters during maximum mouth opening from the interincisal distance present and recorded in that chart section labeled as "Range of Motion."

Step 7. Tooth Contact

Next after relaxation of the patient's mandible, the position of CR can again be attained. The patient is then asked to point to where the teeth first contact during occlusion by having them close their teeth gently together. Ideally all teeth should contact at the same time between the arches with closure. Any tooth or teeth having a **premature contact** will limit the allowance for maximal intercuspation of the teeth. Articulation paper can also be used to observe any premature contact. Any premature contact is recorded in the chart by circling the involved teeth in red in that chart section labeled as "Centric Relation and Occlusion."

Step 8. Centric Occlusion

Next have the patient clench the teeth together to determine the amount of **functional shift** in millimeters from jaw position in CR to jaw position in **centric occlusion (CO)** as well as its direction. The CO or habitual occlusion is the voluntary position of the dentition that allows maximal contact when the teeth occlude. Record the amount of functional shift in millimeters in that chart section; record also the direction of the shift as "Anterior," "Right," "Left," or "Posterior" in that chart section. Ideally, no major shift or small amount is noted such as 1 mm or less for comparison. This is because ideally the position of the teeth is CR = CO so then that is circled instead in that chart section.

Step 9. Lateral Occlusion

Next it is necessary to observe the patient's **lateral occlusion** during **lateral deviation** or *lateral excursion* by moving the mandible to either the right or the left until the canines on that side are in **canine rise**. The patient's mandible is supported with the operating hand and then the mandible is gently moved into CR or even CO. Then slowly guide the mandible to the patient's right or left until the opposing canines are edge-to-edge.

The side to which the mandible has been moved is the **working side**. There are two working sides noted: right lateral and left lateral. Before the opposing canines come into contact on each side, other individual teeth that make contact on the working side should be recorded as a **working contact** by circling the involved teeth in blue in that chart section labeled as "Left Lateral Occlusion" and "Right Lateral Occlusion."

The side of the arch that is opposite or contralateral to the working side with lateral occlusion is the **balancing side** or nonworking side. If any teeth make contact on the balancing side during lateral deviation, they are recorded as a **balancing interference** and the involved teeth are circled in red in that chart section labeled as "Left Lateral Occlusion" and "Right Lateral Occlusion." Do not allow patients to move freely into lateral deviation because they may choose a convenient path to bypass a balancing interference within the occlusion.

For further confirmation of any balancing interferences during lateral deviation, place floss across the retromolar pads extending out to the labial commissures or place articulating paper over the occlusal surfaces on the appropriate side. After guiding the patient into either right or left lateral occlusion, slip the floss or articulating paper forward, noting any points of contact. Adjust recordings as needed with this further information.

If **group function** is present, most of the entire posterior quadrant of each opposing arch is functioning during lateral occlusion without canine rise so as to share the occlusal stress during function. This should be recorded by circling the involved group of teeth in blue in that chart section labeled as "Left Lateral Occlusion" and "Right Lateral Occlusion."

Step 10. Protrusive Occlusion

Finally, observe the patient's **protrusive occlusion** during **protrusion**. With the patient's teeth in CO, support the mandible with the operating hand and have the patient slowly move the mandible forward so that the two arches are in an edge-to-edge relationship with the most anterior teeth. Record any posterior tooth or canine contacts as well as any **balancing interference** during protrusion and record this information on the chart by circling the involved teeth in red in that chart section labeled as "Protrusive Occlusion." Also record the anterior teeth that are in contact during protrusion or any **working contact** by circling the involved teeth in blue in that chart section labeled as "Protrusive Occlusion."

For further confirmation of working contacts and any balancing interferences during protrusion, place the floss across the retromolar pads extending out to the labial commissures. Then guide the patient into protrusive occlusion and slip the floss forward between the teeth until resistance of contacting teeth is met. Adjust recordings as needed with this further information.

OCCLUSION IDENTIFICATION FORM

Occlusal History _____

_____

Extraoral Findings _____

Intraoral Findings _____

Attrition _____ **Abfraction** _____

Angle Classification _____ **Right** _____ **Left** _____ **Subgroup** _____

Molar Right _____ **Canine Right** _____ **Molar Left** _____ **Canine Left** _____

Interocclusal Clearance _____ mm **Sensitivity** _____

Overjet _____ mm **Overbite** _____ mm

Range of Motion _____ mm

Intra-Arch Form/Alignment _____

_____

Dental Imaging (if available) _____

OCCLUSION IDENTIFICATION CHECKLIST																
Centric Relation and Centric Occlusion	1	2	3	4	5	6	7	8	9	10	11	12	13	14	15	16
	(18	17	16	15	14	13	12	11)	(21	22	23	24	25	26	27	28)
	32	31	30	29	28	27	26	25	24	23	22	21	20	19	18	17
	(48	47	46	45	44	43	42	41)	(31	32	33	34	35	36	37	38)
CR = CO	Shift CR to CO ____ mm								Anterior Right Left Posterior							
Right Lateral Occlusion	1	2	3	4	5	6	7	8	9	10	11	12	13	14	15	16
	(18	17	16	15	14	13	12	11)	(21	22	23	24	25	26	27	28)
	32	31	30	29	28	27	26	25	24	23	22	21	20	19	18	17
	(48	47	46	45	44	43	42	41)	(31	32	33	34	35	36	37	38)
Left Lateral Occlusion	1	2	3	4	5	6	7	8	9	10	11	12	13	14	15	16
	(18	17	16	15	14	13	12	11)	(21	22	23	24	25	26	27	28)
	32	31	30	29	28	27	26	25	24	23	22	21	20	9	18	17
	(48	47	46	45	44	43	42	41)	(31	32	33	34	35	36	37	38)
Protrusive Occlusion	1	2	3	4	5	6	7	8	9	10	11	12	13	14	15	16
	(18	17	16	15	14	13	12	11)	(21	22	23	24	25	26	27	28)
	32	31	30	29	28	27	26	25	24	23	22	21	20	19	18	17
	(48	47	46	45	44	43	42	41)	(31	32	33	34	35	36	37	38)
Attrition	1	2	3	4	5	6	7	8	1	2	3	4	5	6	7	8
	(18	17	16	15	14	13	12	11)	(18	17	16	15	14	13	12	11)
	32	31	30	29	28	27	26	25	32	31	30	29	28	27	26	25
	(48	47	46	45	44	43	42	41)	(48	47	46	45	44	43	42	41)
Wear Facets	1	2	3	4	5	6	7	8	9	10	11	12	13	14	15	16
	(18	17	16	15	14	13	12	11)	(21	22	23	24	25	26	27	28)
	32	31	30	29	28	27	26	25	24	23	22	21	20	19	18	17
	(48	47	46	45	44	43	42	41)	(31	32	33	34	35	36	37	38)
Abfraction	1	2	3	4	5	6	7	8	9	10	11	12	13	14	15	16
	(18	17	16	15	14	13	12	11)	(21	22	23	24	25	26	27	28)
	32	31	30	29	28	27	26	25	24	23	22	21	20	19	18	17
	(48	47	46	45	44	43	42	41)	(31	32	33	34	35	36	37	38)
Mobility	1	2	3	4	5	6	7	8	9	10	11	12	13	14	15	16
	(18	17	16	15	14	13	12	11)	(21	22	23	24	25	26	27	28)
	32	31	30	29	28	27	26	25	24	23	22	21	20	19	18	17
	(48	47	46	45	44	43	42	41)	(31	32	33	34	35	36	37	38)

The following are **terminology exercises** that allow one as a student dental professional to feel more comfortable with the terms used in the associated textbook. Thus they include word jumbles, crossword puzzles, and word searches. If one feels more comfortable with dental terminology, then any concepts concerning them and using them within clinical settings will then come more easily to the student dental professional.

PART 1: CHAPTER WORD JUMBLES

The following are exercises *per chapter* using **word jumble** for associated terms, each with a **related term clue**. Then each term has been **jumbled** by scrambling its letters. One rearranges letters to spell the answer term to the clue and places the term into correctly numbered place holders. The **answer key** can be obtained from your instructor and their Evolve Resources.

Chapter 1: Face and Neck Regions

1. *Lower jaw* LEDIBMAN ⬜⬜⬜⬜⬜⬜⬜
2. *Ramus part* ONORIDCO ⬜⬜⬜⬜⬜⬜⬜⬜
3. *Kisser corner* SUREMISCOM ⬜⬜⬜⬜⬜⬜⬜⬜⬜⬜
4. *Muscle mania* TERSEMAS ⬜⬜⬜⬜⬜⬜⬜⬜
5. *Moveable bone* IHDYO ⬜⬜⬜⬜⬜
6. *Cheeky gland* TIDROPA ⬜⬜⬜⬜⬜⬜⬜
7. *Upper lip thick* UERBCLET ⬜⬜⬜⬜⬜⬜⬜⬜
8. *Upper lip dip* TURIMLPH ⬜⬜⬜⬜⬜⬜⬜⬜
9. *Head joint* MANBTOROPDIULAREM ⬜⬜⬜⬜⬜⬜⬜⬜⬜⬜⬜⬜⬜⬜⬜⬜⬜
10. *Lip product home* LIONMIREV ⬜⬜⬜⬜⬜⬜⬜⬜⬜

Chapter 2: Oral Cavity and Pharynx

1. *Misplaced oil* ODRCYEF ⬜⬜⬜⬜⬜⬜⬜
2. *Dog teeth* NESNICA ⬜⬜⬜⬜⬜⬜⬜
3. *Grinding fun* CASTIMIOATN ⬜⬜⬜⬜⬜⬜⬜⬜⬜⬜⬜
4. *Arch bumps* SESXTOESO ⬜⬜⬜⬜⬜⬜⬜⬜⬜
5. *Tooth padding* VAINGGI ⬜⬜⬜⬜⬜⬜⬜
6. *Entrance walls* UFALAIC ⬜⬜⬜⬜⬜⬜⬜
7. *Tongue specials* LALAPPIE ⬜⬜⬜⬜⬜⬜⬜⬜
8. *Tongue line-up* VALARICTMUCE ⬜⬜⬜⬜⬜⬜⬜⬜⬜⬜⬜⬜
9. *Bony arches* EORVALAL ⬜⬜⬜⬜⬜⬜⬜⬜
10. *Midsized mushroom-shapes* GORMFUNIF ⬜⬜⬜⬜⬜⬜⬜⬜⬜

Chapter 3: Prenatal Development

1. *Cavity fluid* TICNAIMO
2. *Outer skin layer* MEERCODT
3. *First divisions* GEAVECLA
4. *Genetic map* YOKAPRETY
5. *Future embryo* TOYSCBALST
6. *Union result* GOTEYZ
7. *From ectoderm* NETUCREDMOORE
8. *Embryonic tissue* CESHEMENYM
9. *First draft* RORPUDMIMI
10. *Toxic types* EGRAOENTTS

Chapter 4: Face and Neck Development

1. *Nose bump* RACTIEGAL
2. *Pouches with punch* LARPYNHGEA
3. *Disappearance act* KEECLM
4. *Neck bone* DIHOY
5. *Sensory button* DLAPSECO
6. *Outer doughnut half* RATELLA
7. *Opening gives communication* NEEMBARM
8. *Four evaginations* CPHOSUE
9. *Upper facial place* SOOFNTNAARL
10. *Primitive oral landmark* MTOODEMUS

Chapter 5: Orofacial Development

1. *Tight tongue* AAGYOINSSKLOL
2. *Parting palate* LETCF
3. *From fourth swelling* TEIPLIGOCT
4. *Stacked six* IESGLWLNS
5. *Least palatal cleft* AULVU
6. *First partial roof* MAYPRIR

7. *Middle mirror meeting* LESVHSE ☐☐☐☐☐☐☐
8. *Posterior roof from shelves* ACONSEDRY ☐☐☐☐☐☐☐☐☐
9. *Initial tongue blob* RETMCUBUUL ☐☐☐☐☐☐☐☐☐
10. *Right in midline* AIPRM ☐☐☐☐☐

Chapter 6: Tooth Development and Eruption

1. *Empty slot* OOAANDINT ☐☐☐☐☐☐☐☐☐
2. *Leftover cells* ZELSMAAS ☐☐☐☐☐☐☐☐
3. *Twining trouble* NOIEGMIATN ☐☐☐☐☐☐☐☐☐☐
4. *Primary shedders* STOSLAODNTOC ☐☐☐☐☐☐☐☐☐☐☐☐
5. *Early bony-like form* IOMCEETND ☐☐☐☐☐☐☐☐☐
6. *Secretory surface* SMTEO ☐☐☐☐☐
7. *Compressed layer* MMDIUNTREEI ☐☐☐☐☐☐☐☐☐☐☐
8. *Second draft* NUUCDSCEAEOS ☐☐☐☐☐☐☐☐☐☐☐☐
9. *Merry myth* YIFAR ☐☐☐☐☐
10. *Accessory cusps* BEECLSTUR ☐☐☐☐☐☐☐☐☐

Chapter 7: Basic Cell Properties and Processes

1. *Intercellular spaces* VAUCLEOS ☐☐☐☐☐☐☐☐
2. *Splitting up* SOMTIIS ☐☐☐☐☐☐☐
3. *Junction tissue tie* DOSMMEOSE ☐☐☐☐☐☐☐☐☐
4. *Cell center* ULCELOUNS ☐☐☐☐☐☐☐☐☐
5. *Moving out* OSSEYTOXIC ☐☐☐☐☐☐☐☐☐☐
6. *Breaking down* MESYSLOOS ☐☐☐☐☐☐☐☐☐
7. *Chromatin condenses* ROSHAEPP ☐☐☐☐☐☐☐☐
8. *Two chromatids* TEMRONEECR ☐☐☐☐☐☐☐☐☐☐
9. *Rough guys* SRIMBOOES ☐☐☐☐☐☐☐☐☐
10. *Major player* FEMSTOINNOLAT ☐☐☐☐☐☐☐☐☐☐☐☐☐

Chapter 8: Basic Tissue and Processes

1. *Mineral identification* PAAYTHRIODXYTE ☐☐☐☐☐☐☐☐☐☐☐☐☐☐
2. *Nutrition canals* CIALNAULIC ☐☐☐☐☐☐☐☐☐☐

86 TERMINOLOGY EXERCISES

3. *Vessel wrapping* THELENDOMUI ☐☐☐☐☐☐☐☐☐☐
4. *Layered epithelium* EFADISTRTI ☐☐☐☐☐☐☐☐☐
5. *Hard rings* TONESSO ☐☐☐☐☐☐☐
6. *Making fibers* BIABSLFROT ☐☐☐☐☐☐☐☐☐
7. *Taking care of alien* NIOMUMENG ☐☐☐☐☐☐☐☐☐
8. *Replacement clocking* ORVENTUR ☐☐☐☐☐☐☐☐
9. *Clot creation* TELLEPAST ☐☐☐☐☐☐☐☐☐
10. *Nerve tagging* NYSASEP ☐☐☐☐☐☐☐

Chapter 9: Oral Mucosa

1. *Unique tissue* TEZEKPAIRNADAIR ☐☐☐☐☐☐☐☐☐☐☐☐☐☐☐
2. *Waterproofing tactic* RAKTENI ☐☐☐☐☐☐☐
3. *Dark spots* LUGREANS ☐☐☐☐☐☐☐☐
4. *Gum tufting* TIGPIPSLN ☐☐☐☐☐☐☐☐☐
5. *Vessel victory* ACALPRILY ☐☐☐☐☐☐☐☐☐
6. *Down deeper* BOSSAMUUC ☐☐☐☐☐☐☐☐☐
7. *Italy map* PHIRGAEOCG ☐☐☐☐☐☐☐☐☐☐
8. *Membrane with bony down under* SMUMEPOCEIROTU ☐☐☐☐☐☐☐☐☐☐☐☐☐☐
9. *Tongue field* ZISPAEECLID ☐☐☐☐☐☐☐☐☐☐☐
10. *Sometimes dried up* KEPICRL ☐☐☐☐☐☐☐

Chapter 10: Gingival and Dentogingival Junctional Tissue

1. *Between layers* NALAMI ☐☐☐☐☐☐
2. *Facing tooth* LAVDENINGTOGI ☐☐☐☐☐☐☐☐☐☐☐☐☐
3. *Always young* JOUCTIANNL ☐☐☐☐☐☐☐☐☐☐
4. *Periodontal playground* LUULSCRA ☐☐☐☐☐☐☐☐
5. *Future fluid measurement* VUCRRIECLA ☐☐☐☐☐☐☐☐☐☐
6. *Growing gums* HYSAPARLEPI ☐☐☐☐☐☐☐☐☐☐☐
7. *Longer teeth* CORSEESIN ☐☐☐☐☐☐☐☐☐
8. *Sore gums* TIINVSGIGI ☐☐☐☐☐☐☐☐☐☐
9. *Deeper disease depot* KEOPCT ☐☐☐☐☐☐
10. *Continued destruction class* DIREPOONTIITS ☐☐☐☐☐☐☐☐☐☐☐☐☐

Chapter 11: Head and Neck Structures

1. *Group secretion* SANCIU
2. *Gland masses* ELFSOLILC
3. *Node depression* HUISL
4. *Bigger grapes* PYHMDAPELONTYAH
5. *Nasal projections* OCCHENA
6. *Desert place* XOOERASMTI
7. *Head spaces* RANSPALAA
8. *Damp kisser* ILASAV
9. *Making thyroxine* DOLICLO
10. *Lymphoid masses* TALOLNSIR

Chapter 12: Enamel

1. *Breaking crystals* FABTCANRIO
2. *Dark brushes* FUSTT
3. *Rubbed out* BANRAISO
4. *Faulty enamel* PDSSYILAA
5. *Short tubules* NIESDSPL
6. *Named layers* TRIESZU
7. *Hard rock bands* AICTMBRINIO
8. *Worn jewel* NOTATRITI
9. *Between enamel units* DORNITER
10. *Getting outer groovy on* KYMPERATIA

Chapter 13: Dentin and Pulp

1. *Whole hole* MONFRAE
2. *Disturbed appositional growth* TURCONO
3. *Around middle* CUCPIRAUMPLL
4. *First root covering* NETMAL
5. *Around tubes* BUTLERAPIUR
6. *Tubule type* TNADELIN
7. *Lateral with complications* RAOSCECSY

8. *Avoid ice* VEISHYPIERSNITTY ☐☐☐☐☐☐☐☐☐☐☐☐☐☐
9. *Named layers* BERNE ☐☐☐☐☐
10. *Inner pain* TULSPIPI ☐☐☐☐☐☐☐☐

Chapter 14: Periodontium: Cementum, Alveolar Process, and Periodontal Ligament

1. *Trouble with therapy* PURSS ☐☐☐☐☐
2. *No outer layer cells* RACELALUL ☐☐☐☐☐☐☐☐☐
3. *Two kinds* NELMSECTICE ☐☐☐☐☐☐☐☐☐☐☐
4. *Dental nightmare* EUSUDENTOL ☐☐☐☐☐☐☐☐☐☐
5. *Bulk fibers* QUOIBLE ☐☐☐☐☐☐☐
6. *Root padding* ISHTYMERCEPENSO ☐☐☐☐☐☐☐☐☐☐☐☐☐☐☐
7. *Probing junction* MEECLEMENTONA ☐☐☐☐☐☐☐☐☐☐☐☐☐
8. *Between roots* RACDILTERIUARN ☐☐☐☐☐☐☐☐☐☐☐☐☐☐
9. *Supporting team* TERIMOODPINU ☐☐☐☐☐☐☐☐☐☐☐☐
10. *Ninety degrees* YESHARP ☐☐☐☐☐☐☐

Chapter 15: Overview of Dentitions

1. *Meeting place* TACONCT ☐☐☐☐☐☐☐
2. *Floss heaven/hell* INOXTMERPRIAL ☐☐☐☐☐☐☐☐☐☐☐☐☐
3. *Bite me* SOONCLUIC ☐☐☐☐☐☐☐☐☐
4. *Record with boxy view* LEPARM ☐☐☐☐☐☐
5. *Four squares* DANQTUARNS ☐☐☐☐☐☐☐☐☐☐
6. *Linear elevations* GRISED ☐☐☐☐☐☐
7. *Root caves* VITANESCOCI ☐☐☐☐☐☐☐☐☐☐☐
8. *Six slices* XSASENTT ☐☐☐☐☐☐☐☐
9. *More specific* HIRSTD ☐☐☐☐☐☐
10. *Talking points* AUSLNIVER ☐☐☐☐☐☐☐☐☐

Chapter 16: Permanent Anterior Teeth

1. *Traumatic injury* NALVUISO ☐☐☐☐☐☐☐☐
2. *Backside major* CUIMGLUN ☐☐☐☐☐☐☐☐

3. *Dog tooth term* DUCSPI ☐☐☐☐☐☐
4. *Cute space* STIEAMAD ☐☐☐☐☐☐☐☐
5. *Odd incisor* CHONTUSHIN ☐☐☐☐☐☐☐☐☐
6. *Getting depressed* SOAFSE ☐☐☐☐☐☐
7. *Canine retained* PIAMDCET ☐☐☐☐☐☐☐☐
8. *Newer ridge* SIACLIN ☐☐☐☐☐☐☐
9. *Even cuter* LOESMNAM ☐☐☐☐☐☐☐☐
10. *Extra something* EOSEDIMNS ☐☐☐☐☐☐☐☐☐

Chapter 17: Permanent Posterior Teeth

1. *Molar associate tag* SPUDICIB ☐☐☐☐☐☐☐☐
2. *Maxillary special* QOEUBIL ☐☐☐☐☐☐☐
3. *Cute small cusp* CLERIABAL ☐☐☐☐☐☐☐☐☐
4. *Angular distortion* LEDIARTOCAIN ☐☐☐☐☐☐☐☐☐☐☐☐
5. *Elongated depression* TULFGINT ☐☐☐☐☐☐☐☐
6. *Hidden areas* SHERCOTC ☐☐☐☐☐☐☐☐
7. *Odd molar* BUMLYRER ☐☐☐☐☐☐☐☐
8. *Outside deep groove* UFINSO ☐☐☐☐☐☐
9. *Between roots* AURCFINOT ☐☐☐☐☐☐☐☐☐
10. *Three roots* TERICFRATUD ☐☐☐☐☐☐☐☐☐☐☐

Chapter 18: Primary Dentition

1. *Baby smile spaces* MIPERAT ☐☐☐☐☐☐☐
2. *Distinct bulging ridge* CLBUCA ☐☐☐☐☐☐
3. *Large chamber* LUPP ☐☐☐☐
4. *Risky restorative moment* NORSH ☐☐☐☐☐
5. *Early childhood issue* SECAIR ☐☐☐☐☐☐
6. *Stained kiddy smile* NAMTHYS ☐☐☐☐☐☐☐
7. *Good start teeth* MRIYPAR ☐☐☐☐☐☐☐
8. *Kid grinding* XIRSBUM ☐☐☐☐☐☐☐
9. *Worn primary tops* OARNTTITI ☐☐☐☐☐☐☐☐☐
10. *Whiter young smile* EELANM ☐☐☐☐☐☐

Chapter 19: Temporomandibular Joint

1. *Raising mandible* VEAOINLET
2. *Inferior depression* CAARITLUR
3. *Joint fluid* YNOILVSA
4. *Side movement* TELLARA
5. *Working muscle group* MOICTASAITN
6. *Sharper ridge* GLOPOSTEDIN
7. *Partial dislocation* BUIULXATSON
8. *Joint negative change* SRIDDORE
9. *Joint cover* LEAPSCU
10. *Lower jaw backward* TROINRACTE

Chapter 20: Occlusion

1. *Possibly noisy occlusion* MRUIBXS
2. *Mandible facial placement* TROSBSICE
3. *Lateral curve* NOLSIW
4. *Resting mandible* RLEANECAC
5. *Space in kiddie bite* WEEYLA
6. *Major disharmony* MRATAU
7. *Habitually centric* OINCUCLSO
8. *More females have it* ROIVEEBT
9. *Horizontal overhang* JOEVETR
10. *Occlusal classification* GALNE

PART 2: UNIT CROSSWORD PUZZLES

The following are exercises using a **crossword puzzle** that consists of a grid of squares in which to enter the **related clue terms** *per unit* that will then **cross** each other horizontally as in *across* and vertically as in *down*. Each white square is filled with one letter of the word, while the black squares are used to separate entries. The first white square in each entry is numbered to correspond to its clue. The **answer key** can be obtained from your Instructor and their Evolve Resources.

UNIT 1: OROFACIAL STRUCTURES

Crossword Puzzle 1

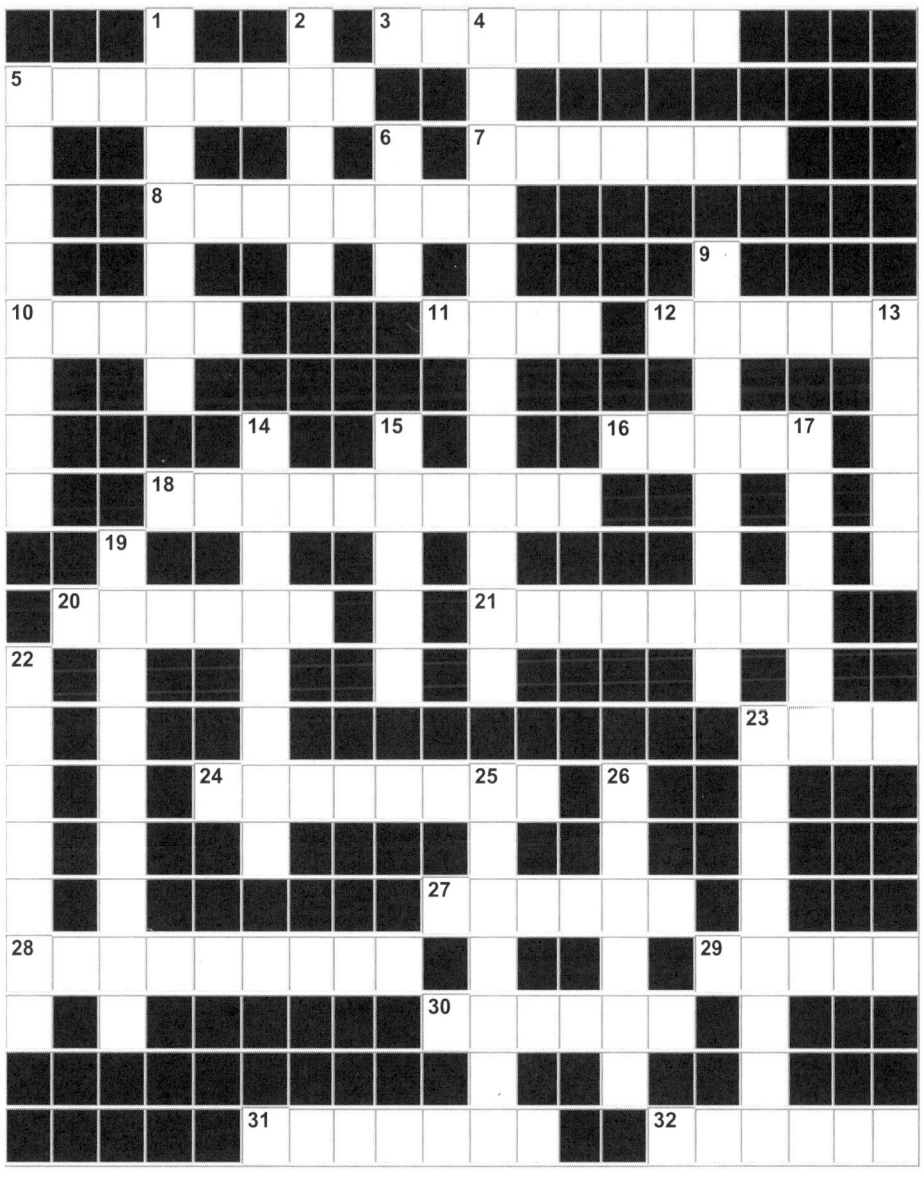

Across

3. Vertical groove noted on midline of upper lip
5. Bony process at anterior border of mandibular ramus
7. Small yellowish oral mucosal bumps from misplaced sebaceous glands
8. Part of maxillae or mandible that supports teeth
10. Nostrils of nose
11. External main feature of nasal region so do not blow it!
12. Structures or facial surfaces of the tooth closest to inner cheek
16. Developmental disturbance for lip that needs to be recorded
18. Part of the face that contains the lips and oral cavity
20. Hard inner crown layer of tooth overlying pulp
21. Surrounding socket of tooth
23. White ridge of raised keratinized epithelial tissue on buccal mucosa
24. Lower jaw
27. Hard outer crown layer of tooth
28. Atypical finding of bone growth on facial surface of maxillary alveolar process
29. Skull socket that contains eyeball and supporting structures
30. Space facing sulcular epithelium
31. Bony projection off posterior and superior border of mandibular ramus
32. Voice box in midline of neck composed of cartilages

Down

1. Opening from the pulp at apex of tooth
2. Keratinization on inner cheek where teeth occlude
4. Facial region located both inferior to orbital region and lateral to nasal region
5. Outermost layer of the root of tooth
6. Winglike cartilaginous structure laterally around each nares
9. Midline thickening of upper lip
13. Extracellular fluid that drains from surrounding region into lymphatic vessels
14. Small elevated structures of specialized mucosa on the tongue
15. Depression at sulcus terminalis points backward toward pharynx
17. Nonencapsulated mass of lymphoid tissue
19. Darker appearance or zone of the lips compared with surrounding skin
22. Anteriors that also third teeth from midline in each quadrant
23. Tooth type that includes incisors and canines located at the front of oral cavity
25. Describes structures or tooth surfaces closest to the tongue
26. Midline tissue fold between ventral surface of the tongue and floor of the mouth

# UNIT 2: DENTAL EMBRYOLOGY

Crossword Puzzle 1

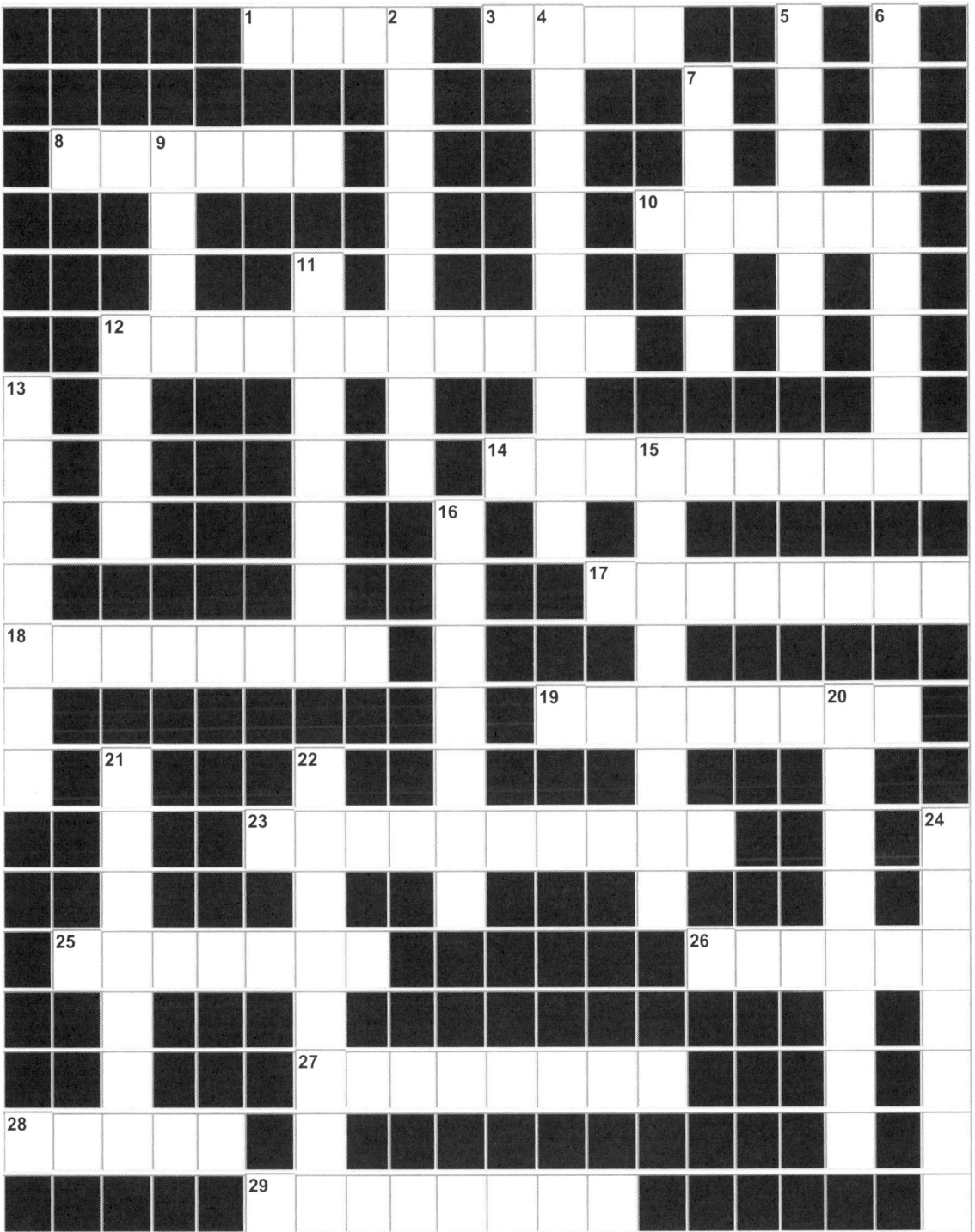

Across

1. Circular plate of bilayer cells developed from blastocyst
3. Depressions in center of each nasal placode that evolve into nasal cavities
8. Structure eliminated between two adjacent swellings during surface fusion
10. Type of tube formed when neural folds meet and fuse superior to neural groove
12. Differentiated cells from preameloblasts during amelogenesis to form enamel
14. Overall form of structure that can undergo change during development
17. Embryonic layer located between ectoderm and endoderm
18. Bilaminar embryonic disc superior layer
19. Ectoderm areas found located at developing special sense organs or teeth on embryo
23. Embryonic disc that includes ectoderm, mesoderm, and endoderm
25. Intermaxillary growth from paired medial nasal processes on internal stomodeum
26. Tail end of structure such as with trilaminar embryonic disc
27. Each half of it mirrors other half of embryo because of primitive streak development
28. Structure of fetal period of prenatal development derived from enlarged embryo
29. Prenatal developmental process when mitosis converts zygote to blastocyst

Down

2. Head end of structure such as with trilaminar embryonic disc
4. Action of one cell group on another leading to establishment of developmental pathway
5. Structure derived from implanted blastocyst
6. Posterior one develops from fourth pharyngeal/branchial arches marking future epiglottis
7. Specialized cells that develop from neuroectoderm that migrate from neural folds
9. Female reproductive cell that can undergo fertilization
11. Paired cuboidal aggregates of cells differentiated from mesoderm
12. Pharyngeal/branchial apparatus part along with grooves, membranes, pouches
13. Cleft lip fusion failure of maxillary one with medial nasal one on each side
15. Processes that occur from start of pregnancy to birth
16. Membrane at caudal end of embryo for future anus
20. Trilaminar embryonic disc layer derived from epiblast layer that lines stomodeum
21. Anterior part of future digestive tract or primitive pharynx forming oropharynx
22. Membrane that disintegrates bringing nasal and oral cavities into communication
24. Process occurring to embryo that places each embryologic tissue in proper position

UNIT 2: DENTAL EMBRYOLOGY

Crossword Puzzle 2

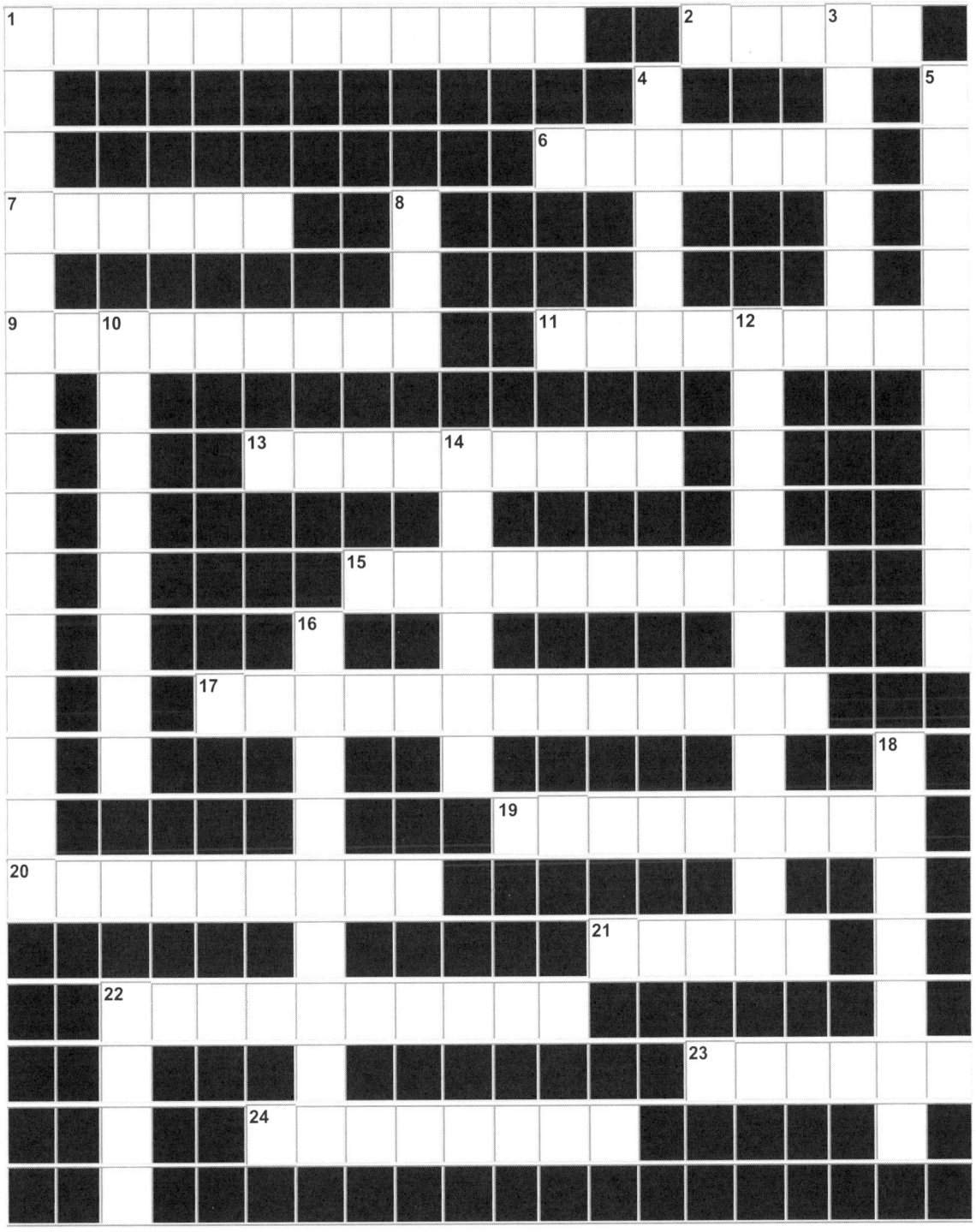

Across

1. Canals that persist after development
2. Fusion failure of palatal shelves with primary palate or with each other
6. Two palatal processes from maxillary processes during prenatal development
7. Part of cervical loop that shape root or roots inducing root dentin formation
9. Cementum matrix laid down by cementoblasts
11. Circular plate of bilayer cells developed from blastocyst
13. One cell group action that leads to developmental pathway in responding tissue
15. Layered formation of tissue such as cartilage, bone, enamel, dentin, cementum
17. Process by which sperm penetrates ovum during preimplantation period
19. Photographic analysis of chromosomes
20. Primitive mouth appearing as shallow depression in embryonic surface
21. Cap or bell-shaped part of tooth germ that produces enamel
22. Prenatal structure of trophoblast cells and inner cell mass that develops into embryo
23. Partially calcified substance that serves as framework for later calcification
24. Layer in trilaminar embryonic disc derived from hypoblast layer

Down

1. Permanent teeth type without primary predecessors as it concerns molars
3. Dental developmental disturbance in which adjacent tooth germs unite
4. Small spherical enamel projection near cementoenamel junction
5. Cellular removal of hard tissue with primary tooth shedding
8. Second stage of tooth development with dental lamina growth into ectomesenchyme
10. Groups of epithelial cells in periodontal ligament after disintegration of sheath
12. Abnormally small teeth
14. Midline swellings from second, third, and fourth pharyngeal/branchial arches associated with hypopharyngeal eminence
16. Dentin matrix laid down through appositional growth by odontoblasts
18. Embryonic process of reproductive cell ensuring correct chromosome number
22. Fourth stage of odontogenesis in which differentiation occurs to its furthest extent

UNIT 3: DENTAL HISTOLOGY

Crossword Puzzle 1

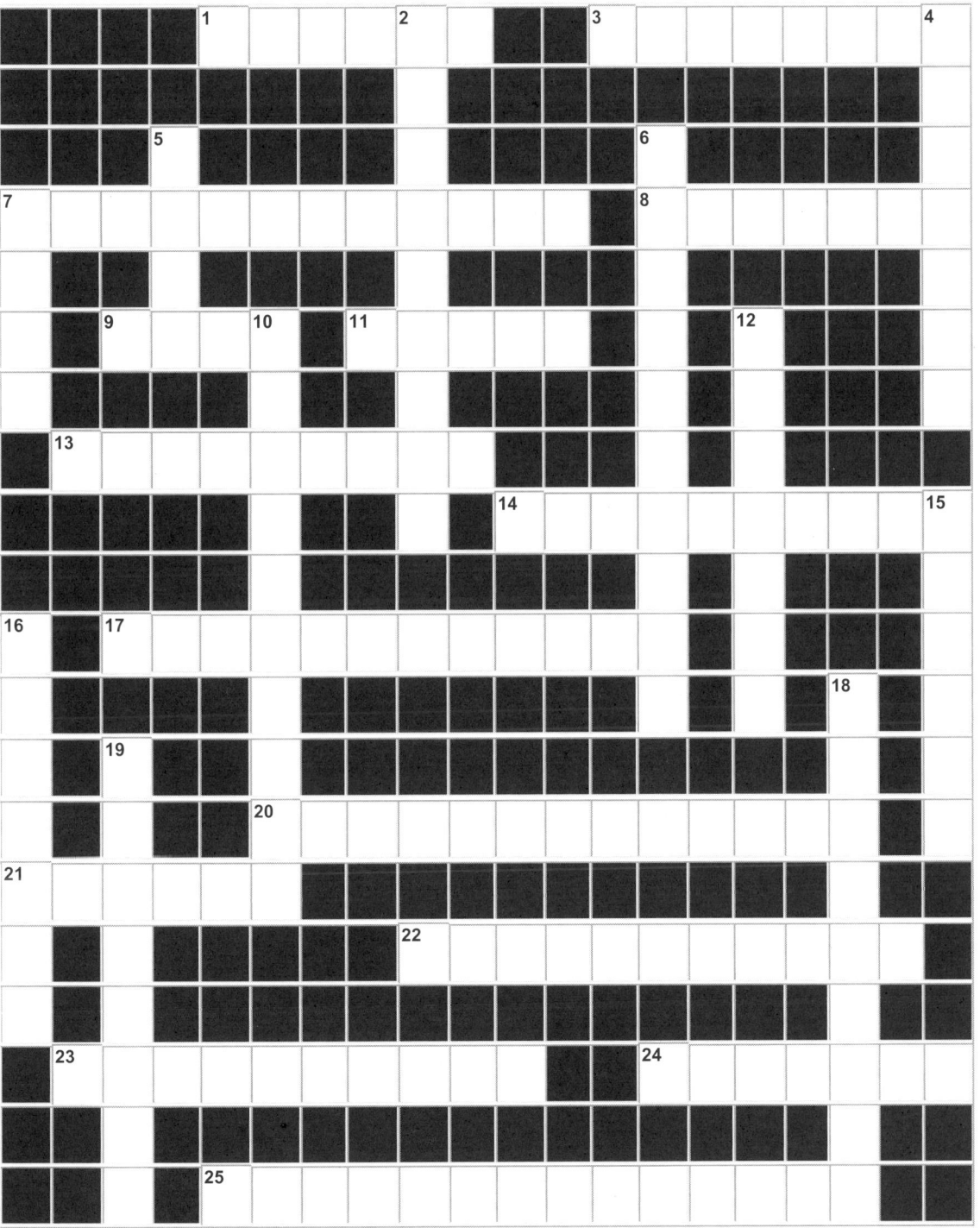

Across

1. Group of organs functioning together
3. Closely apposed sheets of bone tissue in compact bone
7. Organelles associated with manufacture of adenosine triphosphate
8. Largest and most conspicuous organelle in the cell
9. Smallest unit of organization in the body
11. Somewhat independent part that performs specific function or functions
13. Chief nucleoprotein in nondividing nucleoplasm
14. White blood cell that increases in numbers during immune response
17. Three-dimensional cellular system of support
20. Intermediate filament type with major role in intercellular junctions
21. Structure formed by cell groups with similar characteristics of shape and function
22. Immature connective tissue formed during initial repair
23. Filamentous daughter chromosomes joined at centromere during cell division
24. Specialized connective tissue composed of fat, little matrix, adipocytes
25. Along with calcium, main inorganic crystal in enamel, bone, dentin, cementum

Down

2. Superficial skin layers
4. Protein fiber type in connective tissue composed of microfilaments
5. Rigid connective tissue
6. Metabolically inert substances or transient structures within the cell
7. White blood cell similar to basophil that also involved in allergic responses
10. Second most common white blood cell in the blood
12. Part of cell division resulting in two daughter cells identical to parent cell
15. Small space that surrounds chondrocyte or osteocyte
16. Intermediate protein filament that consists of opaque waterproof substance
18. Intercellular junction found between cells
19. Lowest amount white blood cell in blood containing histamine granules

UNIT 3: DENTAL HISTOLOGY

Crossword Puzzle 2

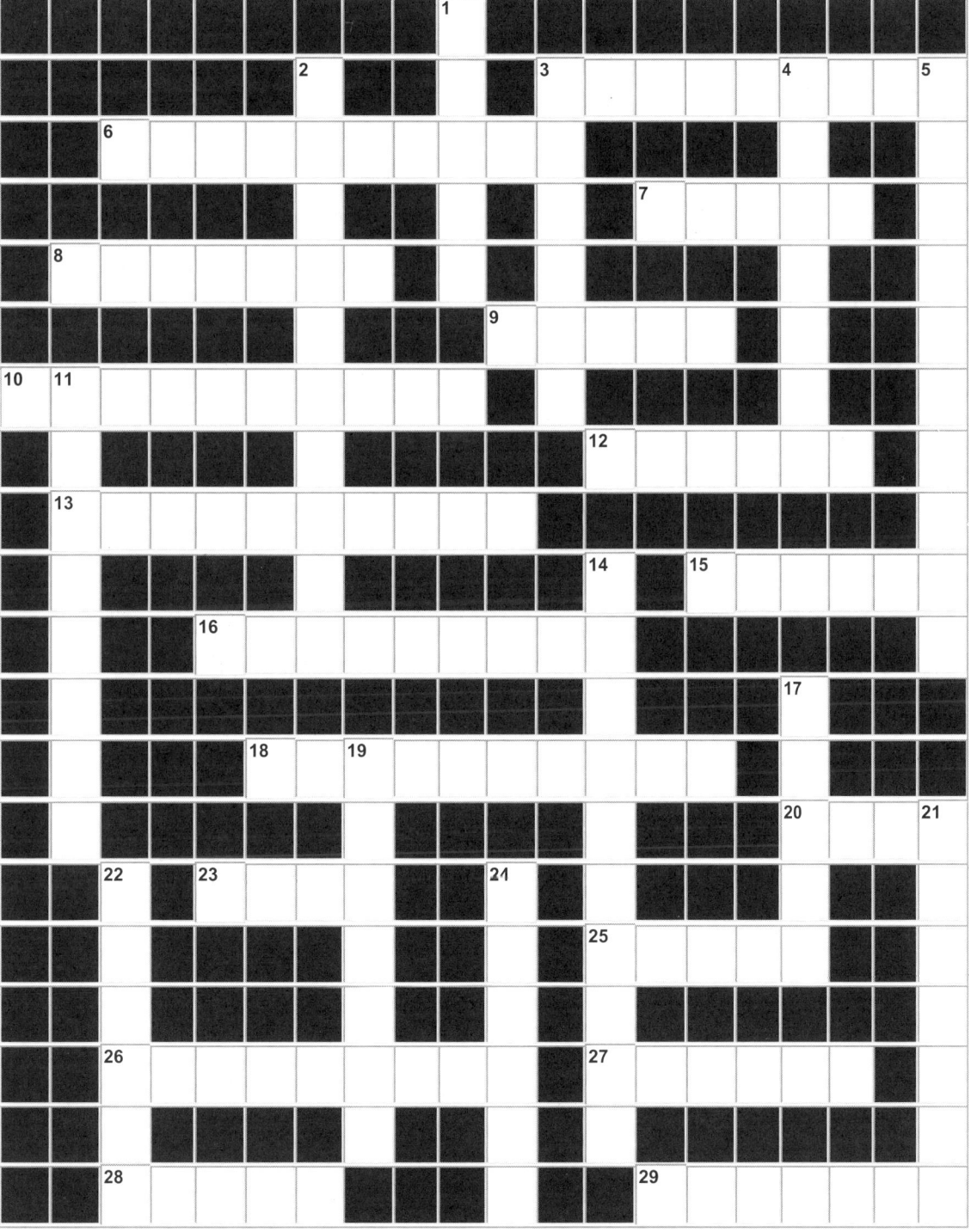

Across

3. Tissue deep to oral mucosa composed of loose connective tissue
6. Joined matrix pieces forming lattice in cancellous bone
7. Extracellular fluid that drains from surrounding region into lymphatic vessels
8. Initially formed bone matrix
9. Central opening where saliva deposited after production by secretory cells
10. Mature osteoblasts entrapped in bone matrix
12. Respiratory mucosal cells that produce mucus to keep mucosa moist
13. Network of vessels that collect and transport lymph linking lymph nodes
15. Hard tooth tissue loss from demineralization by cariogenic bacteria
16. Blood cell fragments that function in clotting mechanism
18. Dense connective tissue layer on outer part of bone
20. Extension of epithelium into connective tissue noted in microscopic section
23. Passageway that allows glandular secretion to be emptied directly into location of use
25. Large inner part of certain glands
26. Dense connective tissue in both dermis and lamina propria
27. Secretion from salivary glands that lubricates and cleanses oral cavity
28. Bundle of neural processes outside central nervous system
29. Localized macules of pigmentation

Down

1. Depression on one side of lymph node
2. Grooves associated with lines of Retzius in enamel
3. Connective tissue that divides inner part of certain glands
4. Connective tissue that surrounds outer part of entire gland or lesion
5. Cells that differentiate from preameloblasts forming enamel during amelogenesis
11. Epithelium that stands away from the tooth creating gingival sulcus
14. Cells that function in resorption of bone
17. Each bilateral structure of nose lined by lined by respiratory mucosa
19. Incremental lines located in histologic sections of mature enamel
21. Hard tooth tissue loss through chemical means not involving bacteria
22. Functional cellular component of nervous system
24. Extracellular substance that serves as framework for later calcification

UNIT 3: DENTAL HISTOLOGY

Crossword Puzzle 3

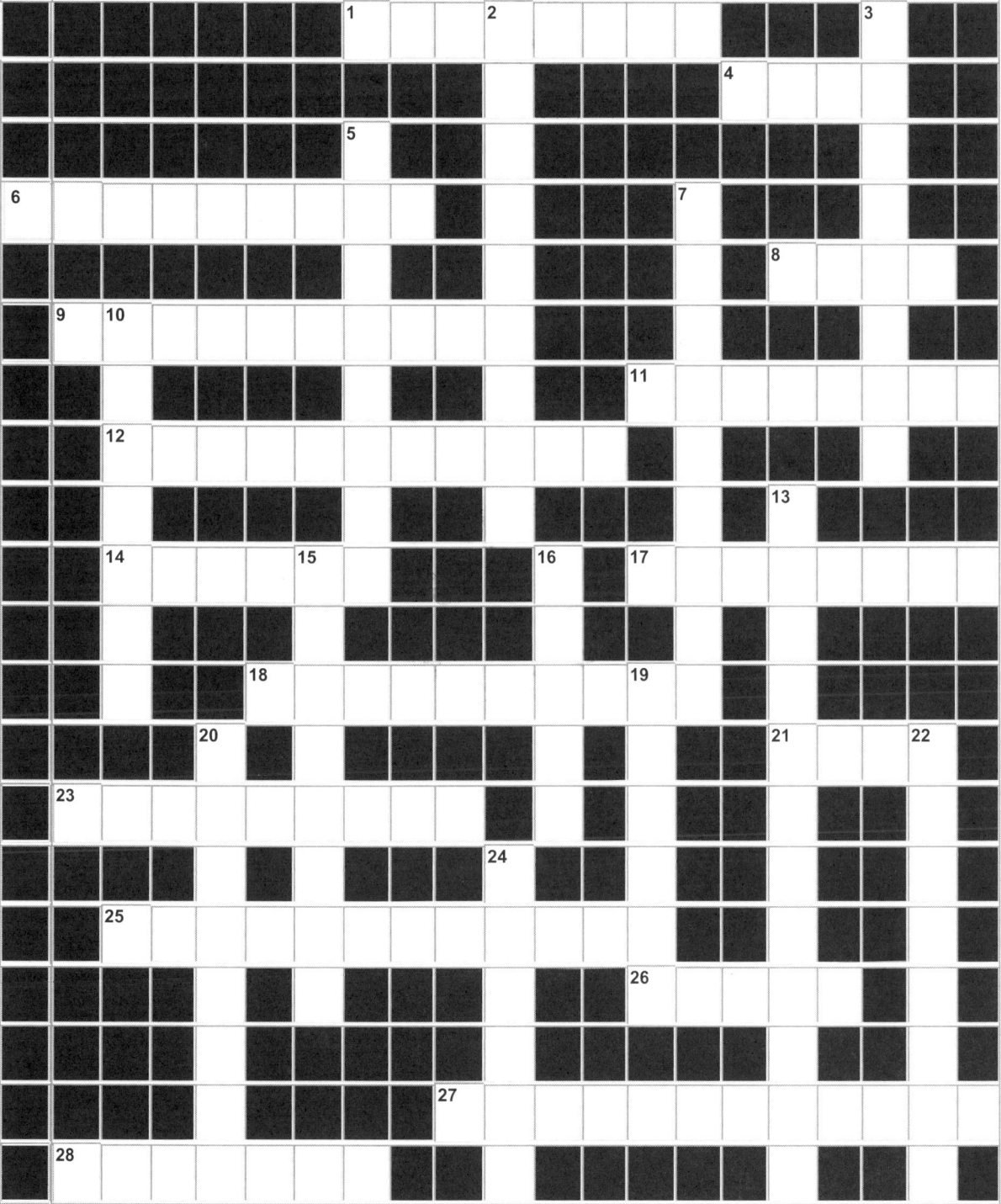

Across

1. Inflammation of pulp
4. Soft innermost connective tissue in both crown and root
6. Hard tooth tissue loss by mastication or orofacial parafunctional habits
8. Crystalline structural units of hardest tissue that give teeth bright white look
9. Layered formation of firm or hard tissue such as enamel, dentin, cementum
11. Surrounds the teeth for support and attaches the teeth to alveoli
12. Incremental lines or bands of von Ebner in mature dentin
14. Foramen from the pulp at root apex
17. Surrounding socket of tooth
18. Cancellous bone located between alveolar bone proper and plates of cortical bone
21. Imbrication lines in dentin demonstrating disturbance in body metabolism
23. Extra openings usually located on lateral parts of the roots
25. Appositional growth of enamel matrix by ameloblasts
26. Microscopic dark brushes in enamel with bases near the dentinoenamel junction
27. Layer of dentin around outer pulpal wall
28. Part of the tooth that contains mass of pulp

Down

2. Dentin matrix laid down by appositional growth by odontoblasts
3. Microscopic enamel feature near dentinoenamel junction of short dentinal tubules
5. Plates of compact bone on facial and lingual surfaces of alveolar process
7. Pup part located in root area of the tooth
10. Dentin formed in tooth before completion of apical foramen
13. Supporting hard or soft dental tissue for the tooth
15. Hard tooth tissue loss by friction from toothbrushing or toothpaste
16. Found within dentinal tubule in dentin
19. Smooth microscopic lines in cartilage, bone, or cementum caused by appositional growth
20. Outermost layer of root of a tooth
22. Accentuated incremental line of Retzius or contour line of Owen from birth process
24. Hard inner layer of the crown of the tooth overlying pulp

UNIT 4: DENTAL ANATOMY

Crossword Puzzle 1

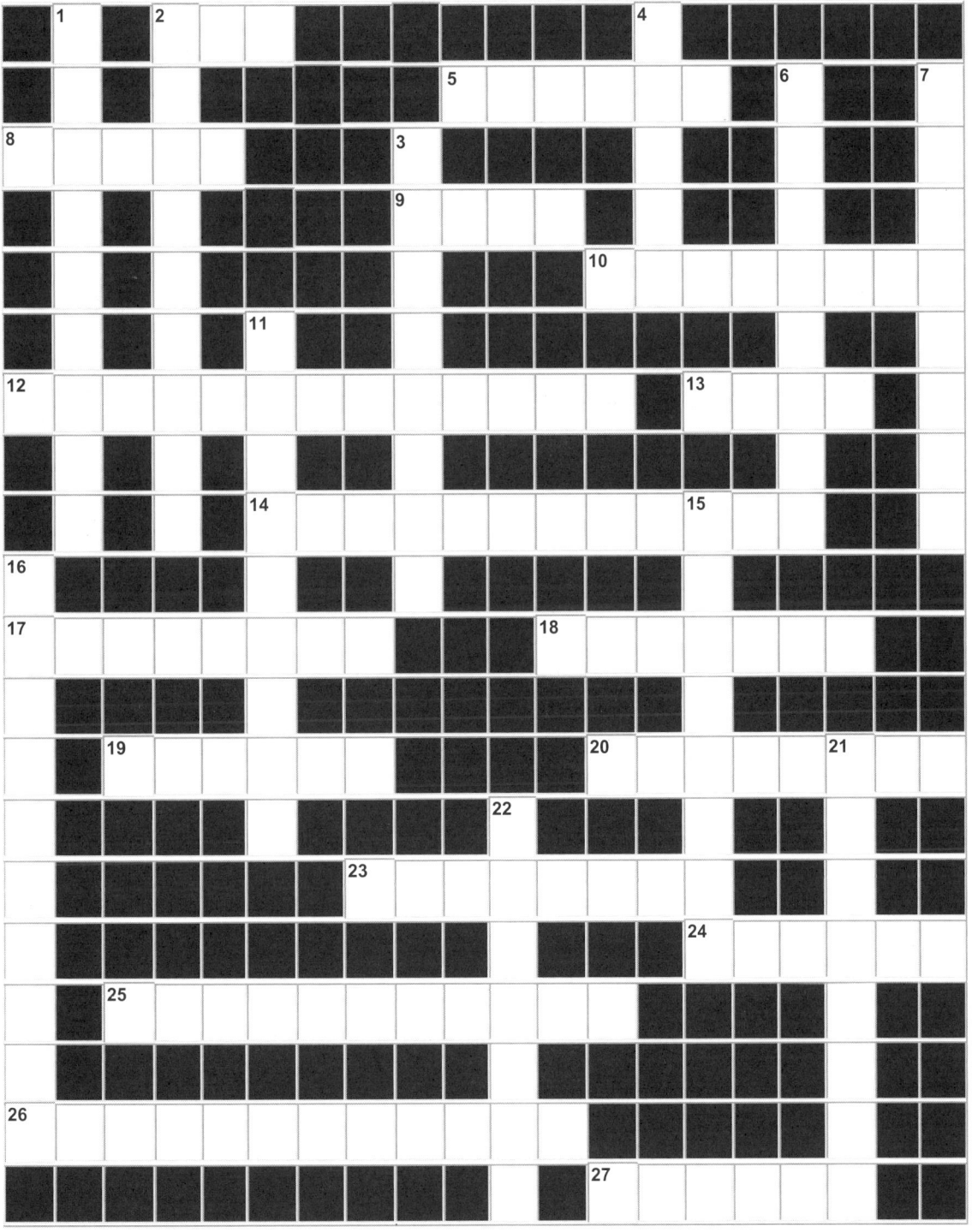

Across

2. Small lateral incisor or third molar crown due to partial microdontia
5. Palmer Notation _____
8. Mythologic nighttime creature that takes shed primary teeth leaving cold hard cash
9. Type of angle formed by lines created at junction of two crown surfaces
10. Rounded enamel extensions on anterior incisal ridge as noted from labial or lingual
12. Tooth designation system using two-digit code
13. Imaginary line representing long line of the tooth that bisects cervical line
14. Crown or root(s) that show angular distortion
17. Rounded raised borders on mesial and distal parts of lingual surface of anteriors
18. Another dental term for canines with much thanks to our tail-wagging friends
19. Surface of the tooth closest to midline
20. Masticatory surface of posteriors
23. Vertically oriented and labially placed bony ridges of alveolar process in both jaws
24. Surface of tooth farthest away from midline
25. Indentations on surface of the root or roots
26. Secondary groove on lingual surface of anteriors and occlusal table on posteriors
27. Division of crown surface or root into three parts

Down

1. Division of each dental arch into two parts with four for entire dentition
2. Second dentition noted in oral cavity; also considered *adult teeth*
3. Part of root visible to the clinician
4. Depression on lingual surface of anteriors or occlusal table of posteriors
6. Complete displacement of the tooth from socket caused by extensive trauma
7. Open contact existing between maxillary central incisors
11. Absence of single tooth or multiple teeth because of lack of initiation
15. Unerupted or partially erupted tooth positioned against an oral structure
16. Spaces formed from curvatures where two teeth in same arch contact
21. Division of each dental arch into three parts based on midline
22. Linear elevation or ridge on masticatory surface of newly erupted incisors

UNIT 4: DENTAL ANATOMY

Crossword Puzzle 2

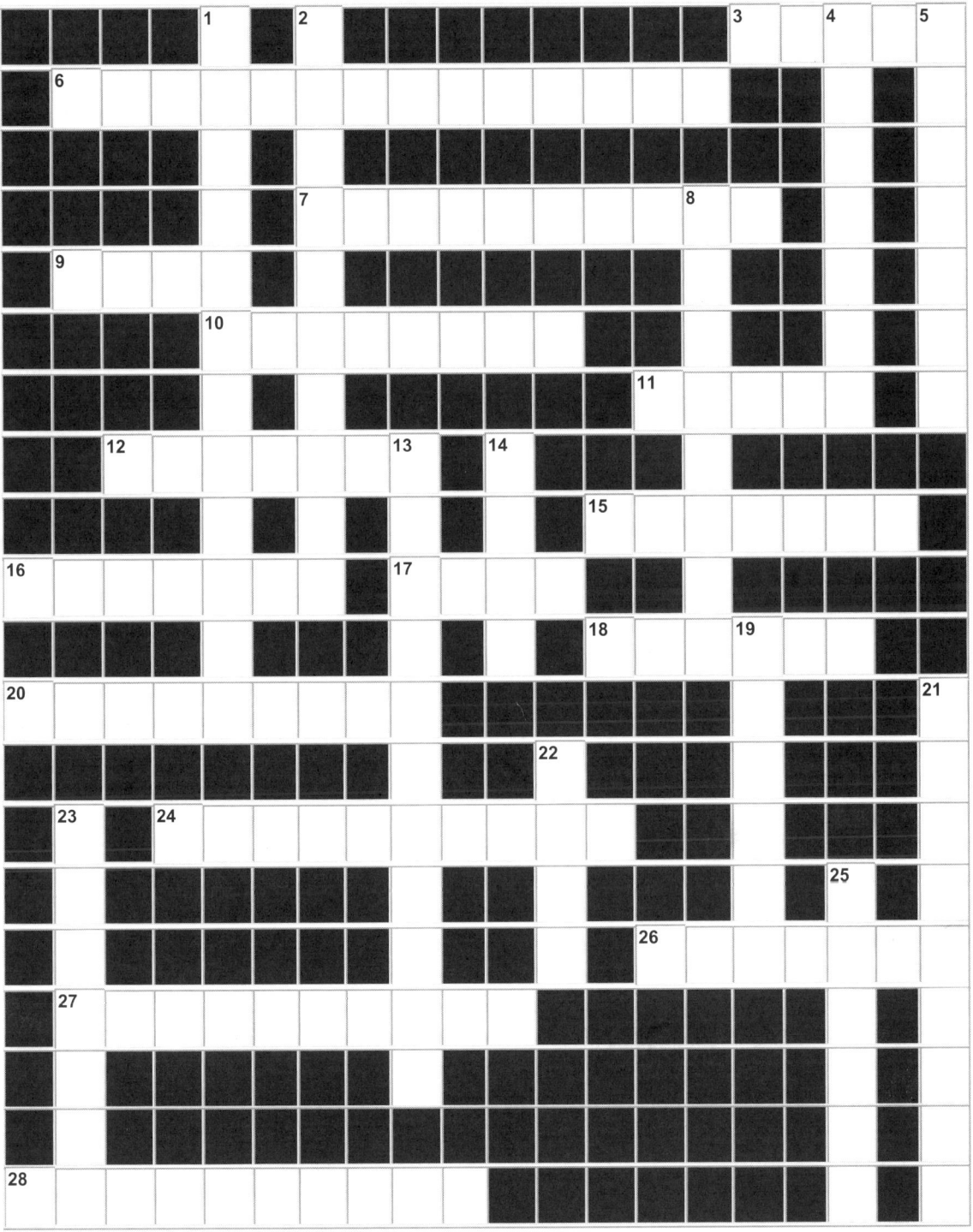

Across

3. Situation in which entire posterior quadrant functions during lateral occlusion
6. Movements of mandible not within usual patterns within orofacial region
7. Moving lower jaw forward
9. Temporomandibular joint part between temporal bone and mandibular condyle
10. Ridge running mesiodistally in the cervical one-third of buccal crown surface
11. Natural movement of all of the teeth over time toward midline of oral cavity
12. Orofacial parafunctional habit of grinding teeth that can sound like jet taking off
15. First dentition; also known as *deciduous dentition*
16. Side to which mandible has been moved during lateral occlusion
17. Terminal plane with primary mandibular second molar mesial to maxillary molar
18. Space created when primary molars shed making room for permanent premolars
20. Contralateral side of arch from working side during lateral occlusion
24. Prominent mandible with normal or even retrusive maxilla and concave profile
26. End point of closure of the mandible with most retruded position
27. Lowering of lower jaw
28. Moving lower jaw backward

Down

1. Failure to have overall ideal form of dentition while in centric occlusion
2. Cusps that function during centric occlusion
4. Maxillary dental arch facially overhangs mandibular arch
5. Specific spaces between certain primary teeth
8. Situation in which maxillary incisors overlap mandibular incisors
13. Facial profile in centric occlusion with slightly protruded jaws
14. Plane where maxillary arch convex occlusally and mandibular arch concave
19. Concave curve that results when section taken through each molar set
21. Orofacial parafunctional habit with teeth held in centric occlusion for long periods
22. Situation in which the canine is only tooth in function during lateral occlusion
23. Bony projection off posterior and superior borders of mandibular ramus
25. What can occur to periodontium and that can result from occlusal disharmony

PART 3: UNIT WORD SEARCHES

The following are exercises that use **word search** that consists of the letters of **hidden related terms** *per unit* placed in a grid with random letters placed around in all directions. One has to **find and circle** the hidden terms listed below. There is *no answer key* to be obtained from your Instructor for this exercise part.

UNIT 1: OROFACIAL STRUCTURES

Words to Find

ALA	INFRAORBITAL	ORBIT	SULCUS
ANGLE	LABIOMENTAL	PAROTID	SYMPHYSIS
APEX	LARYNX	PHILTRUM	TEMPOROMANDIBULAR
ARTICULATING	LYMPH	PROPORTIONS	THYROID
BUCCAL	MANDIBLE	RAMUS	TUBERCLE
COMMISSURE	MASSETER	ROOT	VERMILION
CONDYLE	MENTAL	STERNOCLEIDOMASTOID	ZYGOMATIC
CORONOID	NARIS	SUBLINGUAL	
FRONTAL	NASAL	SUBMANDIBULAR	
HYOID	NOSE	SUBMENTAL	

Word Search Puzzle 1

```
L A R Y N X S K P R O P O R T I O N S I
S R D O G Z H L A T N O R F T O O R D R
I Y A I R E L C R E B U T S Y L W I A Y
S S E L O D I O R Y H T A R A P O L L D
Y S L A U Y H N O S E H Q L O T U A I E
H I Y T G B H P C U S P A A S B T O R S
P R D N E J I I M U Y I L A I I R U U B
M A N E N W T D B Y B A M D B Y S C L M
Y N O M B A J L N A L O N R H S L A Q A
S H C B M A I E L A D A O T I U B V L S
C J U O N N F O L I M A L M S I G A R S
C I G G G K S M E B R O M N O X T B V E
T Y L U E A T L U F I O R M B N E X B T
Z E A Z N N C S N L C D E O E U P P J E
L L V F K O U I U A A N N M P A C X A R
M D I O N O R O C M T S B A R M Y C Y R
A M U R T L I H P A A U A O M I E M A L
P I E A X Q M E L I S R T N J A N T U L
E T C Z E R A H A R T I C U L A T I N G
S N O I L I M R E V D T I B R O G P Z V
```

UNIT 1: OROFACIAL STRUCTURES

Words to Find

- ALVEOLAR
- ALVEOLUS
- ANTERIOR
- CARUNCLE
- CECUM
- DORSAL
- EXOSTOSES
- FACIAL
- FAUCES
- FAUCIAL
- FILIFORM
- FIMBRIATA
- FOLIATE
- FORDYCE
- FORNIX
- FUNGIFORM
- GINGIVA
- INCISORS
- LABIAL
- LINGUAL
- MASTICATION
- MELANIN
- MOLARS
- MUCOBUCCAL
- MUCOGINGIVAL
- MUCOSA
- NASOPHARYNX
- OROPHARYNX
- PAROTID
- PERIODONTAL
- PERMANENT
- POSTERIOR
- PREMOLARS
- PRIMARY
- PTERYGOMANDIBULAR
- PULP
- RAPHE
- RETROMOLAR
- SUBMANDIBULAR
- TASTE
- TERMINALIS
- TONSIL
- TORUS
- TUBEROSITY
- UVULA
- VENTRAL
- VESTIBULES

Word Search Puzzle 2

```
T S R O S I C N I F P R I M A R Y F V T
S L D E G N L M I L V S A Q R R R O E O
R H A G L A O M R E A S U O W A A L N N
A N O V I C B I S O O U I L L L P I T S
L Y U B I R N T T C F R G U O O H A R I
O Y A L I G I U U A E I B N U E E T A L
M L T A A B N M R T C I L X I V V E L S
E X T I U C L I N A D I W I S L U L I O
R A N L S A C A G N C N T U F A J L A L
P T E Y I O D U A O A E B S A T A S A R
Z S N C R O R M B S C M C W A N X T A M
F R U E R A O E O O A U E U I M N L R Y
P A O S N G H P B N C X M M M O O O F R
F G A I Y A H P D U O U R U D M F O P M
F L I R R A M I O S T E M O O I R A F E
W A E N R E B R T R T S I R G D R O A L
F T U Y G U T O E A O R T N Y O R P C A
P A N C L I S S S P E E U C T N U E I N
O X T A E E V T O P R F E I I L N F A I
T O R U S S E A T P H S D X P I J H L N
```

UNIT 2: DENTAL EMBRYOLOGY

Words to Find

AMNIOCENTESIS
BILAMINAR
BLASTOCYST
CAUDAL
CEPHALIC
CLEAVAGE
CLOACAL
DISC
ECTODERM
EMBRYO
ENDODERM
EPIBLAST
FERTILIZATION
FETUS
FOLDING
FUSION
HYPOBLAST
INDUCTION
KARYOTYPE
MATURATION
MEIOSIS
MESODERM
MITOSIS
MORPHOLOGY
NEUROECTODERM
PRENATAL
PRIMORDIUM
SOMITES
SYMMETRY
TERATOGENS
TRILAMINAR
ZYGOTE

Word Search Puzzle 1

```
Q F E V U D C L L S F D C L E A V A G E
A B P T X S F L M E S O D E R M S M L S
Q E I R S Y M M E T R Y B I H N R A I N
C C B I B L A S T O C Y S T E E T S O S
L T L L M I T O S I S G R G D I E I U W
O O A A W R C L V S J S O O N T T T E P
A D S M Y J A N I A E T T E N C E T R H
C E T I W D G S G T A C G E U F F D P Z
A R M N U B O D I R E N C D E P E Q R C
L M E A C I L M E O O O N C H I R J E R
M G C R E U O T R C I I P M Y D T K N O
J A B M F S Y U C N H K R O P S I U A E
F C T I X O E W M U U A I R O A L E T M
U E M U L N L A J H R R M P B B I N A B
S P D R R A Z D O Q I Y O H L X Z D L R
I H J H A A M Y I U Y O R O A S A O U Y
O A D G L Z T I G N U T D L S F T D H O
N L J I R D L I N O G Y I O T F I E Z T
K I U J S S V F O A T P U G C L O R Q B
B C Q T O C K O H N R E M Y L K N M X V
```

UNIT 2: DENTAL EMBRYOLOGY

Words to Find

- APPOSITION
- BELL
- BUD
- CEMENTOBLASTS
- CEMENTOCYTES
- CEMENTOID
- DILACERATION
- ECTODERM
- ECTOMESENCHYME
- FUSION
- GEMINATION
- INDUCTION
- INITIATION
- MACRODONTIA
- MALASSEZ
- MATRIX
- MEMBRANE
- MICRODONTIA
- MORPHOGENESIS
- NONSUCCEDANEOUS
- ODONTOBLASTS
- ODONTOCLASTS
- ORGAN
- PEARL
- PREAMELOBLASTS
- PREDENTIN
- REPOLARIZATION
- RESORPTION
- SHEATH
- SUCCEDANEOUS
- SUPERNUMERARY

Word Search Puzzle 2

```
W C X O O X X L C E M E N T O C Y T E S
M M A L A S S E Z E N N N N S N S S V X
I B S F U S I O N I O O O I O T U K I E
C R E S Y G K A T I I I S I S O Y R O S
R Z X L P J R N T T T E T A E F T O T O
O F P Q L B E A I A N A L N O A S S B L
D C C L M D N S I E Z B A E M N A X R N
O E Z E E I O T G I O D V C H L W A A S
N M M R M P I O R L E E N T B F E G O U
I E P E P N II A E C Z O A O M P R I D P
I N G A I P L M C G I E T M A O R N O E
A T D D R O A U Q T H N K E C C E D N R
R O U O P E S J A S O O B S R E S U T N
O B M E R N L R H D E H M E O M O C O U
E L R P O Q E S O T Y Q R N D E R T C M
K A W N E C E B M Q N D M C O N P I L E
I S R C A E C T O D E R M H N T T O A R
R T U L N E Q L J M D F B Y T O I N S A
A S I S D P B I O Y P C U M I I O F T R
C D J A S U W R V E E R T E A D N H S Y
```

UNIT 3: DENTAL HISTOLOGY

Words to Find

CELL
CENTROMERE
CENTROSOME
CHROMATIDS
CHROMATIN
CHROMOSOMES
CYTOSKELETON
DESMOSOME
ENDOCYTOSIS
EXOCYTOSIS
HEMIDESMOSOME
HISTOLOGY
INCLUSIONS
INTERPHASE
KERATIN
LYSOSOMES
METAPHASE
MICROFILAMENTS
MICROTUBULES
MITOCHONDRIA
MITOSIS
NUCLEOLUS
NUCLEOPLASM
NUCLEUS
ORGAN
PHAGOCYTOSIS
PROPHASE
RIBOSOMES
SYSTEM
TELOPHASE
TISSUE
TONOFILAMENTS
VACUOLES

Word Search Puzzle 1

M	I	M	E	K	W	Q	Q	P	H	A	G	O	C	Y	T	O	S	I	S
I	J	E	X	K	U	N	W	E	E	M	S	S	S	S	S	S	E	A	A
T	G	T	D	B	E	U	U	S	S	I	E	I	D	S	T	S	E	I	E
O	D	A	I	I	K	S	A	A	S	M	S	I	U	N	A	Q	R	M	S
S	M	P	K	K	S	H	L	O	O	O	T	L	E	H	S	D	O	E	M
I	M	H	L	I	P	P	T	S	T	A	O	M	P	E	N	S	L	S	J
S	J	A	T	O	O	Y	O	Y	M	E	A	O	M	O	O	O	A	E	S
M	I	S	L	T	C	M	C	O	L	L	R	O	H	R	U	L	M	T	N
I	N	E	Y	O	O	O	R	C	I	P	S	C	T	C	P	O	N	I	S
C	T	C	X	R	D	H	U	F	Y	O	O	N	A	O	S	E	T	N	V
R	E	E	H	N	C	N	O	X	M	T	E	V	E	O	M	A	O	W	E
O	R	C	E	P	H	R	G	S	I	C	O	L	M	A	R	I	L	R	C
T	P	I	C	F	C	I	E	M	N	U	C	S	L	E	S	L	E	T	H
U	H	G	B	I	N	D	S	A	U	U	F	I	K	U	L	M	N	Z	U
B	A	S	M	O	I	U	G	T	N	D	F	I	L	E	O	S	S	T	O
U	S	M	S	M	S	R	C	B	O	O	L	C	C	R	L	F	Y	O	M
L	E	R	E	W	O	O	M	L	N	L	N	R	T	H	P	E	S	A	A
E	V	H	O	O	Q	Z	M	O	E	I	O	N	M	B	N	H	T	D	T
S	D	D	Z	D	I	Q	T	E	C	U	E	G	R	T	H	J	E	O	I
L	Y	S	O	S	O	M	E	S	S	C	S	X	Y	Z	N	V	M	O	N

UNIT 3: DENTAL HISTOLOGY

Words to Find

- ADIPOSE
- APPOSITIONAL
- BASOPHIL
- BONE
- CANALICULI
- CARTILAGE
- CHONDROBLASTS
- CHONDROCYTES
- COLLAGEN
- DERMIS
- ELASTIC
- ENDOSTEUM
- ENDOTHELIUM
- EOSINOPHIL
- EPIDERMIS
- EPITHELIUM
- FIBROBLAST
- GRANULATION
- HAVERSIAN
- HEMIDESMOSOMES
- HYDROXYAPATITE
- IMMUNOGEN
- IMMUNOGLOBULIN
- INTERSTITIAL
- KERATIN
- LACUNA
- LAMELLAE
- LYMPHOCYTE
- MACROPHAGE
- MAST

Word Search Puzzle 2

```
N E S J X J V B O N E C A R T I L A G E
M A S T E P I T H E L I U M L A C U N A
U J E I J C B D L M X B D R O Z T Z I C
W I L M J H E I U L A M E L L A E L F W
I J A M O O I M M U N O G L O B U L I N
H Z S U E N Q K V M M E P I D E R M I S
I C T N A D D E R M I S D R O K X Y G H
T L I O P R C B F O F I B R O B L A S T
G D C G P O I I F A M A C R O P H A G E
G B G E O C H E M I D E S M O S O M E S
E B R N S Y Q I W E N D O T H E L I U M
O U A H I T W C H O N D R O B L A S T S
S B N A T E Q C P V A J C O L L A G E N
I A U V I S J A D I P O S E Z S V P U C
N S L E O Y G J D S D D R K E R A T I N
O O A R N Q E W U F L Y M P H O C Y T E
P P T S A W Z S I N T E R S T I T I A L
H H I I L K C U O B I E N D O S T E U M
I I O A R F H Y D R O X Y A P A T I T E
L L N N W J Q B B I C A N A L I C U L I
```

UNIT 3: DENTAL HISTOLOGY

Words to Find

ENDOCHONDRAL
INTRAMEMBRANOUS
MATRIX
MONOCYTE
NERVE
NEURON
NEUTROPHIL

ODONTOCLAST
OSSIFICATION
OSTEOBLASTS
OSTEOCLAST
OSTEOCYTES
OSTEOID
OSTEONS

PAPILLARY
PERICHONDRIUM
PERIOSTEUM
PLASMA
PLATELETS
RETE
RETICULAR

SQUAMES
SUBMUCOSA
SYNAPSE
TONOFILAMENTS
TRABECULAE

Word Search Puzzle 3

```
U S P L A S M A E L L I C O I O H X L Z
B U T F Z M F W P Y R X F Z A T C D N L
J B O Y Y W N D L H W F J R S T I O A X
I M N R V S Y N A P S E F A H O I R S M
V U O E F K F O T J I W L O E T D K U B
P C F T L I B X E S H C T T A N U E A K
L O I I Z N S O L D O W S C O A T W B U
T S L C G T P F E E I O I H W S V T P Z
L A A U V R G W T E P F C H O O S F E G
B C M L O A S S S C I O S I E A E P R X
L T E A S M O P V S D C R T L V O A I N
E R N R T E N L S N K E Y C R N S P C E
W A T G E M B O E R P C O E O Z T I H U
O B S S O B D R I D O T N Z O F E L O T
N E X Q B R R G X N N C W M S B O L N R
E C K U L A P P O O M V K A T V C A D O
U U B A A N K M D A V E C T E K Y R R P
R L R M S O M O D J T P E R O G T Y I H
O A J E T U N K W E A J S I N K E W U I
N E T S S S F K R I C U H X S B S X M L
```

UNIT 3: DENTAL HISTOLOGY

Words to Find

- AFFERENT
- CAPSULE
- COLLOID
- DENTOGINGIVAL
- DUCT
- EFFERENT
- ENDOCRINE
- EXOCRINE
- FIBROBLAST
- FOLLICLES
- GERMINAL
- GINGIVITIS
- GOBLET
- GOITER
- GRANULATION
- HILUS
- HYPERKERATINIZED
- JUNCTIONAL
- KERATIN
- KERATOHYALIN
- LOBES
- LOBULES
- LUMEN
- LYMPH
- MASTICATORY
- MELANIN
- MUCOGINGIVAL
- MUCOPERIOSTEUM
- MUCOSA
- NODES
- PERIODONTITIS
- PRICKLE
- RECESSION
- STIPPLING
- SULCULAR
- SULCUS
- TASTE

Word Search Puzzle 4

```
N O D E S E G V K Y Q K A O S U L C U S
A P C K O N P E H K A U R F E L E I T P
H R O H D D M Z R G E E S N F N Y S Y T
A I L H K O U U D M T R I L I E A M C D
E C L Z L C H D C I I R A L O L R U P G
T K O U I R Y E O O C N A T B B D E N H
A L I T S I P G G O P Y A O I S E I N N
P E D D T N E Y X O H E R L E N L S O T
E S W E A E R C C O B B R I M P R I Z L
R E M N S M K Z T A I L C I P G S S A N
I G A T T U E A M F T I E I O S T V O S
O I S O E D R L P S L E T T E S I I E Z
D N T G I E A V A L U S Z C N G T L W A
O G I I K C T V O N I L E L N A U E S V
N I C N E A I F X G I R C I L B Z O U V
T V A G X P N I A J A N G U O A C L Y M
I I T I V S I M O M J O N L L U P U U N
T T O V F U Z S H N C A M W M A I M Z L
I I R A D L E P B U R M E F F E R E N T
S S Y L X E D Z M G J U N C T I O N A L
```

UNIT 3: DENTAL HISTOLOGY

Words to Find

- ABFRACTION
- ABRASION
- AMELOBLAST
- AMELOGENESIS
- ATTRITION
- CARIES
- DEMILUNE
- EROSION
- LYMPHADENOPATHY
- LYMPHATICS
- MUCOCELE
- MUCOSEROUS
- MYOEPITHELIAL
- NARIS
- PARATHYROID
- PERIKYMATA
- RANULA
- RETZIUS
- SALIVA
- SECRETORY
- SINUSITIS
- THYROGLOSSAL
- THYROID
- THYROXINE
- TONSILS
- TRABECULAE
- XEROSTOMIA

Word Search Puzzle 5

I	B	W	S	T	H	Y	R	O	X	I	N	E	T	T	P	E	Z	P	B
S	A	B	F	R	A	C	T	I	O	N	N	K	F	S	K	Z	E	S	S
L	C	A	R	I	E	S	I	L	H	O	G	X	Z	V	I	A	U	I	A
P	A	R	A	T	H	Y	R	O	I	D	Y	E	U	Y	L	O	S	T	T
F	G	Y	L	S	I	N	U	S	I	T	I	S	H	U	R	E	A	S	N
G	D	Y	W	H	G	I	A	M	P	S	K	T	C	E	N	M	A	O	W
Y	E	D	M	U	U	R	X	L	R	N	A	E	S	E	Y	L	I	A	S
M	M	S	S	U	B	U	M	E	Y	P	B	O	G	K	B	T	D	C	D
U	I	A	E	A	J	C	Y	R	O	A	C	O	I	O	I	S	I	I	S
C	L	L	P	N	Z	W	O	N	R	U	L	R	L	R	V	T	O	U	N
O	U	I	T	I	W	T	E	T	M	E	E	E	T	D	A	R	I	O	C
C	N	V	U	U	E	D	P	E	M	P	M	T	F	H	Y	Z	I	D	L
E	E	A	M	R	A	Q	I	A	U	A	A	R	P	H	T	S	K	Q	F
L	H	T	C	H	U	R	T	Z	U	B	P	M	T	E	O	W	M	M	X
E	G	E	P	Y	G	A	H	R	F	R	Y	U	R	R	U	Q	I	G	W
P	S	M	F	Z	X	N	E	O	Y	L	W	G	E	R	G	D	A	N	T
X	Y	U	B	Z	A	U	L	E	F	X	E	R	O	S	T	O	M	I	A
L	K	N	S	F	L	I	C	Q	L	L	E	T	O	N	S	I	L	S	
I	E	U	V	W	F	A	A	T	H	Y	R	O	G	L	O	S	S	A	L
P	H	T	B	F	V	N	L	N	A	R	I	S	B	F	W	H	S	U	Q

UNIT 3: DENTAL HISTOLOGY

Words to Find

ACCESSORY
ALVEOLUS
APICAL
APPOSITION
ARREST
ATTRITION
CANALICULI
CEMENTICLES
CEMENTOBLASTS
CEMENTOCYTES
CEMENTOGENESIS
CEMENTOID
CEMENTUM
CHAMBER
CIRCUMPULPAL
DENTIN
DENTINOGENESIS
EDENTULOUS
FLUID
GLOBULAR
HYPERCEMENTOSIS
HYPERSENSITIVITY
IMBRICATION
INTERGLOBULAR
INTERTUBULAR
MANTLE
NEONATAL
ODONTOBLASTS
OWEN
PERIODONTIUM
PERITUBULAR
PREDENTIN
PRIMARY
PRINCIPAL
PULP
PULPITIS
RADICULAR
SECONDARY
STONES
TERTIARY
TRABECULAR
TUBULES

Word Search Puzzle 6

```
A T T A T Q M P N T G K O I B S A D C C
R E U L C P A U E R D A W M P T T B E H
R R B V E R N L O A E P E B R O T U M A
E T U E M I T P N B N I N R I N R B E M
S I L O E N L I A E T C H I M E I H N B
T A E L N C E T T C I A Y C A S T Z T E
C R S U T I C I A U N L P A R H I C U R
E Y P S O P E S L L O I E T Y Y O E M C
M P E C I A M E I A G N R I O P N M P E
E E R I D L E V N R E T S O D E K E R M
N R I R K C N E T Z N E E N O C A N E E
T I O C S A T D E R E R N A N E P T D N
I T D U E N O E R A S G S C T M P O E T
C U O M C A G N T D I L I C O E O C N O
L B N P O L E T U I S O T E B N S Y T B
E U T U N I N U B C F B I S L T I T I L
S L I L D C E L U U L U V S A O T E N A
U A U P A U S O L L U L I O S S I S W S
I R M A R L I U A A I A T R T I O Q R T
Y Q X L Y I S S R R D R Y Y S S N E Q S
```

UNIT 4: DENTAL ANATOMY

Words to Find

ANATOMIC
AXIS
CEMENTOENAMEL
CLINICAL
CONCAVITIES
CONTACT
CONTOUR
CUSP
DECIDUOUS
DENTITION
DISTAL
EMBRASURES
INCISAL
INTERNATIONAL
INTERPROXIMAL
MASTICATORY
MESIAL
MIDLINE
OCCLUSAL
OCCLUSION
PALMER
PERMANENT
PRIMARY
PROXIMAL
QUADRANTS
SEXTANTS
THIRDS
UNIVERSAL

Word Search Puzzle 1

```
A I A J G I N T E R P R O X I M A L O Q
T H I R D S T L T L R V F L Y R V S B L
P K L N B C F N T M X U A L U C T H E L
N S O Z A A E G Y D A I O O T N A M B L
I F S T K N V W M C S S T C A C A X A J
C S N Z A A U E O E O N T T C N K N I L
T O V M B T N T M K O N X I E L O X A S
C C R P S O I G E C V E C O C I U M L C
H E U Q K M V S J N S O T A T A I S Y E
P N W S K I E D J Q D N C A V X T Q A L
L R L R P C R B U E E I N C O I N O A L
W V I E R A S Q K M M R S R L B T C R S
Z C N M D L A U E R E B P T C U I I U Y
B J C V A H L C C T M P R V A N S O E R
K M I F X R F K N P F C Y A I L U I E S
Q A S F U V Y I A I Z S V L S D U M O I
Z W A U X O N R J M S J C Q I U L E E N
O M L Q U A D R A N T S Z C F A R K D T
X W D E N T I T I O N D E K P Q Z E D D
O H M I D L I N E J H D T W N U Q X S P
```

UNIT 4: DENTAL ANATOMY

Words to Find

ANODONTIA
AVULSION
BICUSPID
BIFURCATED
CARABELLI
CENTRAL
CINGULUM
CUSPIDS
DENTIGEROUS
DIASTEMA
DILACERATION
EMINENCE
FLUTTING
FOSSA
FURCATION
IMPACTED
MAMELONS
MARGINAL
MESIODENS
MULBERRY
MULTIROOTED
PEG
SUPERNUMERARY
SUPPLEMENTAL
TRANSVERSE
TRIANGULAR
TRIFURCATED
TUBERCLES

Word Search Puzzle 2

```
P K A C B B I F U R C A T E D E U F F M
U O A I B T O S T Y E N L W D T D X R D
S I Z N N B I J U S W A U E D I O A E A
F M C G K A D M R P T S T D P Y L T A Q
L P J U T G K E A N E O N S Q U A S Y H
U A K L L Z V I E I O R U P G C S G E F
T C W U Y S T M G R S C N N R O R M F V
T T S M N N E L I L I K A U F O V F X E
I E U A O L H T L B H I F D M F X A R I
N D R D P W L Q D U R I Z I Z E X I Y Q
G T O P D U Y A E T N D X L Z I R G Q N
R N U R M F B T N T P C M A M S H A P P
A S M M E U K U T D E A A C P E A I R S
V C U A S R N B I I G R R E N M V C F Y
A U L M I C D E G A S A G R G I U E J L
P S B E O A H R E S L B I A O N L N X C
P P E L D T L C R T Z E N T D E S T D C
X I R O E I C L O E X L A I P N I R D O
I D R N N O B E U M K L L O S C O A D Y
U S Y S S N O S S A B I P N T E N L V X
```

UNIT 4: DENTAL ANATOMY

Words to Find

- ABFRACTION
- ARTICULAR
- BALANCING
- BRUXISM
- CAPSULE
- CENTRIC
- CLENCHING
- CONDYLE
- CROSSBITE
- DEPRESSION
- DEVIATION
- DISC
- DRIFT
- ELEVATION
- GROUP
- INTEROCCLUSAL
- LEEWAY
- MALOCCLUSION
- MESOGNATHIC
- OCCLUSION
- OVERBITE
- OVERJET
- PARAFUNCTIONAL
- PREMATURE
- PRIMARY
- PRIMATE
- PROGNATHIC
- PROTRUSION
- RETRACTION
- RETROGNATHIC
- RISE
- SPEE
- STEP
- SUBLUXATION
- SUPPORTING
- SYNOVIAL
- TEMPOROMANDIBULAR
- TERMINAL
- TRAUMA
- WILSON
- WORKING

Word Search Puzzle 3

```
A U F P R I M A T E R E T R A C T I O N
R I N T E R O C C L U S A L W I L S O N
T O N T E M P O R O M A N D I B U L A R
I P G X E L E V A T I O N P R I M A R Y
C O N D Y L E M A L O C C L U S I O N J
U S P M D S U B L U X A T I O N R I S E
L P W O R K I N G B P R O G N A T H I C
A W R X M E S O G N A T H I C D R I F T
R R A E V V C E I U P M T E R M I N A L
H C E O M L E E W A Y D E V I A T I O N
D L P T M A P A R A F U N C T I O N A L
E E B R R X T T O V E R B I T E S T E P
P N A S O O Z U C R O S S B I T E O T J
R C L B C T G Q R T F O C C L U S I O N
E H A R T E R N C E R V I C A L S P E E
S I N U R G N U A V A B F R A C T I O N
S N C X A R D T S T S U P P O R T I N G
I G I I U O I X R I H H S Y N O V I A L
O H N S M U S D Y I O I X O V E R J E T
N W G M A P C Q L I C N C C A P S U L E
```

The following are tooth drawing exercises that emphasize **basic principles of comprehensive tooth design**, which later have direct application in clinical coursework of the student dental professional. While presentations to the whole class by student groups working together on one tooth is worthwhile, it is felt by many past students that they really only learned about one tooth in depth. Instead with this exercise, the student will be able to better visualize the entire dentition.

The student should not overly worry about this exercise since it is understood that these initial drawings are most likely to be the student's first attempts at capturing any tooth likeness; therefore the overriding goal is only to encourage accuracy and judgment about the important features of the teeth and hopefully assist with the recognition of these tooth details. Thus any overwhelming artistic inclinations are not what is being exercised with these basic drawings of the teeth.

It is important to also note that these drawings are only 2D and are somewhat limited to basic outlines and proportions; real specimens in patients' mouths vary considerably. However, these drawings will serve to help create mental pictures of the teeth in their ideal form and composite state using each standard view of the individual tooth. Later, these mental images can be called upon during clinical situations. The specific tooth anatomy discussions *are located* in **Unit 4** of the associated textbook and measurements used throughout are noted in millimeters (mm) as adapted from Nelson SJ: *Wheeler's Dental Anatomy, Physiology, and Occlusion.* Ed. 11, Elsevier, 2020 as well as being located in its **Appendix B**.

Exercise Directions

Step 1. Locate the two blank gridded worksheets in the student workbook. Any additional gridded worksheets can be easily scanned and printed for the correct spacing of the grid needed. Correctly label the worksheet with the tooth that will be drawn at the bottom of the page, as shown in the smaller professionally drawn figures.

Step 2. Using the included table of tooth measurements (also in the associated textbook's Appendix B), mark off the overall bordering tooth measurements for each of the gridded view boxes of the tooth. Note that the grid of the blank worksheet is larger than that shown with the professionally drawn tooth outlines to better enable the student to have room to work. Each square of grid equates to 1 mm of actual dimension, so count off as many squares for each bordering measurement (such as the mesiodistal diameter) as indicated from the table onto the proper area of the gridded worksheet.

Step 3. To establish crown and root proportions, divide each gridded view box into two parts corresponding to these two measurements, except of course for the incisal or occlusal view.

Step 4. To indicate the height of contour, locate the approximate area of contact between the adjacent teeth and the area of greatest convexity on the labial or buccal, lingual, mesial, and distal surfaces (as mentioned in the associated textbook's Unit 4 on dental anatomy).

Step 5. To locate the root axis line (RAL), draw a line that exactly bisects the whole gridded box showing the overall crown and root measurements. The cementoenamel junction (CEJ) will then be bisected by the RAL. The root apex may or may not be located on this RAL, depending on the tooth's apex traits.

Step 6. To locate the center of the cingulum, the midpoint of the incisal ridge, the center of the occlusal table, root apex, or other important basic feature as needed, divide the crown and root (if included in that particular view box) into imaginary thirds. Then place the cingulum, incisal ridge, occlusal table, or root apex into proper perspective with respect to the other overall bordering tooth measurements such as the mesiodistal diameter.

Step 7. To complete the crown outline, connect the heights of contour to the incisal ridge or occlusal table, to the CEJ, and to the other heights of contour. Any additional anatomic features such as marginal ridges, depressions, and others can then be indicated upon completion of the crown outline.

Step 8. To complete the root outline, follow the same directions for developing the crown outline with the understanding that the cervical one-third to one-half of the root width generally approximates the cervical width of the crown before it starts to narrow considerably to form the root apex.

Step 9. Shading or light stippling of the features may now be added, if desired.

Step 10. A drawing evaluation checklist is also included and can be used by both the student and instructor. Multiple copies of the form may be scanned and printed if needed.

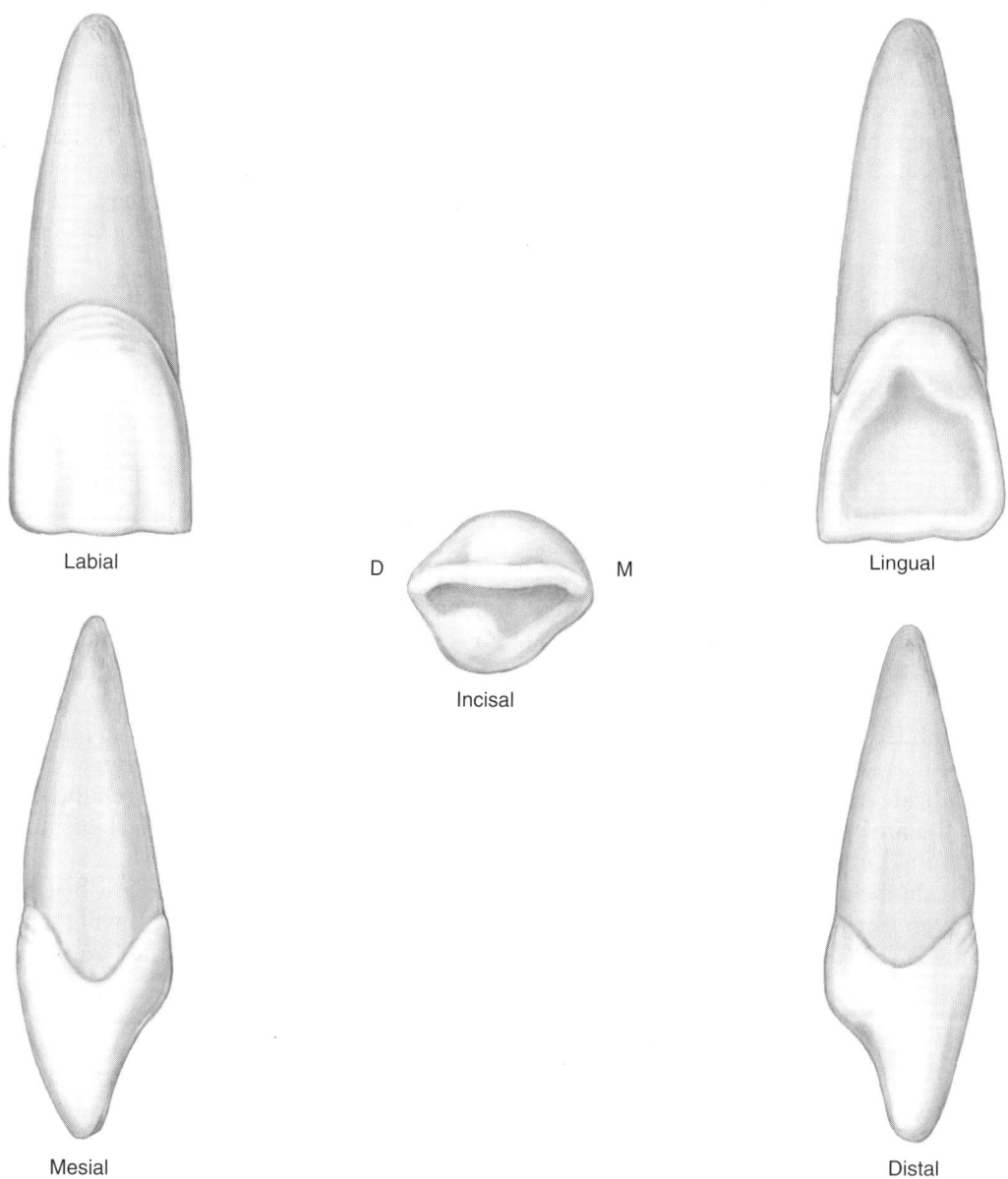

Views of Permanent Maxillary Right Central Incisor

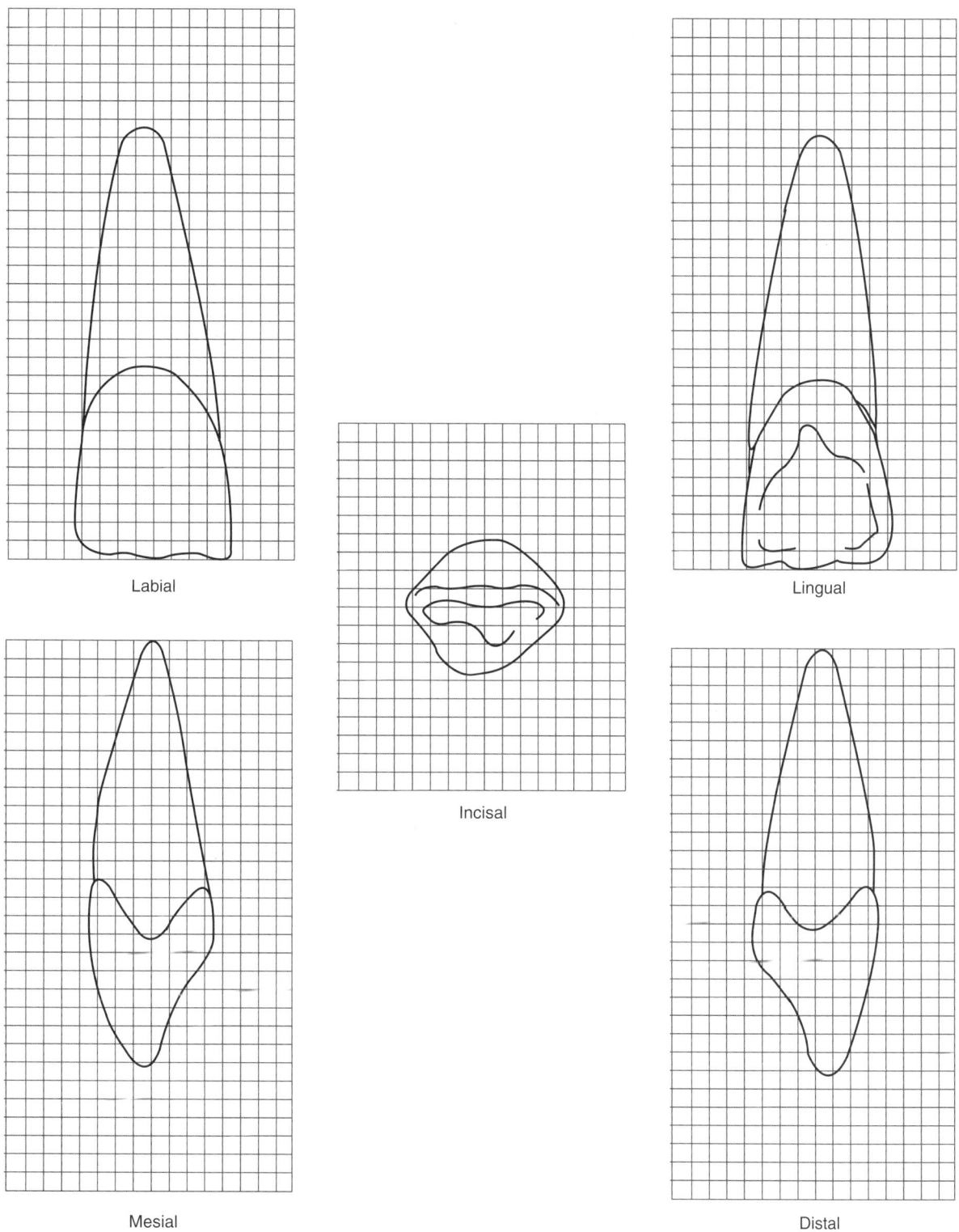

Outline Views of Permanent Maxillary Right Central Incisor

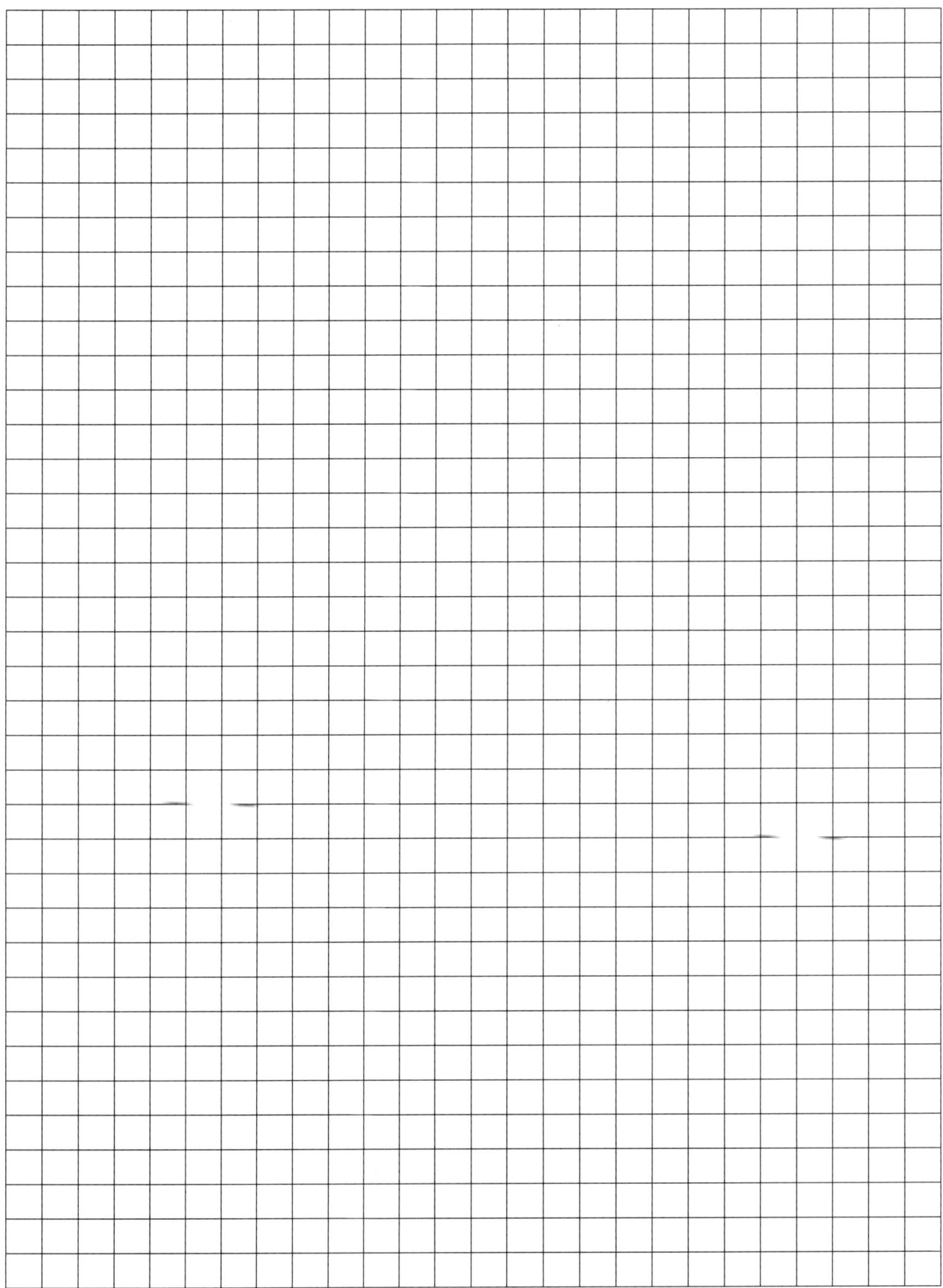

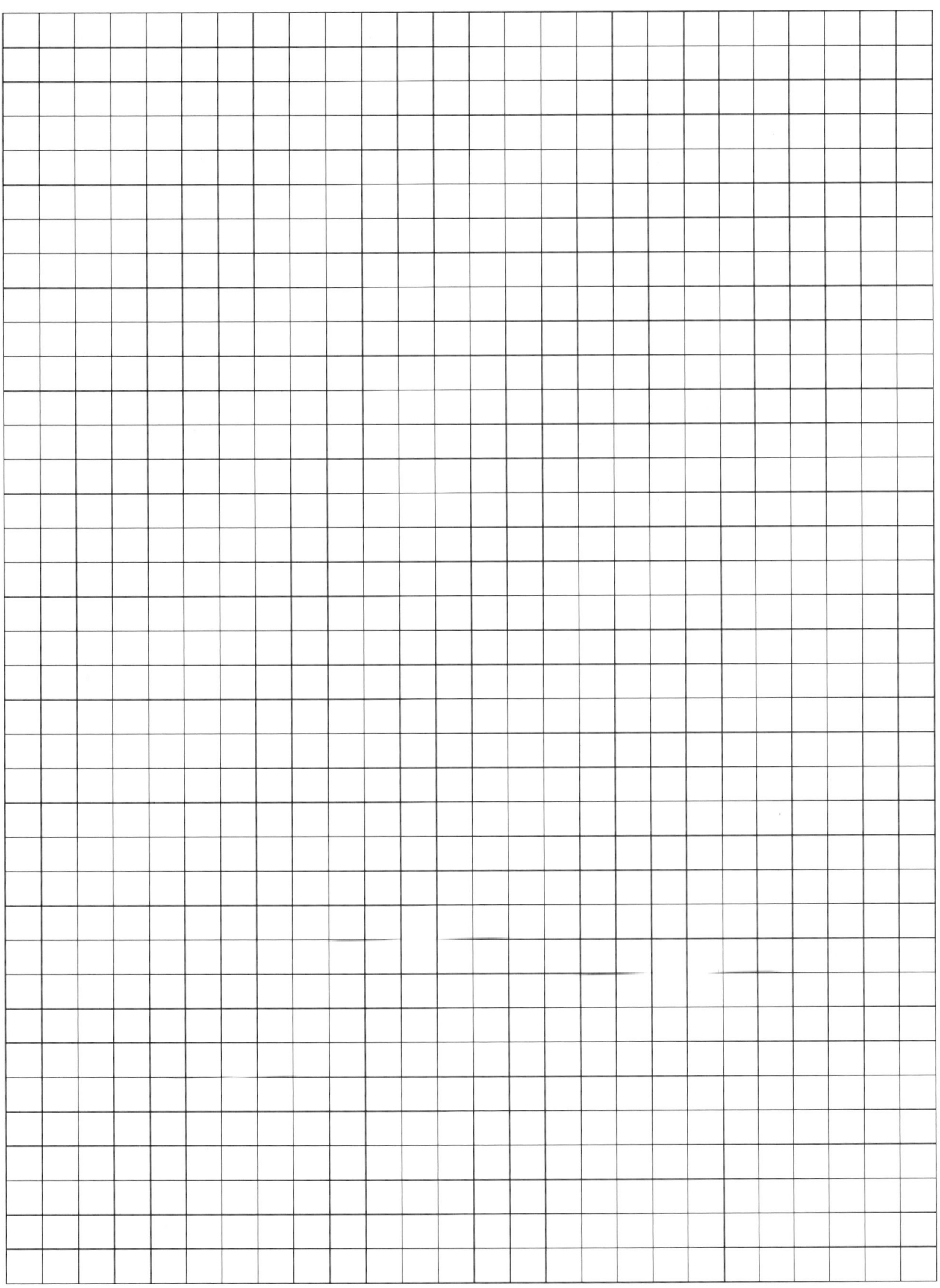

MEASUREMENTS FOR PERMANENT MAXILLARY CENTRAL INCISOR

Cervico-incisal Length of Crown	10.5
Length of Root	13.0
Mesiodistal Diameter of Crown	8.5
Mesiodistal Diameter of CEJ	7.0
Labiolingual Diameter	7.0
Labiolingual Diameter of CEJ	6.0
Curvature of CEJ at Mesial	3.5
Curvature of CEJ at Distal	2.5

CHECKLIST FOR PERMANENT MAXILLARY CENTRAL INCISOR

Features Noted	Features Present
Crown Features	
Incisal ridge, incisal angles, cingulum, marginal ridges, lingual fossa	
Pronounced distal offset wide cingulum and marginal ridges with wide lingual fossa of various depths	
Sharper mesio-incisal angle and rounder disto-incisal angle and more pronounced mesial CEJ curvature	
Height of contour in cervical third	
Mesial contact at incisal third	
Distal contact at junction of incisal and middle thirds	
Root Features	
Single root	
Overall conical shape with no proximal root concavities and rounded apex	

Name _____   Tooth Number/Name _____

Date _____   Instructor Rating _____

DRAWING EVALUATION CHECKLIST

RATING SCALE

Completely Correct = 2 points   Major Error = 0 points
Minor Error = 1 point   Note = NA (Not Applicable)

SELF-EVALUATION RATING

Five Views	Clearly Drawn	Accurate Sizing	General Features Included	Specific Features Included
1. Facial View				
2. Lingual View				
3. Mesial View				
4. Distal View				
5. Incisal View				

Self-Evaluation Rating = $\dfrac{\text{Points received}}{\text{Points possible}}$ = _____ = _____ %

INSTRUCTOR EVALUATION RATING

Five Views	Clearly Drawn	Accurate Sizing	General Features Included	Specific Features Included
1. Facial View				
2. Lingual View				
3. Mesial View				
4. Distal View				
5. Incisal View				

Instructor Evaluation Rating = $\dfrac{\text{Points received}}{\text{Points possible}}$ = _____ = _____ %

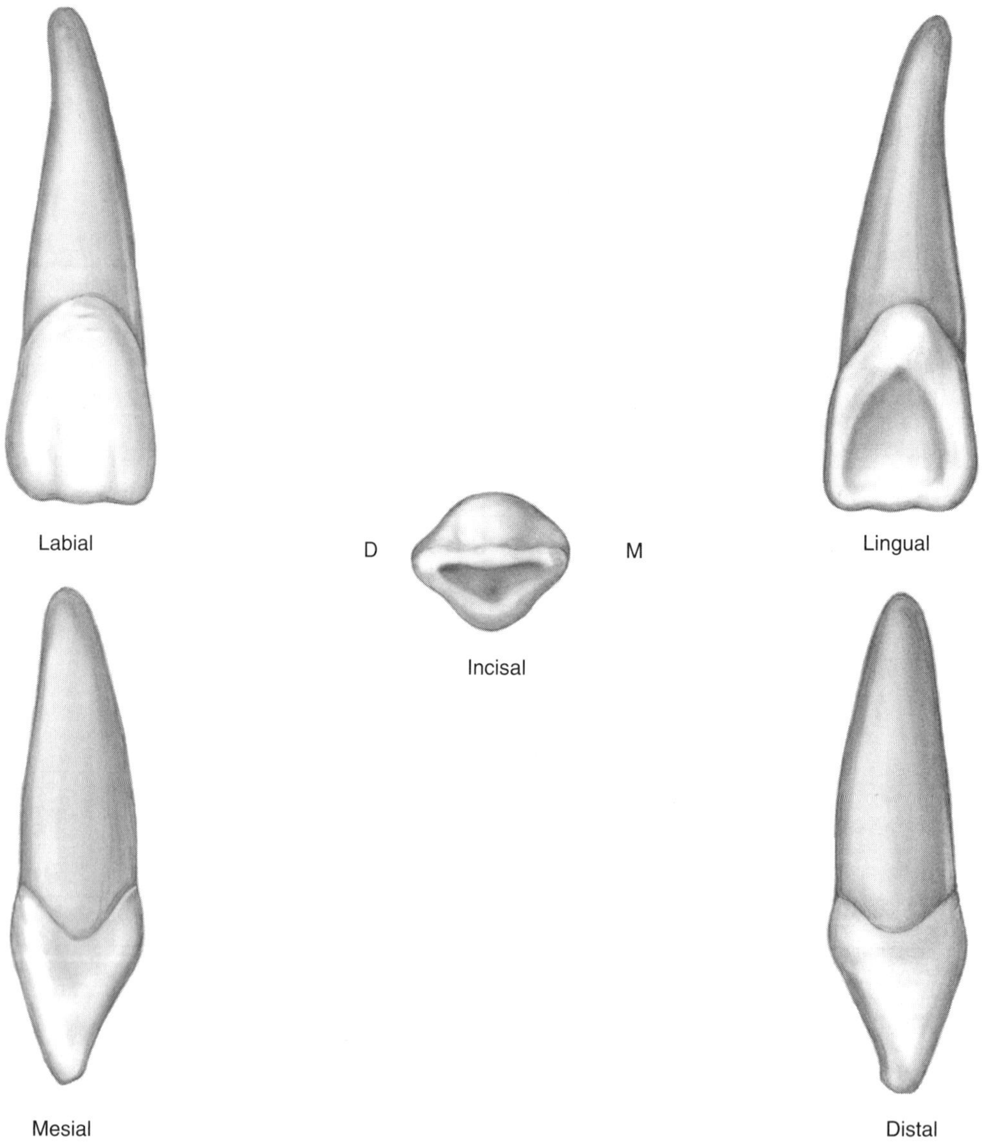

Labial

D M
Incisal

Lingual

Mesial

Distal

Views of Permanent Maxillary Right Lateral Incisor

TOOTH DRAWING EXERCISES **129**

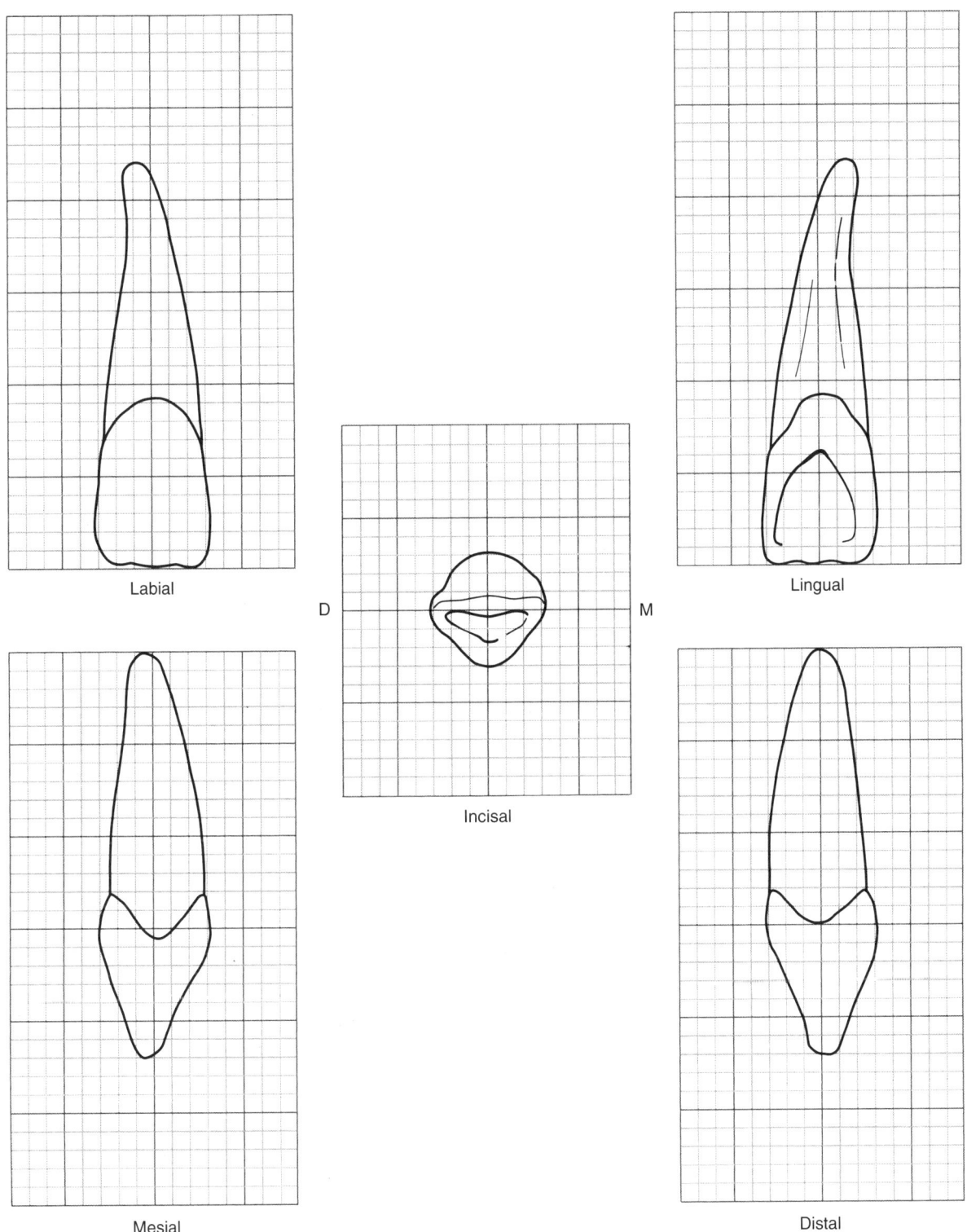

Outline Views of Permanent Maxillary Right Lateral Incisor

Copyright © 2026 by Elsevier Inc. All rights are reserved, including those for text and data mining, AI training, and similar technologies.

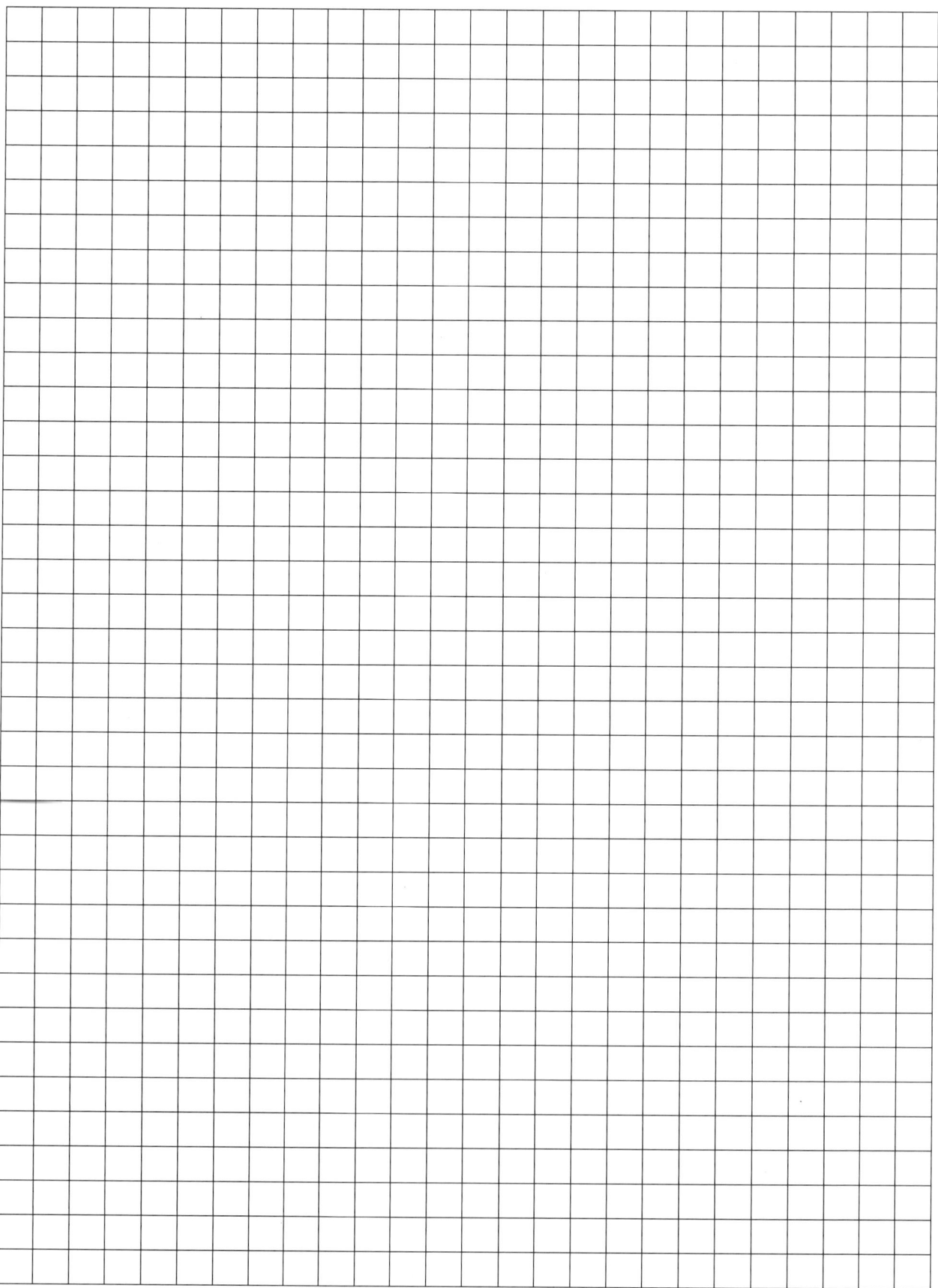

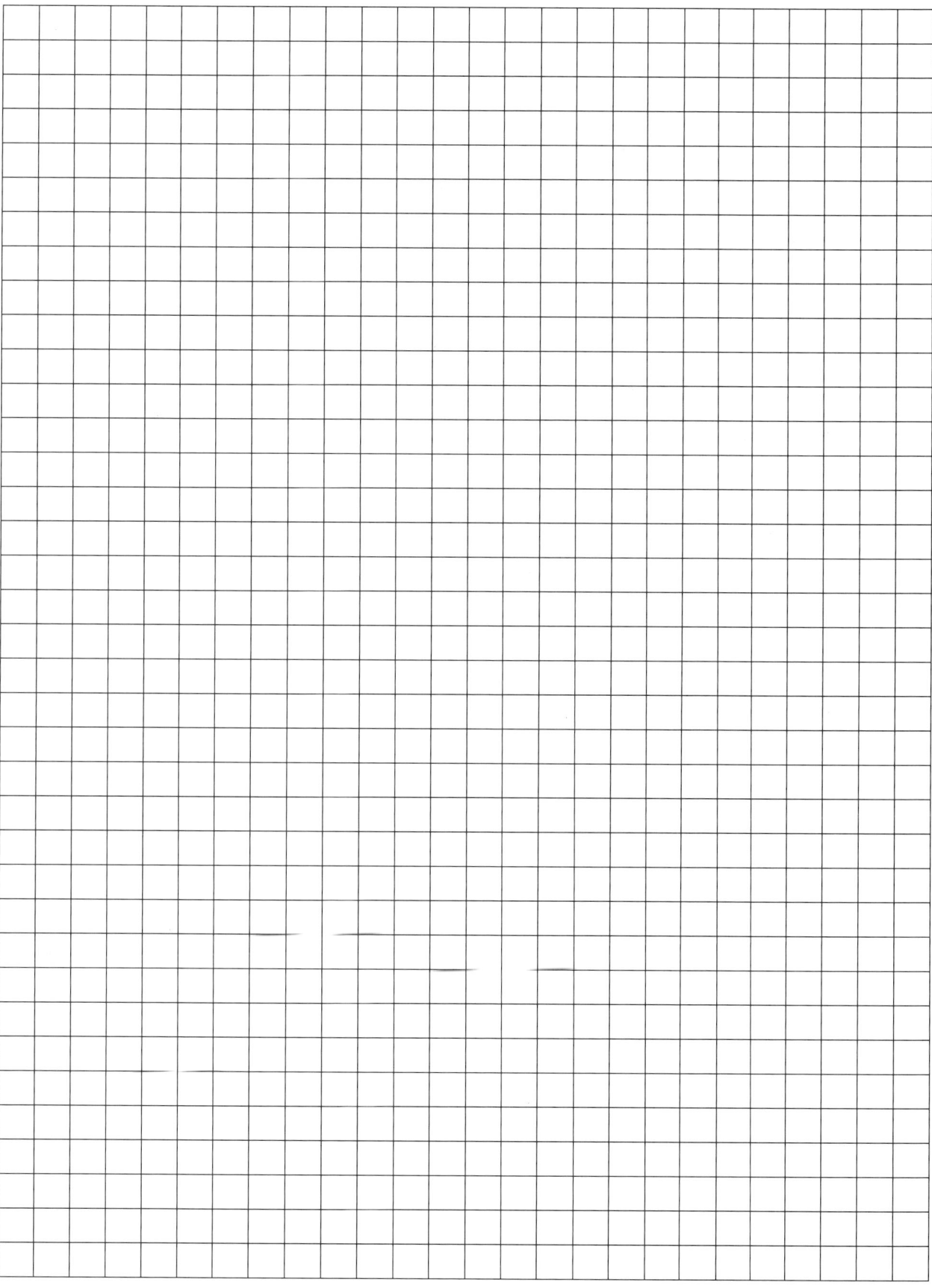

MEASUREMENTS FOR PERMANENT MAXILLARY LATERAL INCISOR	
Cervico-incisal Length of Crown	9.0
Length of Root	13.0
Mesiodistal Diameter of Crown	6.5
Mesiodistal Diameter of CEJ	5.0
Labiolingual Diameter	6.0
Labiolingual Diameter of CEJ	5.0
Curvature of CEJ at Mesial	3.0
Curvature of CEJ at Distal	2.0

CHECKLIST FOR PERMANENT MAXILLARY LATERAL INCISOR	
Features Noted	**Features Present**
Crown Features	
Incisal ridge, incisal angles, cingulum, marginal ridges, lingual fossa	
Pronounced lingual surface with centered narrower cingulum and more pronounced marginal ridges with deeper lingual fossa	
Sharper mesio-incisal angle and rounder disto-incisal angle with more pronounced mesial CEJ curvature	
Height of contour in cervical third	
Mesial contact at incisal third	
Distal contact at middle third	
Root Features	
Single root	
Overall conical shape with no proximal root concavities and root curves distally with sharp apex	

Name _____   Tooth Number/Name _____

Date _____   Instructor Rating _____

DRAWING EVALUATION CHECKLIST

RATING SCALE

Completely Correct = 2 points   Major Error = 0 points
Minor Error = 1 point   Note = NA (Not Applicable)

SELF-EVALUATION RATING

Five Views	Clearly Drawn	Accurate Sizing	General Features Included	Specific Features Included
1. Facial View				
2. Lingual View				
3. Mesial View				
4. Distal View				
5. Incisal View				

Self-Evaluation Rating = $\dfrac{\text{Points received}}{\text{Points possible}}$ = _____ = _____ %

INSTRUCTOR EVALUATION RATING

Five Views	Clearly Drawn	Accurate Sizing	General Features Included	Specific Features Included
1. Facial View				
2. Lingual View				
3. Mesial View				
4. Distal View				
5. Incisal View				

Instructor Evaluation Rating = $\dfrac{\text{Points received}}{\text{Points possible}}$ = _____ = _____ %

Copyright © 2026 by Elsevier Inc. All rights are reserved, including those for text and data mining, AI training, and similar technologies.

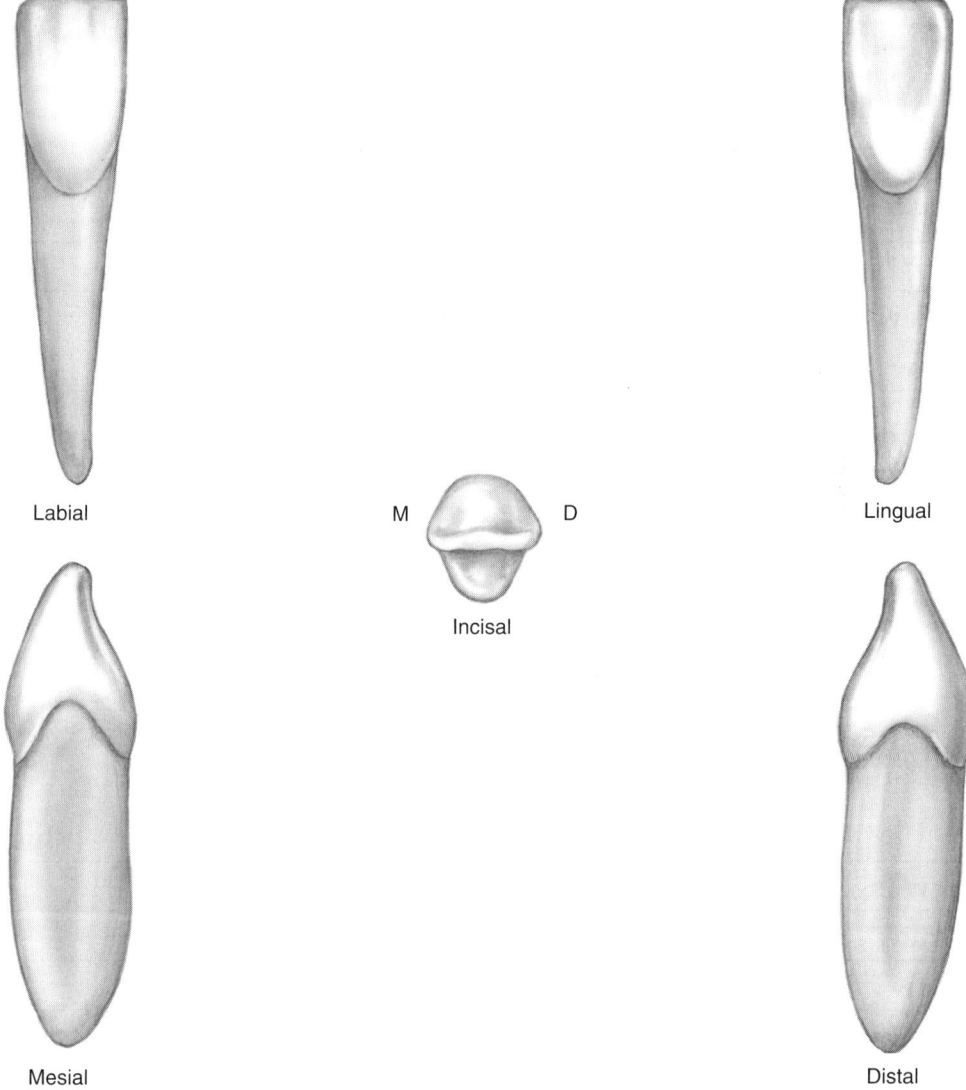

Views of Permanent Mandibular Right Central Incisor

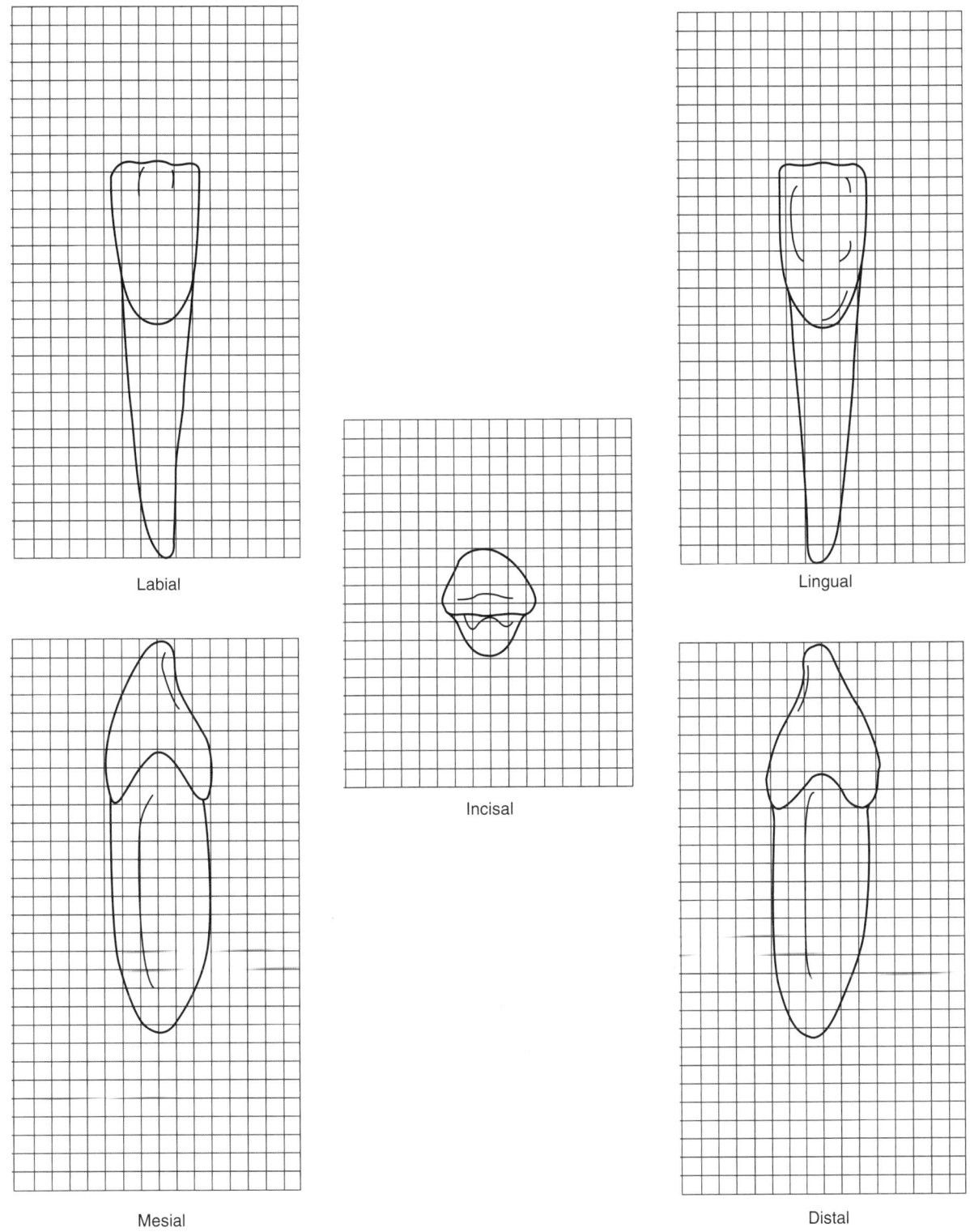

Outline Views of Permanent Mandibular Right Central Incisor

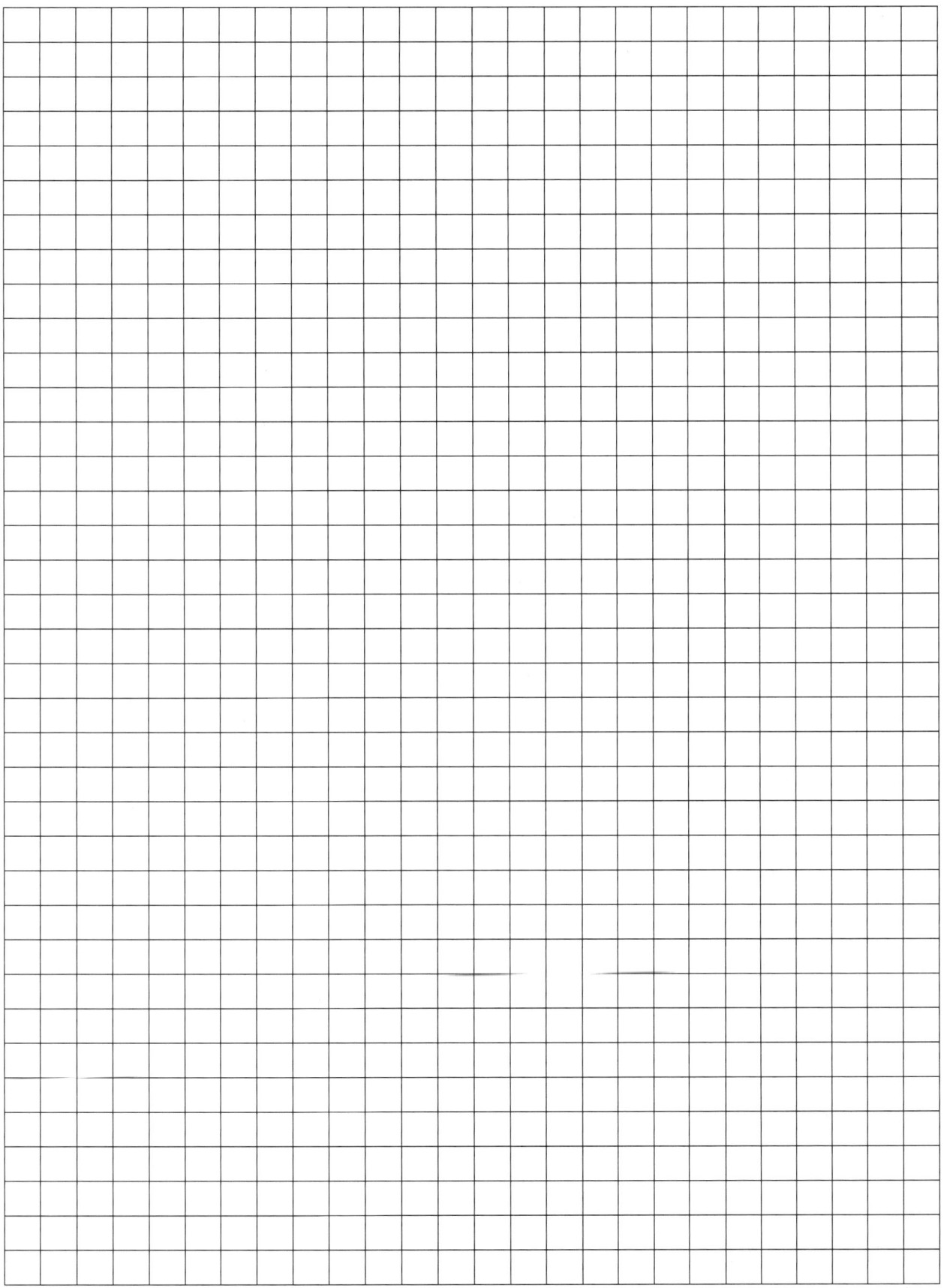

MEASUREMENTS FOR PERMANENT MANDIBULAR CENTRAL INCISOR	
Cervico-incisal Length of Crown	9.0
Length of Root	12.5
Mesiodistal Diameter of Crown	5.0
Mesiodistal Diameter of CEJ	3.5
Labiolingual Diameter	6.0
Labiolingual Diameter of CEJ	5.3
Curvature of CEJ at Mesial	3.0
Curvature of CEJ at Distal	2.0

CHECKLIST FOR PERMANENT MANDIBULAR CENTRAL INCISOR	
Features Noted	Features Present
Crown Features	
Incisal ridge, incisal angles, cingulum, marginal ridges, lingual fossa	
Symmetrical with small centered cingulum and less pronounced marginal ridges and less deep lingual fossa	
Sharper mesio-incisal angle and rounder disto-incisal angle with more pronounced mesial CEJ curvature	
Height of contour in cervical third	
Mesial contact at incisal third	
Distal contact at incisal third	
Root Features	
Single root	
Root longer than crown and deeper proximal root concavities	

Name _____   Tooth Number/Name _____
Date _____   Instructor Rating _____

DRAWING EVALUATION CHECKLIST

RATING SCALE

Completely Correct = 2 points   Major Error = 0 points
Minor Error = 1 point   Note = NA (Not Applicable)

SELF-EVALUATION RATING

Five Views	Clearly Drawn	Accurate Sizing	General Features Included	Specific Features Included
1. Facial View				
2. Lingual View				
3. Mesial View				
4. Distal View				
5. Incisal View				

Self-Evaluation Rating $= \dfrac{\text{Points received}}{\text{Points possible}} =$ _____ $=$ _____ %

INSTRUCTOR EVALUATION RATING

Five Views	Clearly Drawn	Accurate Sizing	General Features Included	Specific Features Included
1. Facial View				
2. Lingual View				
3. Mesial View				
4. Distal View				
5. Incisal View				

Instructor Evaluation Rating $= \dfrac{\text{Points received}}{\text{Points possible}} =$ _____ $=$ _____ %

Copyright © 2026 by Elsevier Inc. All rights are reserved, including those for text and data mining, AI training, and similar technologies.

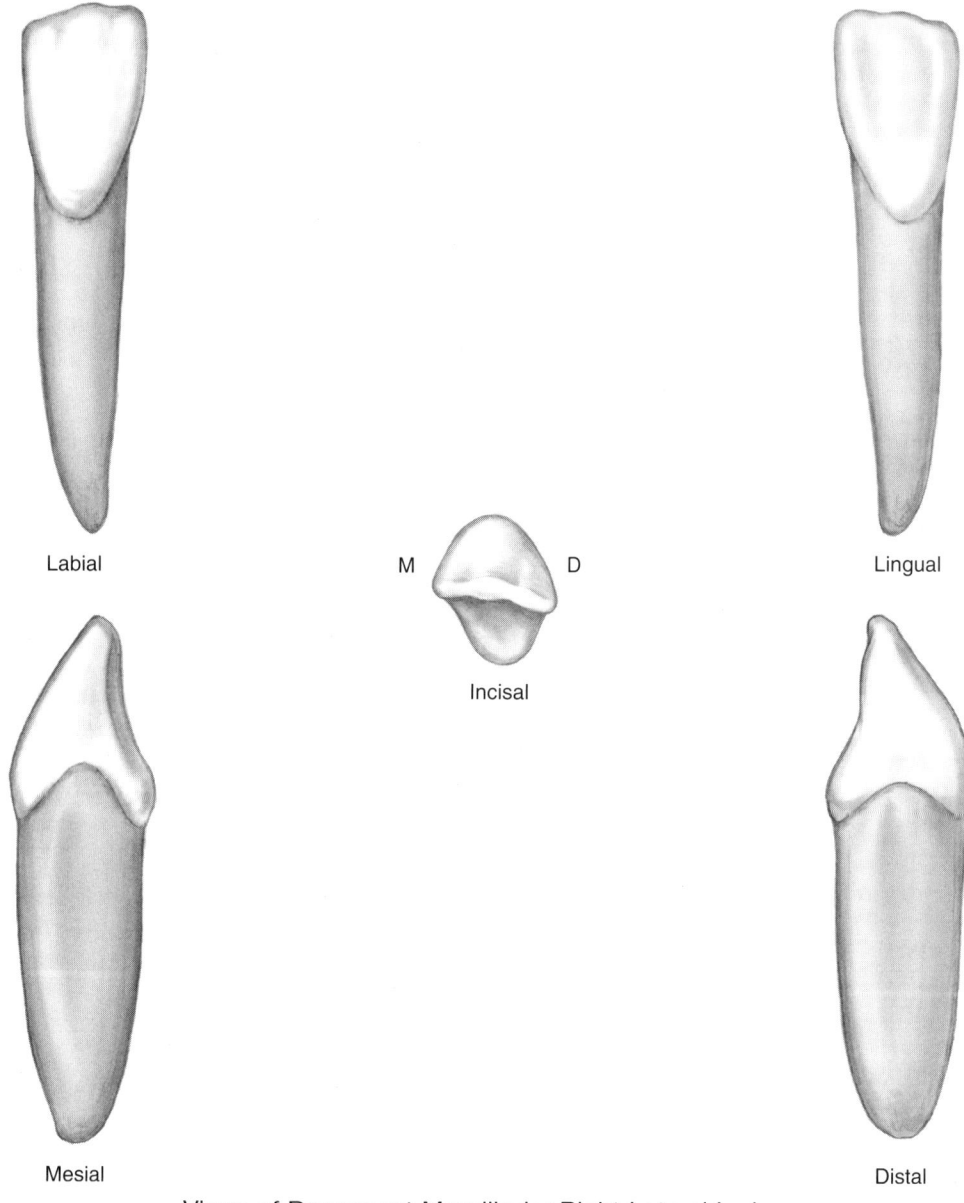

Views of Permanent Mandibular Right Lateral Incisor

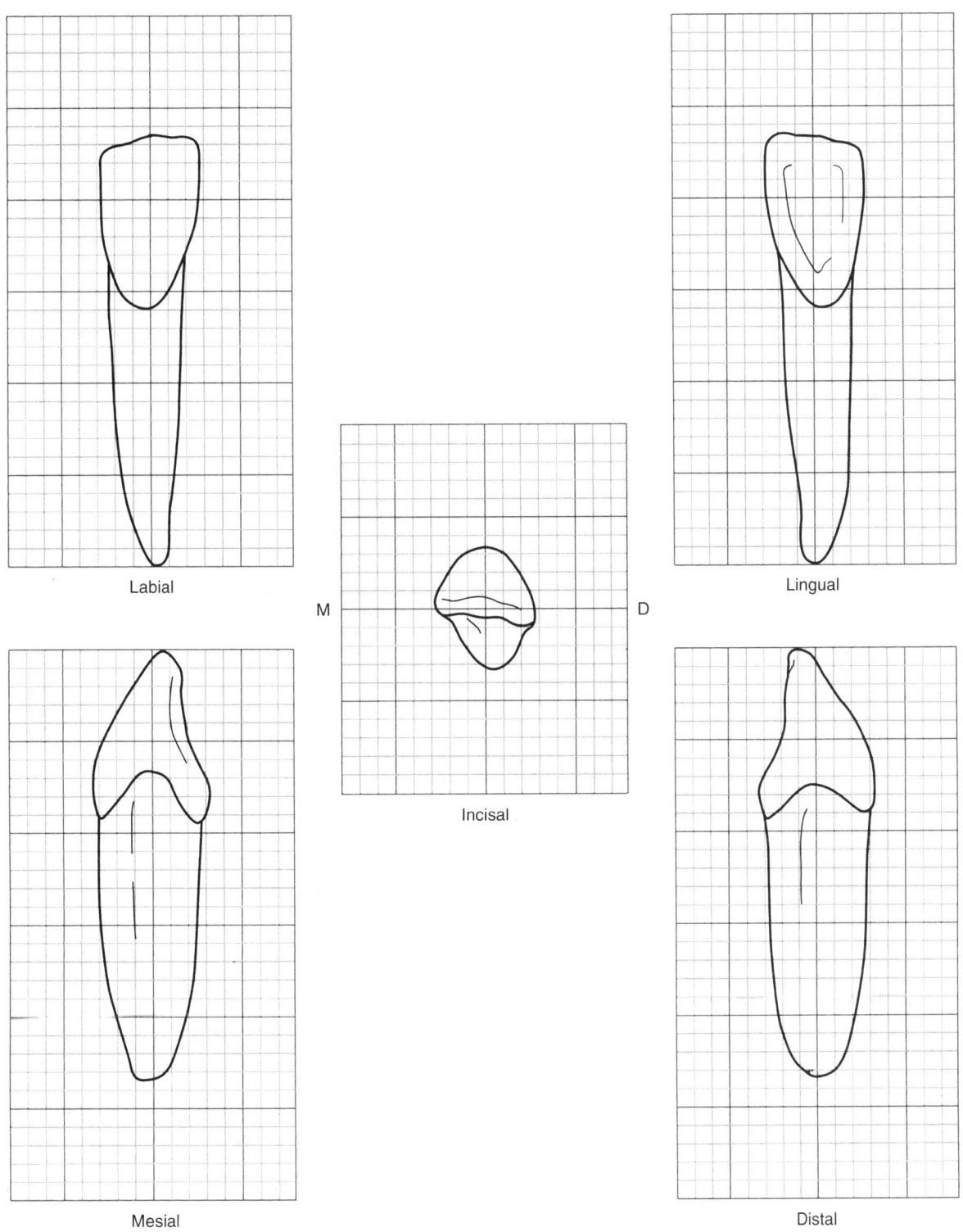

Outline Views of Permanent Mandibular Right Lateral Incisor

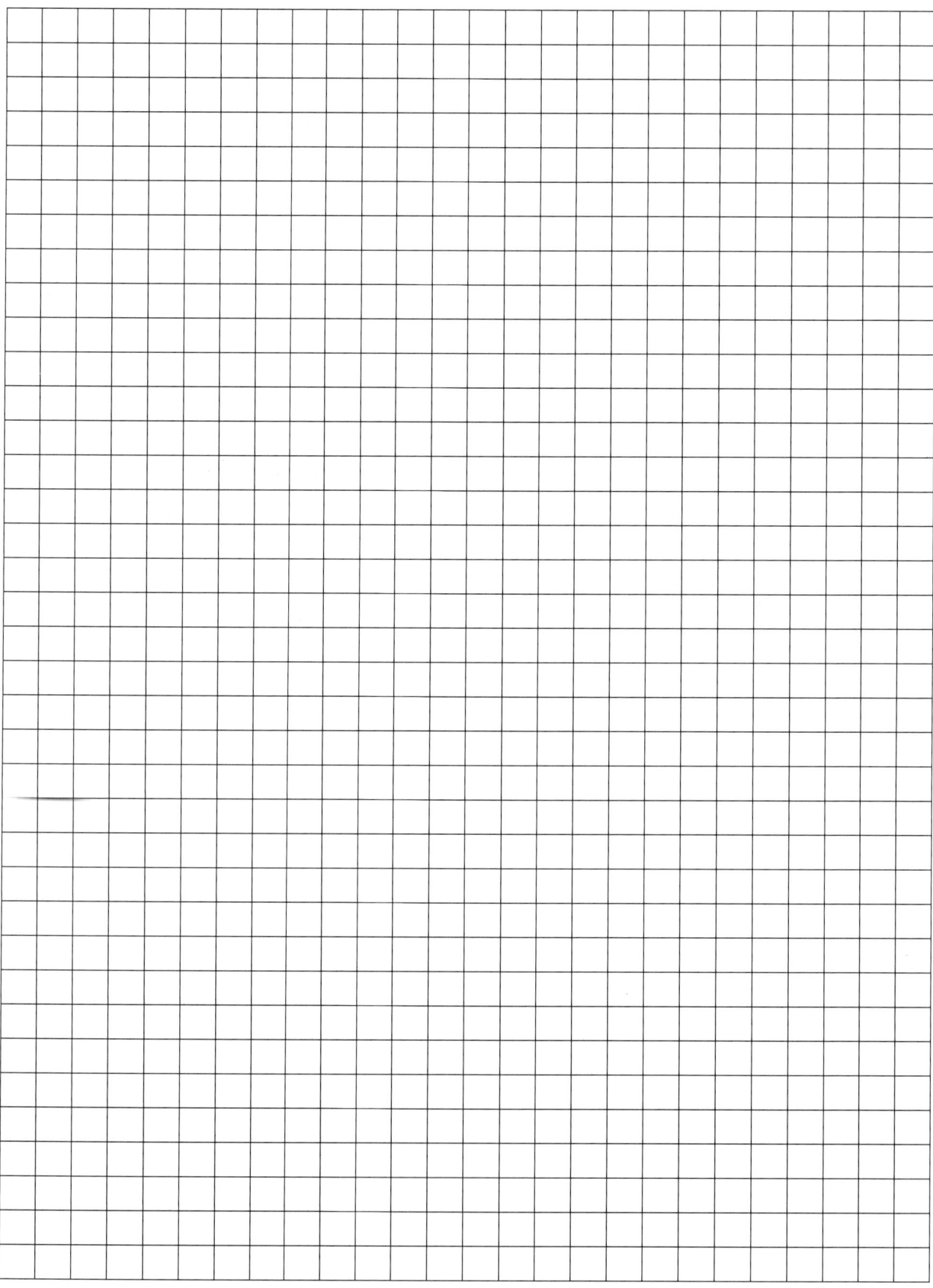

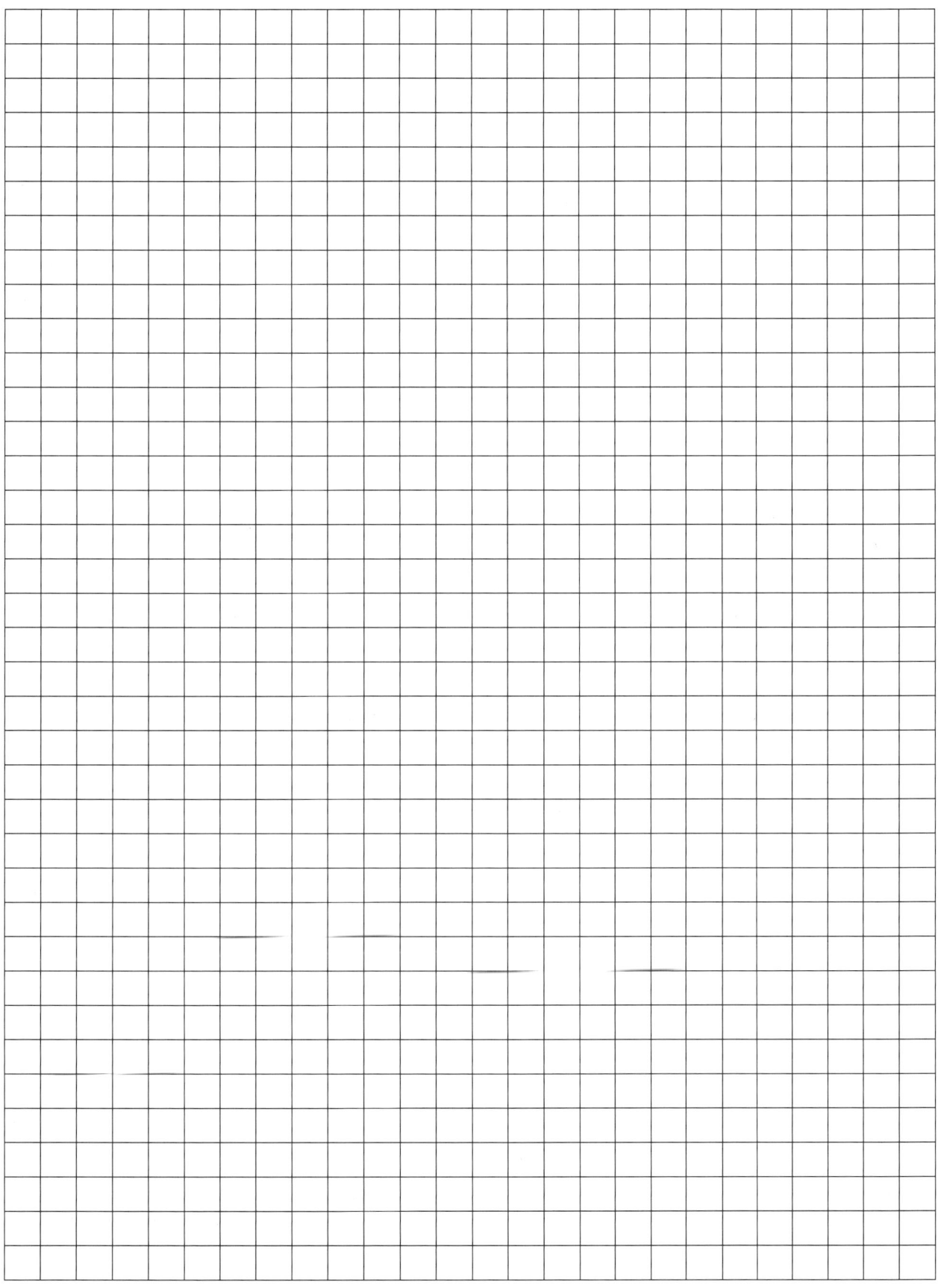

MEASUREMENTS FOR PERMANENT MANDIBULAR LATERAL INCISOR	
Cervico-Incisal Length of Crown	9.5
Length of Root	14.0
Mesiodistal Diameter of Crown	5.5
Mesiodistal Diameter of CEJ	4.0
Labiolingual Diameter	6.5
Labiolingual Diameter of CEJ	5.8
Curvature of CEJ at Mesial	3.0
Curvature of CEJ at Distal	2.0

CHECKLIST FOR PERMANENT MANDIBULAR LATERAL INCISOR	
Features Noted	Features Present
Crown Features	
Incisal ridge, incisal angles, cingulum, marginal ridges, lingual fossa	
Not symmetrical and appears twisted distally	
Small distally placed cingulum with mesial marginal ridge longer than distal marginal ridge and more pronounced marginal ridges and deeper lingual fossa	
Sharper mesio-incisal angle and rounder disto-incisal angle with more pronounced mesial CEJ curvature	
Height of contour in cervical third	
Mesial contact at incisal third	
Distal contact at incisal third	
Root Features	
Single root	
Root longer than crown and deeper proximal root concavities	

Name _____ Tooth Number/Name _____

Date _____ Instructor Rating _____

DRAWING EVALUATION CHECKLIST

RATING SCALE

Completely Correct = 2 points Major Error = 0 points
Minor Error = 1 point Note = NA (Not Applicable)

SELF-EVALUATION RATING

Five Views	Clearly Drawn	Accurate Sizing	General Features Included	Specific Features Included
1. Facial View				
2. Lingual View				
3. Mesial View				
4. Distal View				
5. Incisal View				

Self-Evaluation Rating = $\dfrac{\text{Points received}}{\text{Points possible}}$ = _____ = _____ %

INSTRUCTOR EVALUATION RATING

Five Views	Clearly Drawn	Accurate Sizing	General Features Included	Specific Features Included
1. Facial View				
2. Lingual View				
3. Mesial View				
4. Distal View				
5. Incisal View				

Instructor Evaluation Rating = $\dfrac{\text{Points received}}{\text{Points possible}}$ = _____ = _____ %

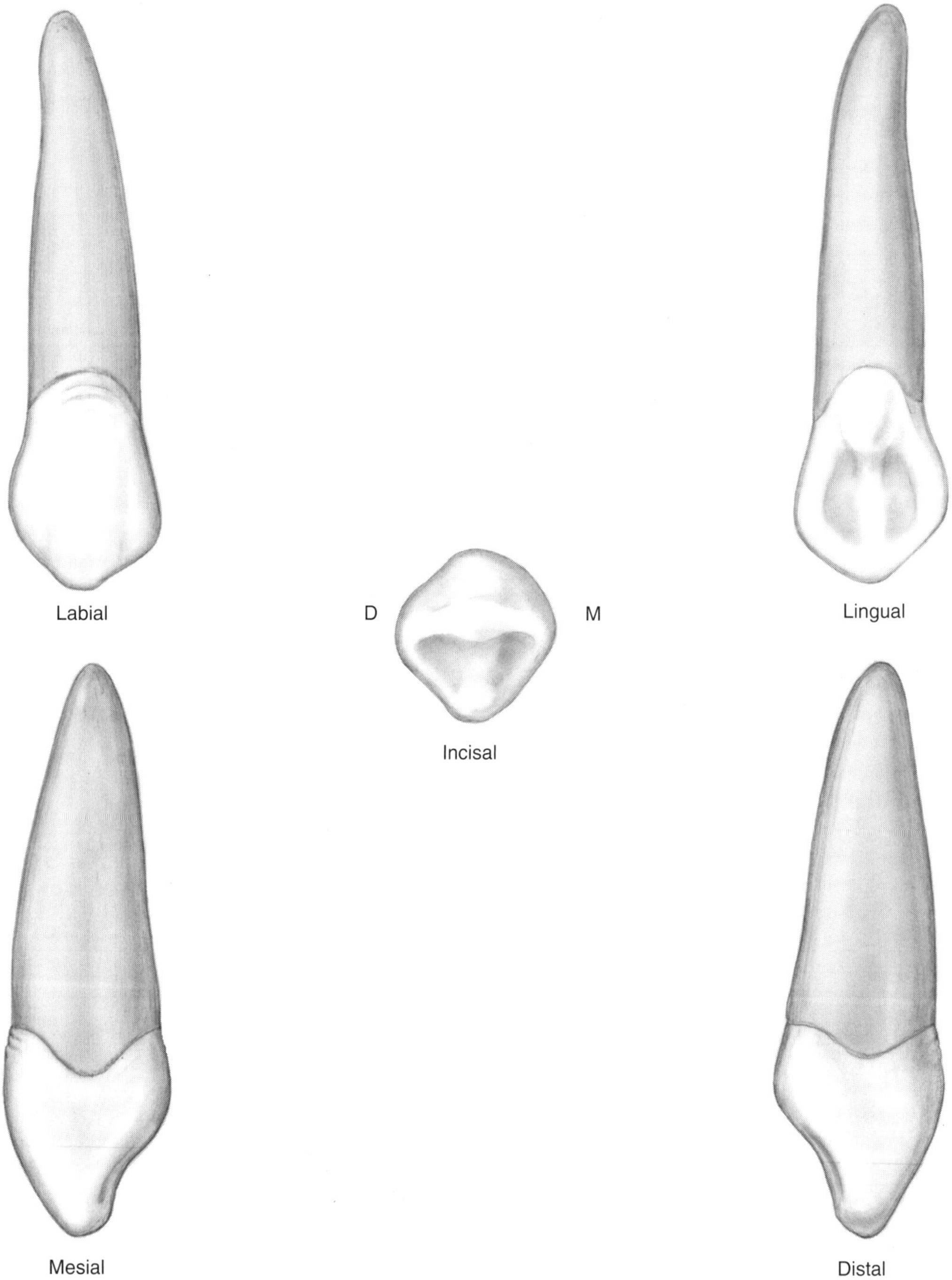

146 TOOTH DRAWING EXERCISES

Labial

D M

Incisal

Lingual

Mesial

Distal

Views of Permanent Maxillary Right Canine

TOOTH DRAWING EXERCISES 147

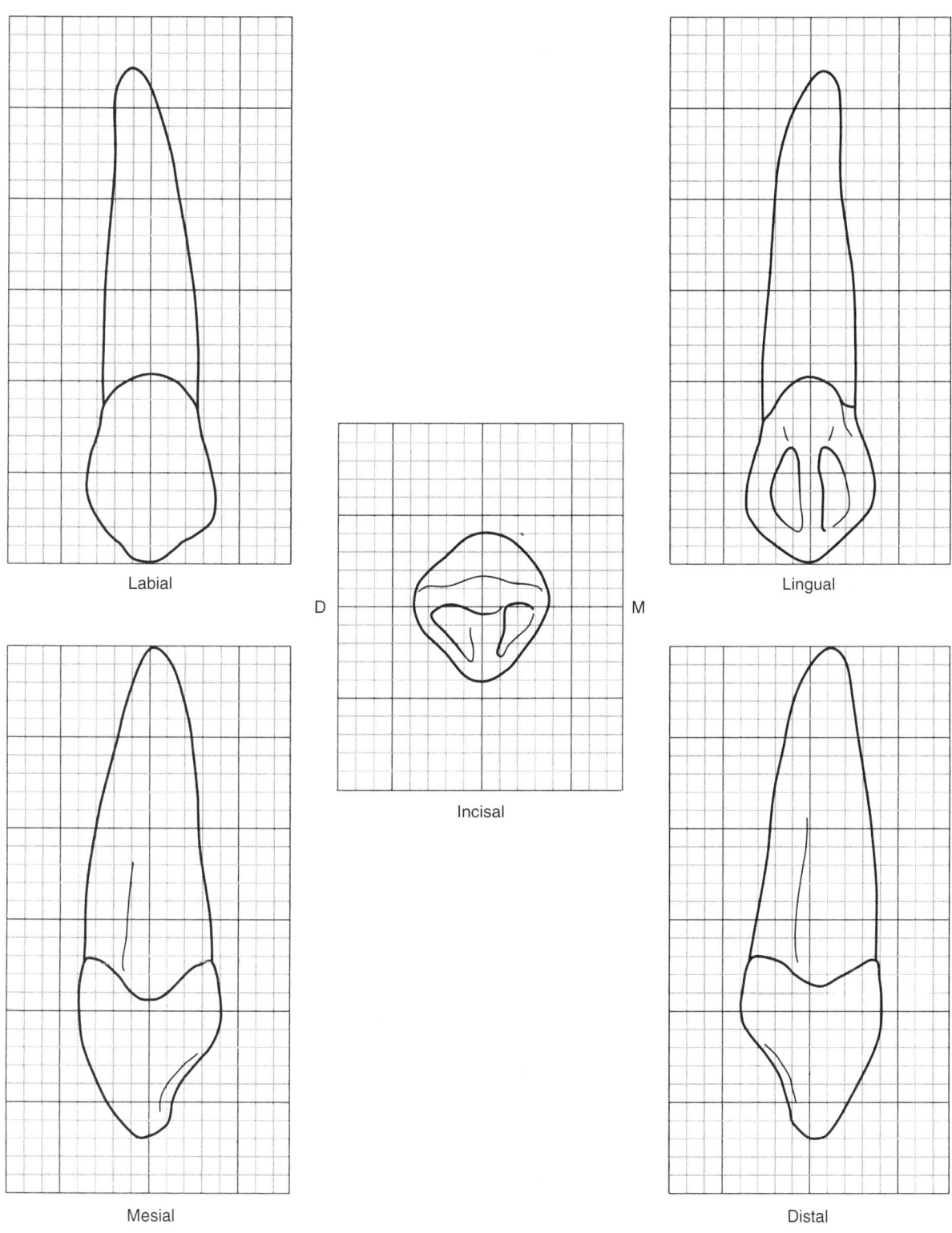

Outline Views of Permanent Maxillary Right Canine

Copyright © 2026 by Elsevier Inc. All rights are reserved, including those for text and data mining,
AI training, and similar technologies.

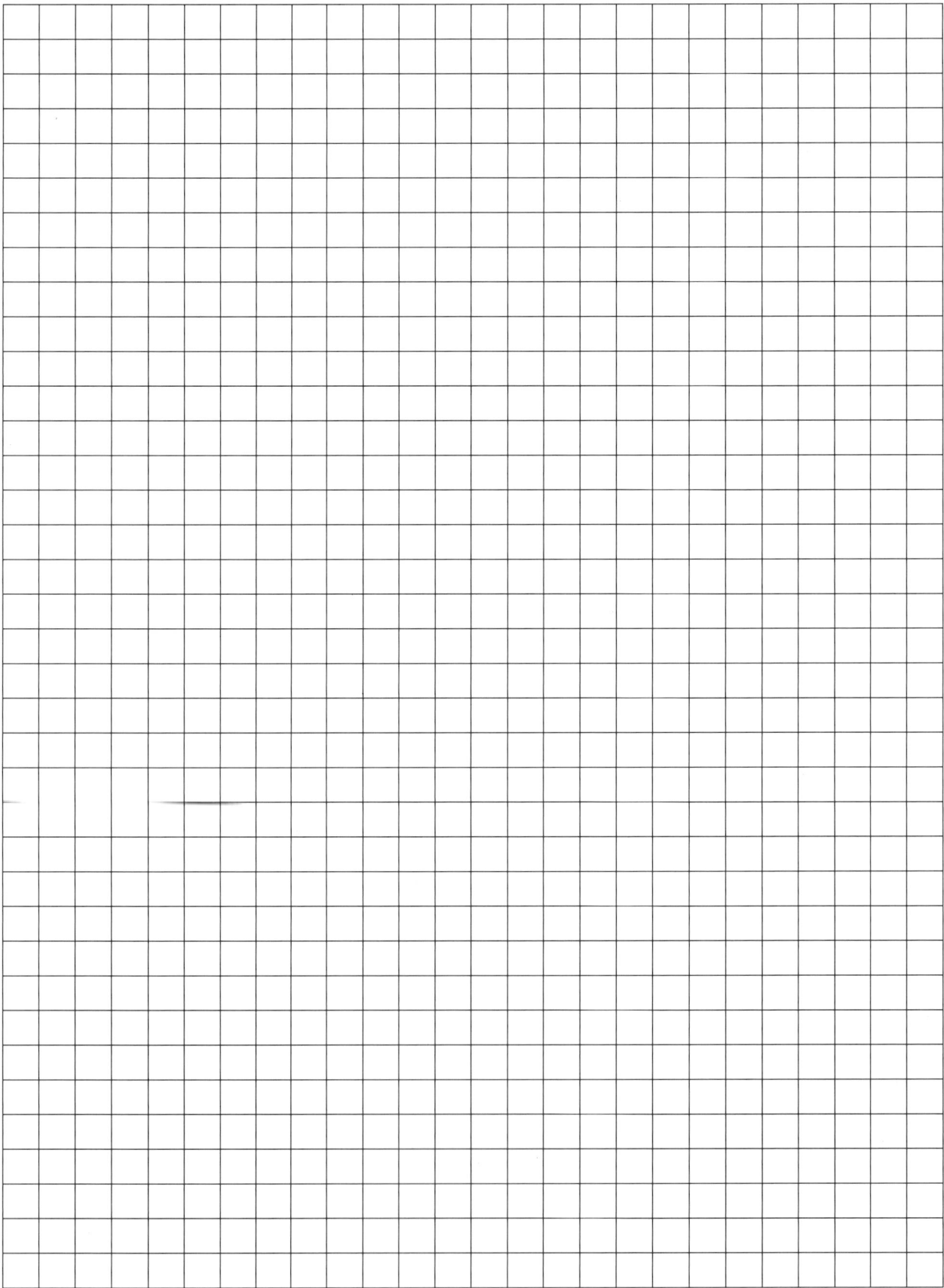

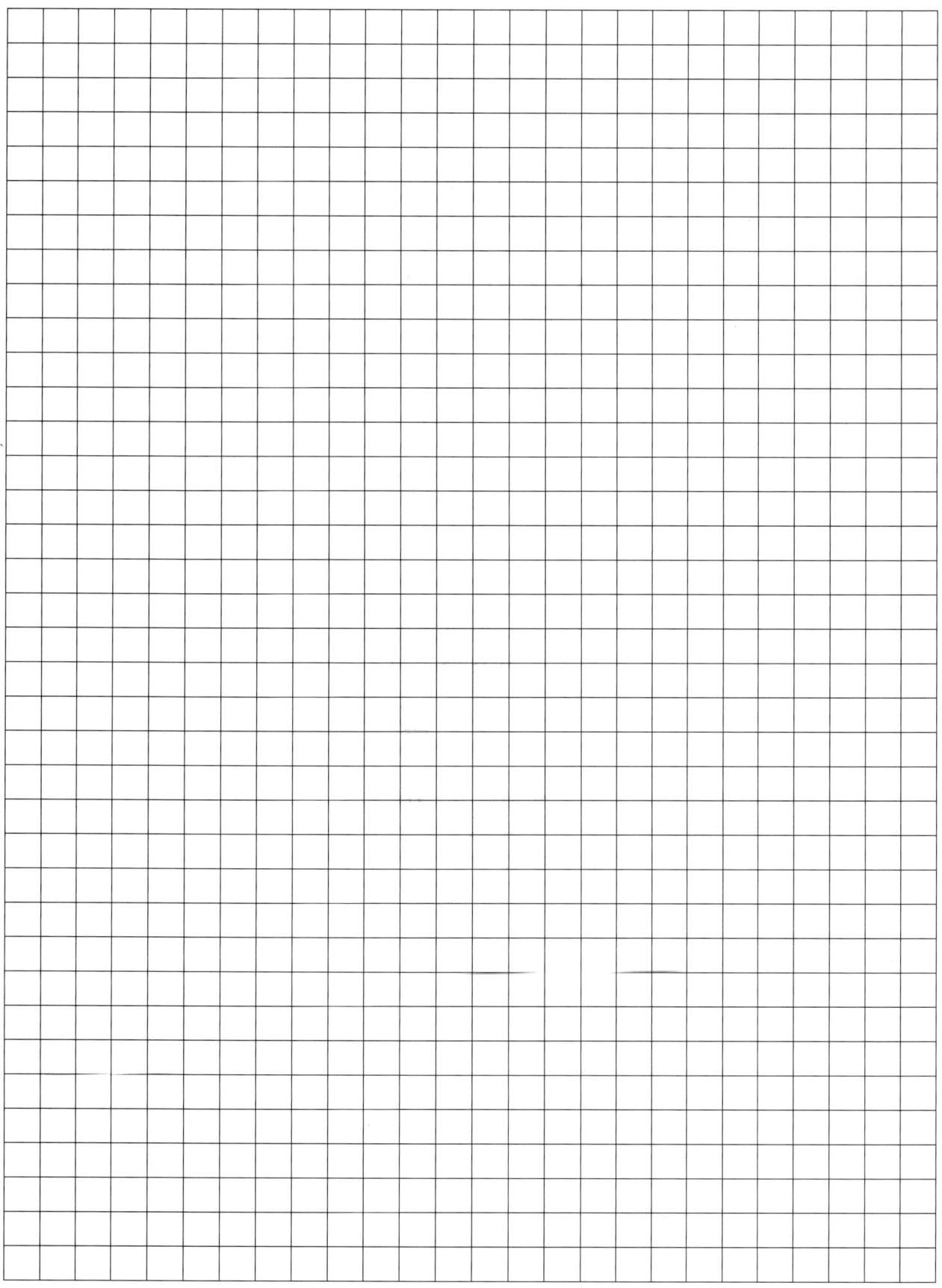

MEASUREMENTS FOR PERMANENT MAXILLARY CANINE	
Cervico-incisal Length of Crown	10.0
Length of Root	17.0
Mesiodistal Diameter of Crown	7.5
Mesiodistal Diameter of CEJ	5.5
Labiolingual Diameter	8.0
Labiolingual Diameter of CEJ	7.0
Curvature of CEJ at Mesial	2.5
Curvature of CEJ at Distal	1.5

CHECKLIST FOR PERMANENT MAXILLARY CANINE	
Features Noted	Features Present
Crown Features	
Single cusp with tip, slopes, labial ridge, cingulum, lingual ridge, marginal ridges, lingual fossae	
More pronounced lingual surface with sharp cusp tip	
Shorter mesial cusp slope with more pronounced mesial CEJ curvature	
More cervical contact on distal with shorter distal outline than mesial on labial with depression between distal contact and CEJ	
Height of contour for labial in cervical third and for lingual in middle third	
Mesial contact at junction of incisal third and middle thirds	
Distal contact at middle third	
Root Features	
Long thick single root	
Proximal root concavities and blunt root apex	

Name _____   Tooth Number/Name _____

Date _____   Instructor Rating _____

DRAWING EVALUATION CHECKLIST

RATING SCALE

Completely Correct = 2 points   Major Error = 0 points
Minor Error = 1 point   Note = NA (Not Applicable)

SELF-EVALUATION RATING

Five Views	Clearly Drawn	Accurate Sizing	General Features Included	Specific Features Included
1. Facial View				
2. Lingual View				
3. Mesial View				
4. Distal View				
5. Incisal View				

Self-Evaluation Rating = $\dfrac{\text{Points received}}{\text{Points possible}}$ = _____ = _____ %

INSTRUCTOR EVALUATION RATING

Five Views	Clearly Drawn	Accurate Sizing	General Features Included	Specific Features Included
1. Facial View				
2. Lingual View				
3. Mesial View				
4. Distal View				
5. Incisal View				

Instructor Evaluation Rating = $\dfrac{\text{Points received}}{\text{Points possible}}$ = _____ = _____ %

Copyright © 2026 by Elsevier Inc. All rights are reserved, including those for text and data mining, AI training, and similar technologies.

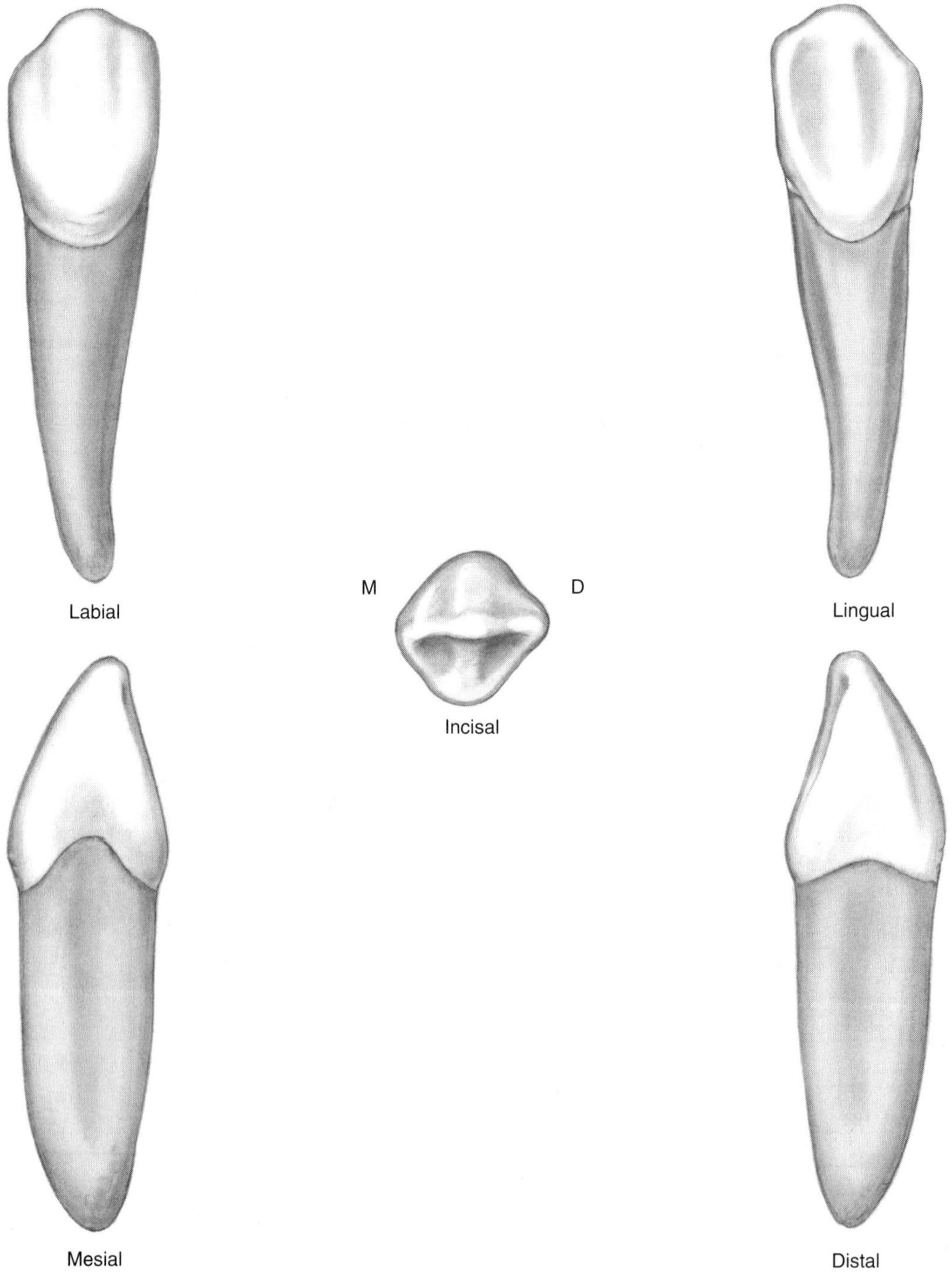

Labial

M D

Incisal

Lingual

Mesial

Distal

Views of Permanent Mandibular Right Canine

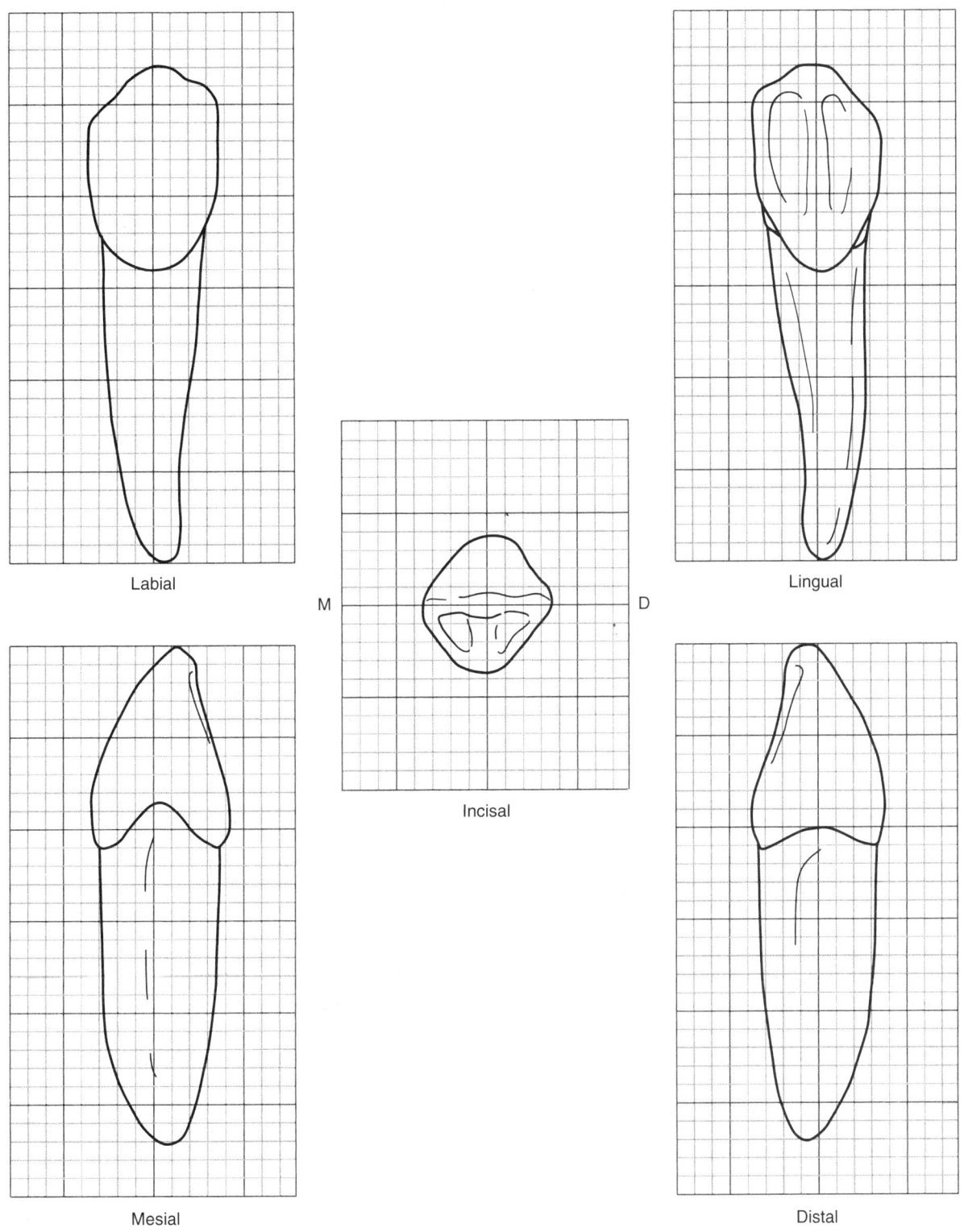

Outline Views of Permanent Mandibular Right Canine

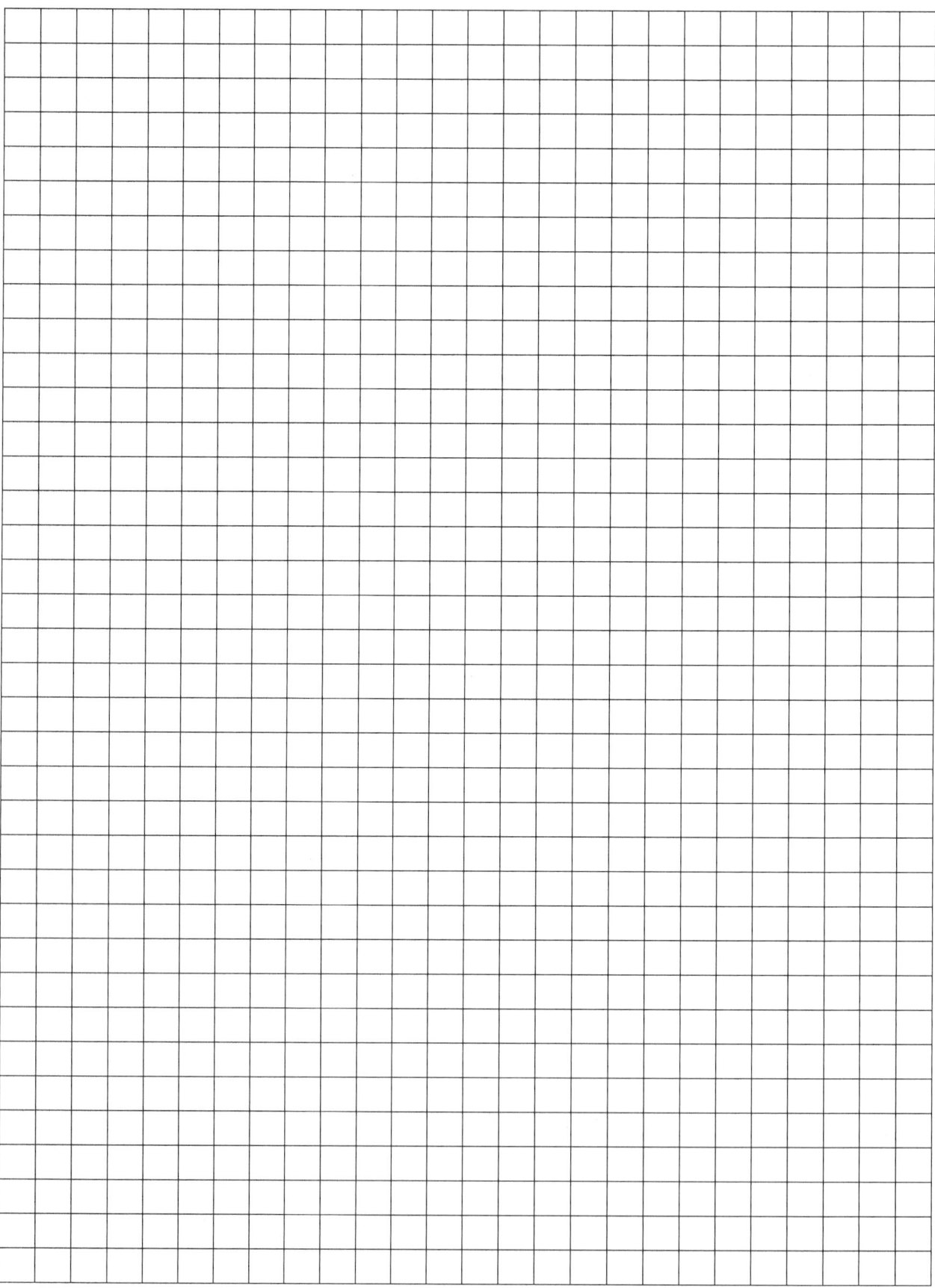

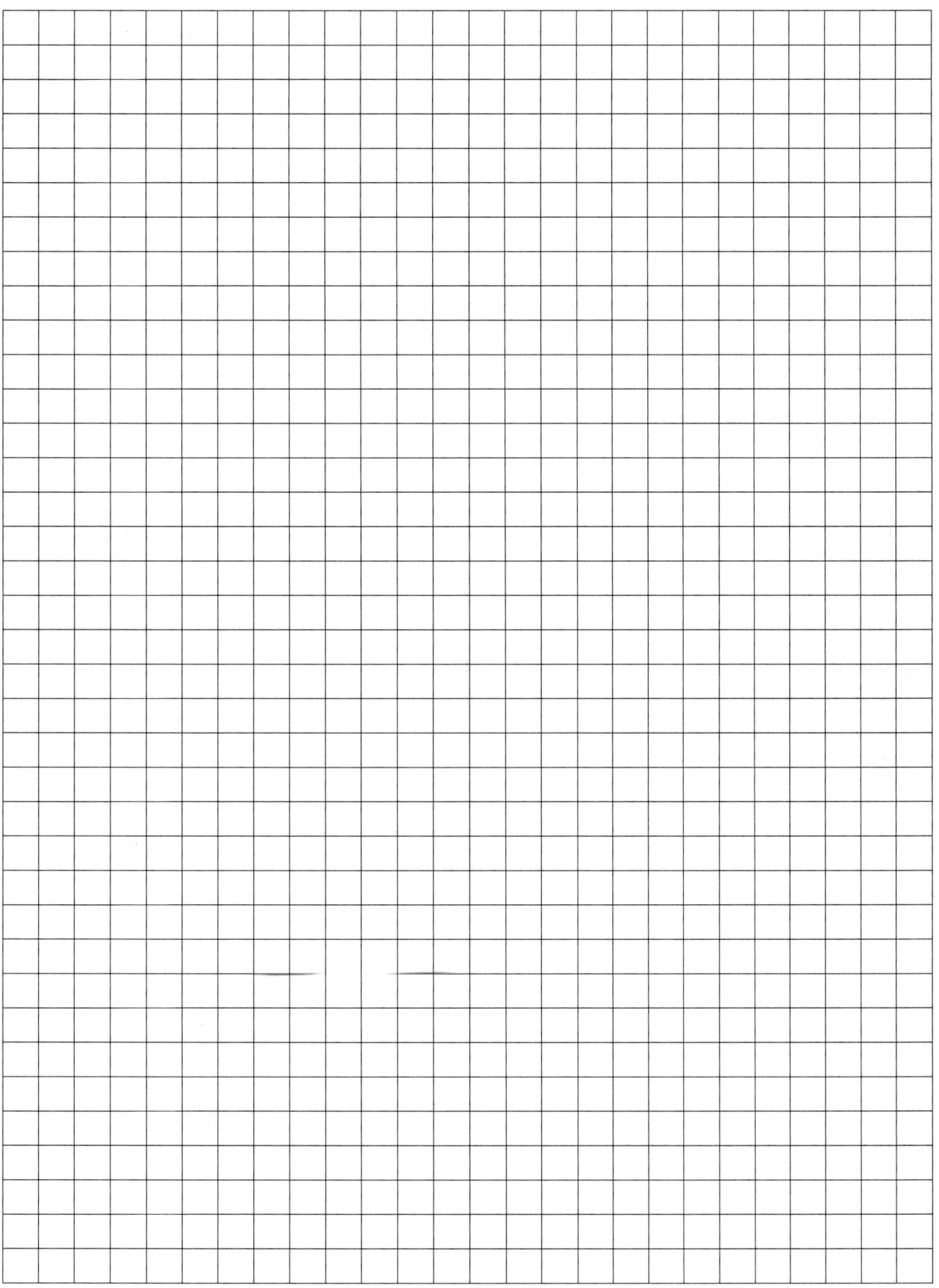

MEASUREMENTS FOR PERMANENT MANDIBULAR CANINE	
Cervico-incisal Length of Crown	11.0
Length of Root	16.0
Mesiodistal Diameter of Crown	7.0
Mesiodistal Diameter of CEJ	5.5
Labiolingual Diameter	7.5
Labiolingual Diameter of CEJ	7.0
Curvature of CEJ at Mesial	2.5
Curvature of CEJ at Distal	1.0

CHECKLIST FOR PERMANENT MANDIBULAR CANINE	
Features Noted	**Features Present**
Crown Features	
Single cusp with tip, slopes, labial ridge, cingulum, lingual ridge, marginal ridges, lingual fossae	
Less pronounced lingual surface with less sharp cusp tip	
Shorter mesial cusp slope with more pronounced mesial CEJ curvature	
More cervical contact on distal with shorter and rounder distal outline than mesial on labial with shorter mesial slope than distal	
Height of contour for labial in cervical third and for lingual in middle third	
Mesial contact at incisal third	
Distal contact at junction of incisal and middle thirds	
Root Features	
Long thick single root	
Proximal root concavities with developmental depressions on mesial and distal and pointed apex	

Name _____   Tooth Number/Name _____
Date _____   Instructor Rating _____

DRAWING EVALUATION CHECKLIST

RATING SCALE

Completely Correct = 2 points   Major Error = 0 points
Minor Error = 1 point   Note = NA (Not Applicable)

SELF-EVALUATION RATING

Five Views	Clearly Drawn	Accurate Sizing	General Features Included	Specific Features Included
1. Facial View				
2. Lingual View				
3. Mesial View				
4. Distal View				
5. Incisal View				

$$\text{Self-Evaluation Rating} = \frac{\text{Points received}}{\text{Points possible}} = \underline{\hspace{2cm}} = \underline{\hspace{2cm}}\%$$

INSTRUCTOR EVALUATION RATING

Five Views	Clearly Drawn	Accurate Sizing	General Features Included	Specific Features Included
1. Facial View				
2. Lingual View				
3. Mesial View				
4. Distal View				
5. Incisal/View				

$$\text{Instructor Evaluation Rating} = \frac{\text{Points received}}{\text{Points possible}} = \underline{\hspace{2cm}} = \underline{\hspace{2cm}}\%$$

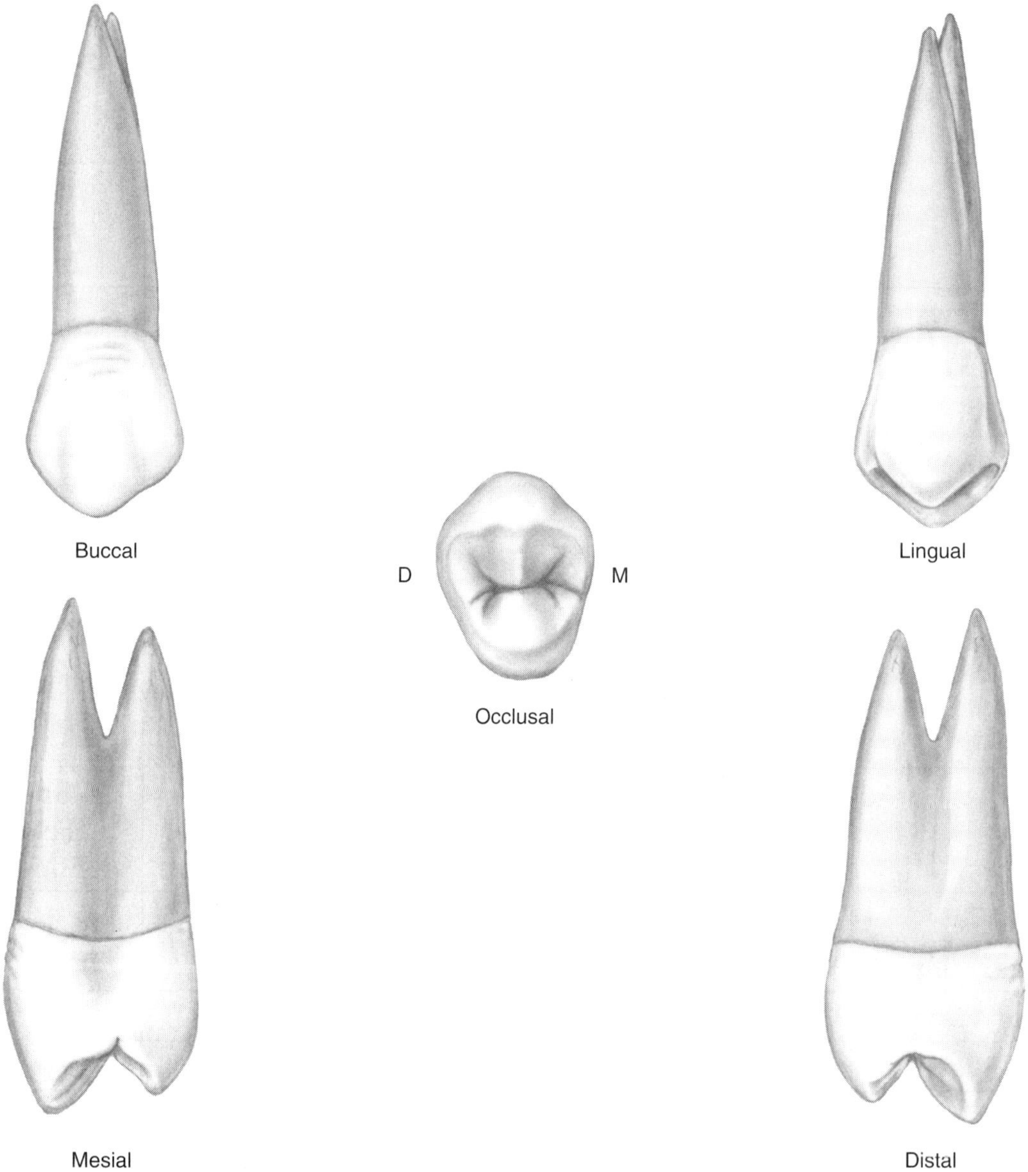

Buccal
D M
Occlusal
Lingual
Mesial
Distal

Views of Permanent Maxillary Right First Premolar

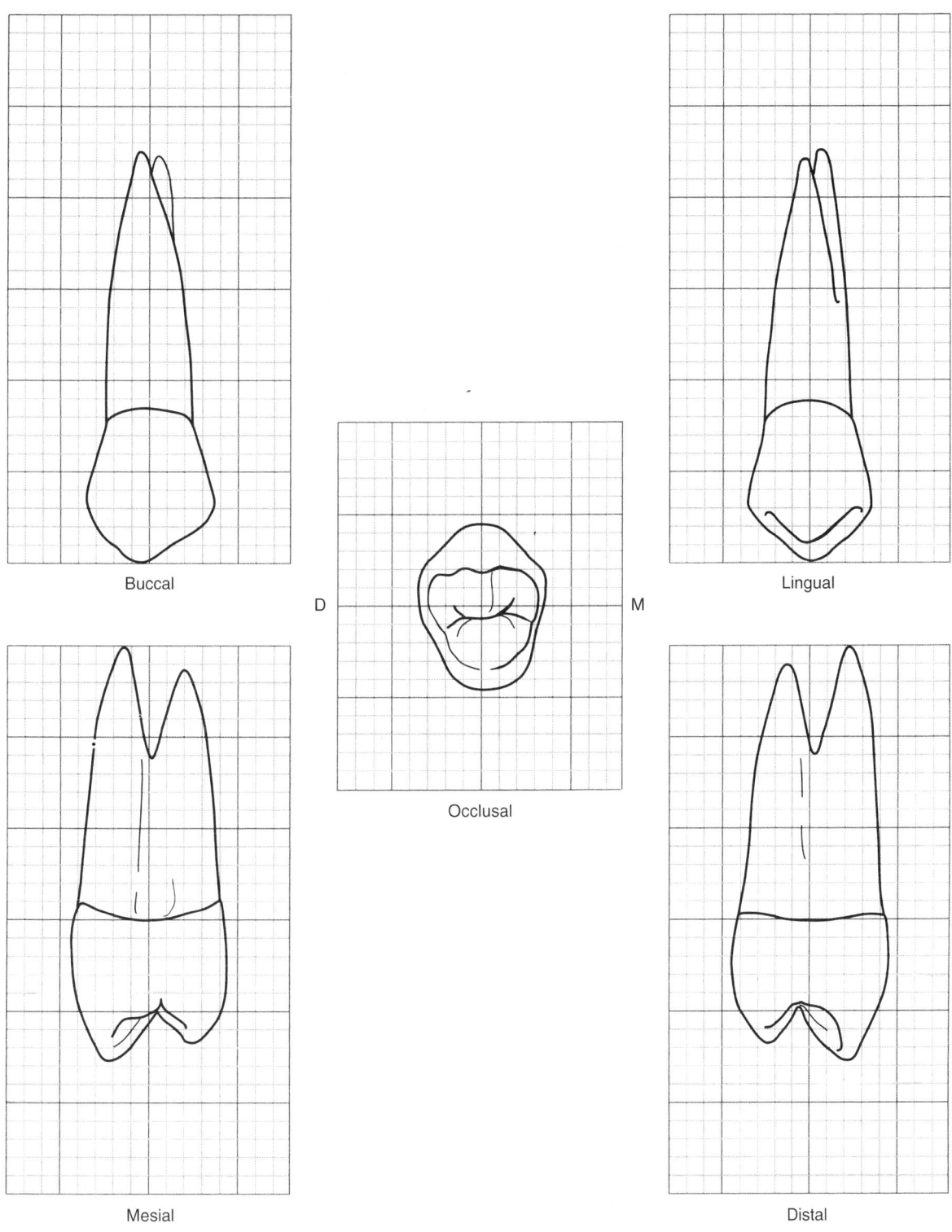

Outline Views of Permanent Maxillary Right First Premolar

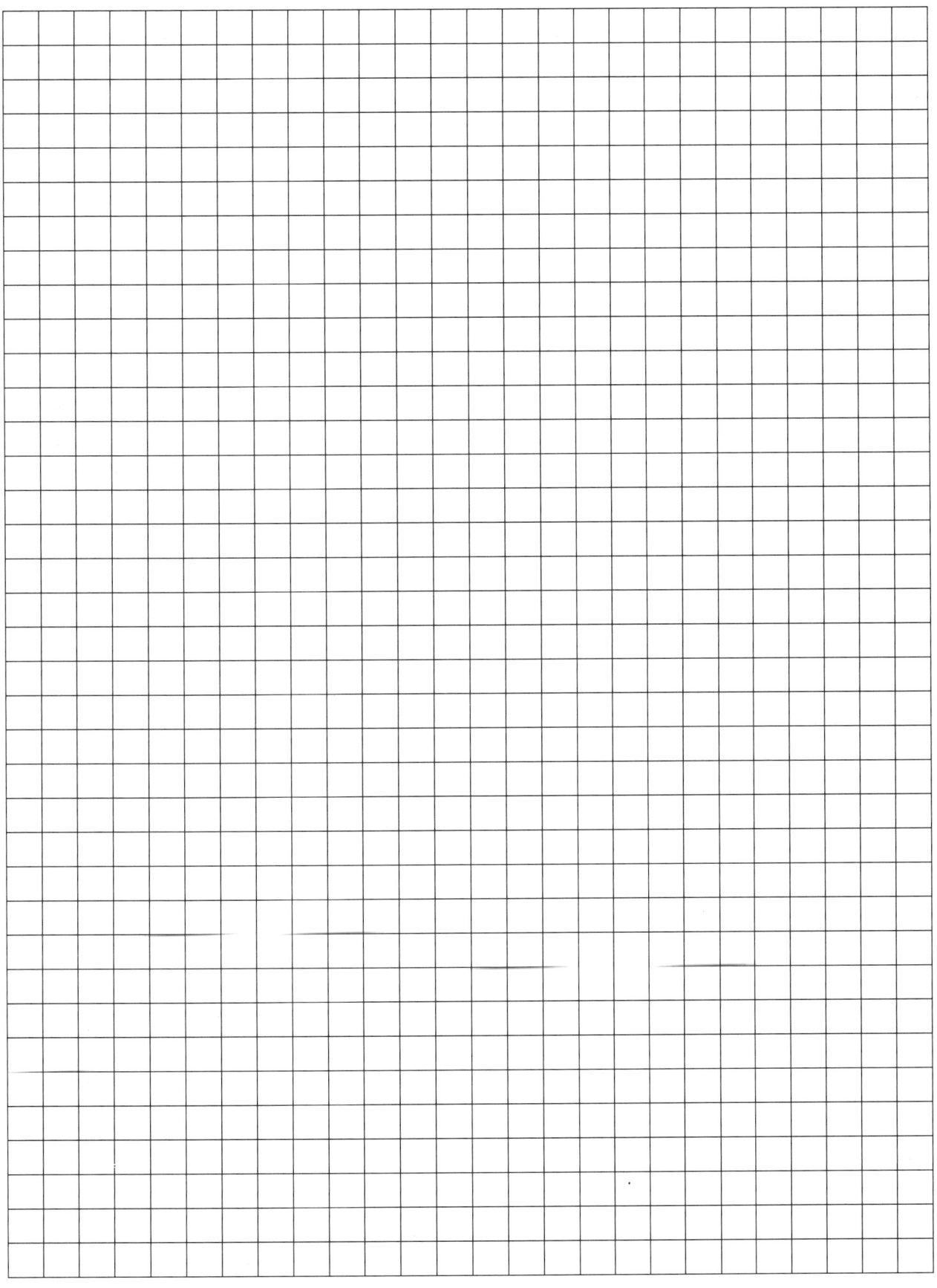

MEASUREMENTS FOR PERMANENT MAXILLARY FIRST PREMOLAR	
Cervico-occlusal Length of Crown	8.5
Length of Root	14.0
Mesiodistal Diameter of Crown	7.0
Mesiodistal Diameter of CEJ	5.0
Buccolingual Diameter	9.0
Buccolingual Diameter of CEJ	8.0
Curvature of CEJ at Mesial	1.0
Curvature of CEJ at Distal	0.0

CHECKLIST FOR PERMANENT MAXILLARY FIRST PREMOLAR	
Features Noted	Features Present
Crown Features	
Occlusal table with marginal ridges and cusps with tips, ridges, inclined planes, grooves, fossae, pits	
Buccal cusp longer of two cusps with long central groove	
Longer mesial cusp slope than distal cusp slope and with distinct mesial features: deeper CEJ curvature, marginal groove, developmental depression	
Buccal ridge	
Mesial and distal contact just cervical to junction of occlusal and middle thirds with height of contour for buccal in cervical third and lingual in middle third	
Root Features	
Two roots with root trunk	
Proximal root concavities with especially deep mesial root concavity	

Name _____   Tooth Number/Name _____
Date _____   Instructor Rating _____

DRAWING EVALUATION CHECKLIST

RATING SCALE

Completely Correct = 2 points   Major Error = 0 points
Minor Error = 1 point   Note = NA (Not Applicable)

SELF-EVALUATION RATING

Five Views	Clearly Drawn	Accurate Sizing	General Features Included	Specific Features Included
1. Facial View				
2. Lingual View				
3. Mesial View				
4. Distal View				
5. Occlusal View				

Self-Evaluation Rating = $\dfrac{\text{Points received}}{\text{Points possible}}$ = _____ = _____ %

INSTRUCTOR EVALUATION RATING

Five Views	Clearly Drawn	Accurate Sizing	General Features Included	Specific Features Included
1. Facial View				
2. Lingual View				
3. Mesial View				
4. Distal View				
5. Occlusal View				

Instructor Evaluation Rating = $\dfrac{\text{Points received}}{\text{Points possible}}$ = _____ = _____ %

Copyright © 2026 by Elsevier Inc. All rights are reserved, including those for text and data mining, AI training, and similar technologies.

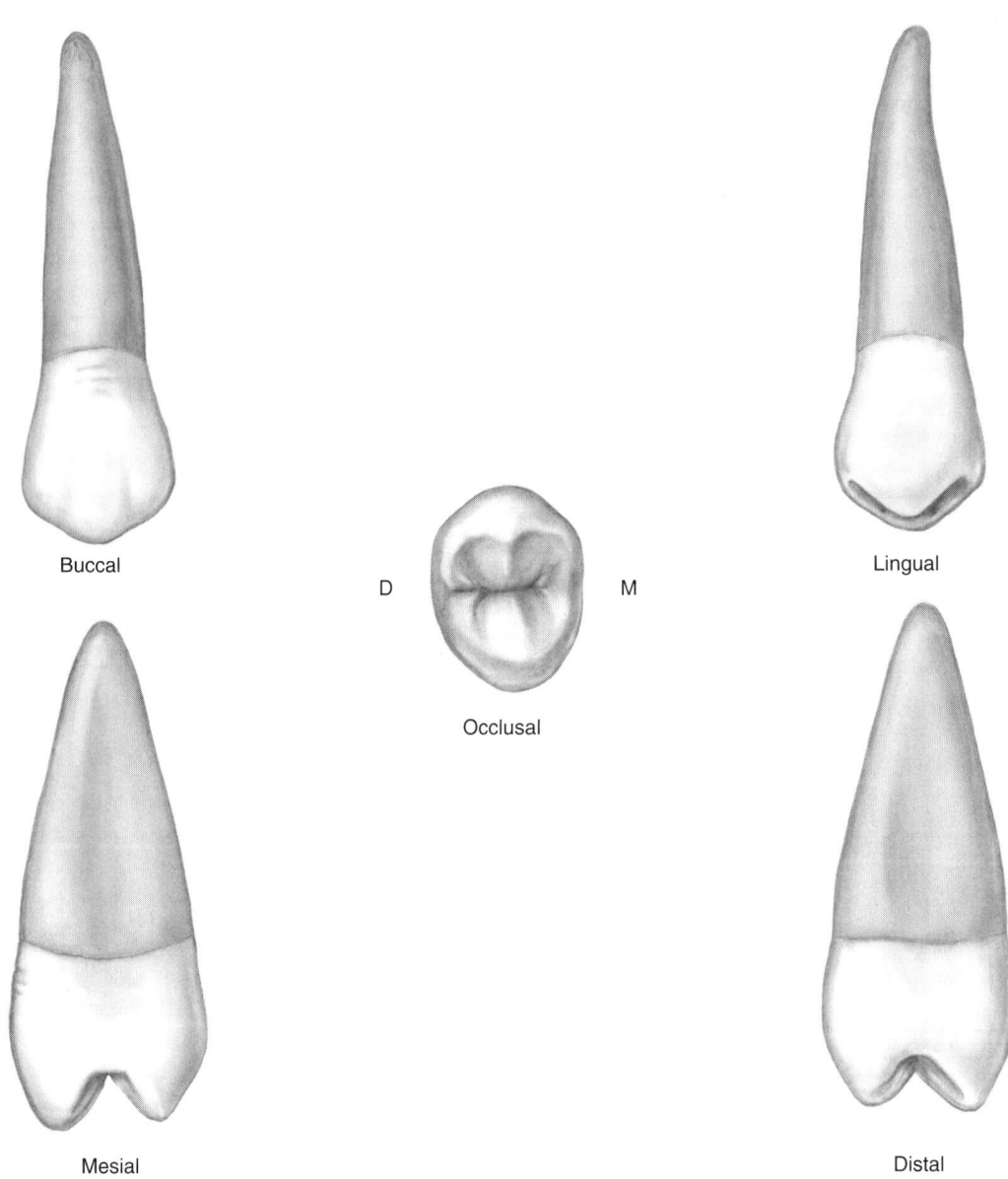

Views of Permanent Maxillary Right Second Premolar

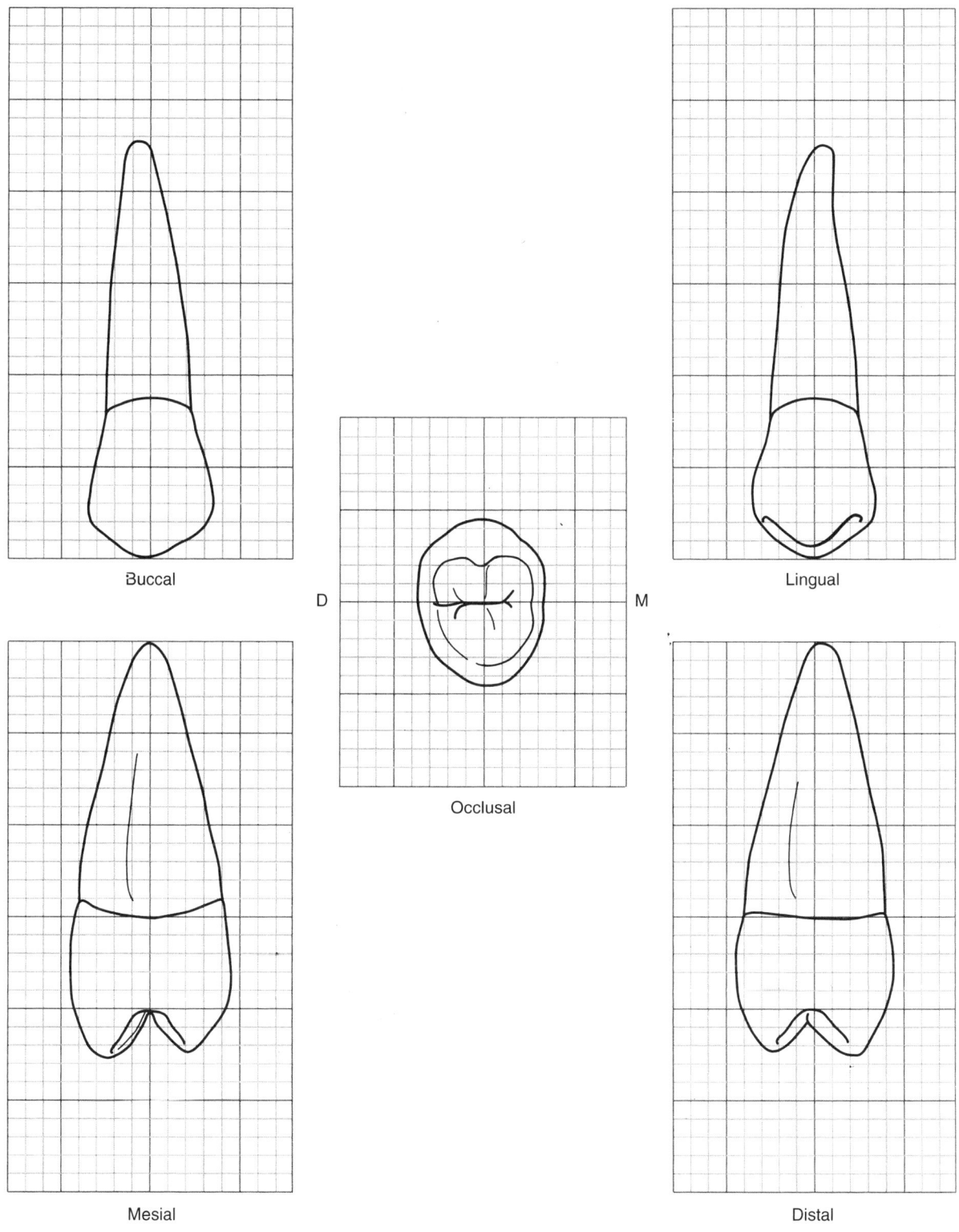

Outline Views of Permanent Maxillary Right Second Premolar

TOOTH DRAWING EXERCISES

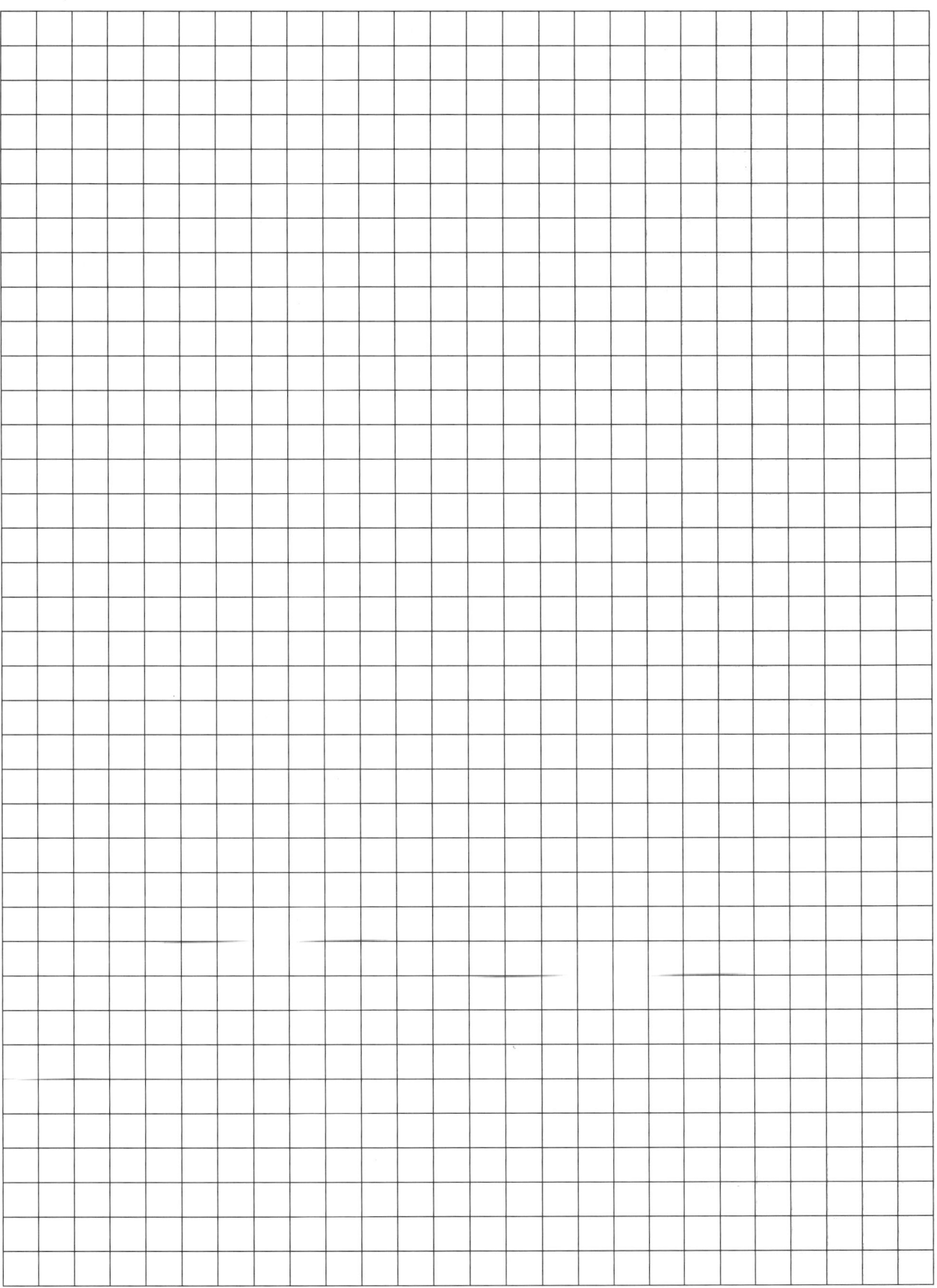

MEASUREMENTS FOR PERMANENT MAXILLARY SECOND PREMOLAR

Cervico-occlusal Length of Crown	8.5
Length of Root	14.0
Mesiodistal Diameter of Crown	7.0
Mesiodistal Diameter of CEJ	5.0
Buccolingual Diameter	9.0
Buccolingual Diameter of CEJ	8.0
Curvature of CEJ at Mesial	1.0
Curvature of CEJ at Distal	0.0

CHECKLIST FOR PERMANENT MAXILLARY SECOND PREMOLAR

Features Noted	Features Present
Crown Features	
Occlusal table with marginal ridges and cusps with tips, ridges, inclined planes, grooves, fossae, pits	
Two cusps same length with short central groove	
Lingual cusp offset to mesial	
Buccal ridge	
Mesial and distal contact just cervical to junction of occlusal and middle thirds with height of contour for buccal in cervical third and lingual in middle third	
Root Features	
Single root	
Proximal root concavities	

Name _____   Tooth Number/Name _____

Date _____   Instructor Rating _____

DRAWING EVALUATION CHECKLIST

RATING SCALE

Completely Correct = 2 points   Major Error = 0 points
Minor Error = 1 point   Note = NA (Not Applicable)

SELF-EVALUATION RATING

Five Views	Clearly Drawn	Accurate Sizing	General Features Included	Specific Features Included
1. Facial View				
2. Lingual View				
3. Mesial View				
4. Distal View				
5. Occlusal View				

Self-Evaluation Rating = $\dfrac{\text{Points received}}{\text{Points possible}}$ = _____ = _____ %

INSTRUCTOR EVALUATION RATING

Five Views	Clearly Drawn	Accurate Sizing	General Features Included	Specific Features Included
1. Facial View				
2. Lingual View				
3. Mesial View				
4. Distal View				
5. Occlusal View				

Instructor Evaluation Rating = $\dfrac{\text{Points received}}{\text{Points possible}}$ = _____ = _____ %

Copyright © 2026 by Elsevier Inc. All rights are reserved, including those for text and data mining, AI training, and similar technologies.

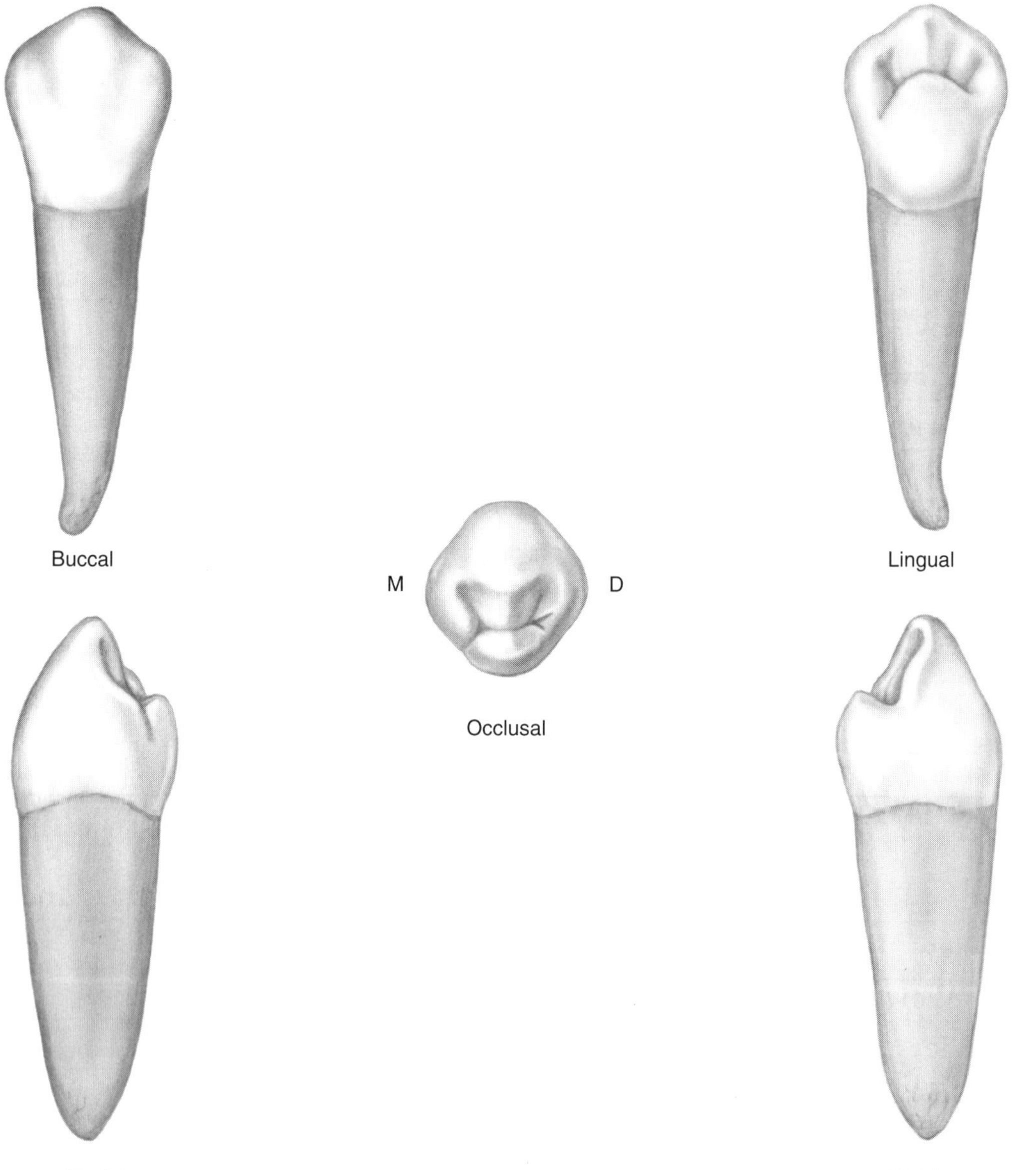

Buccal
Lingual
M   D
Occlusal
Mesial
Distal

Views of Permanent Mandibular Right First Premolar

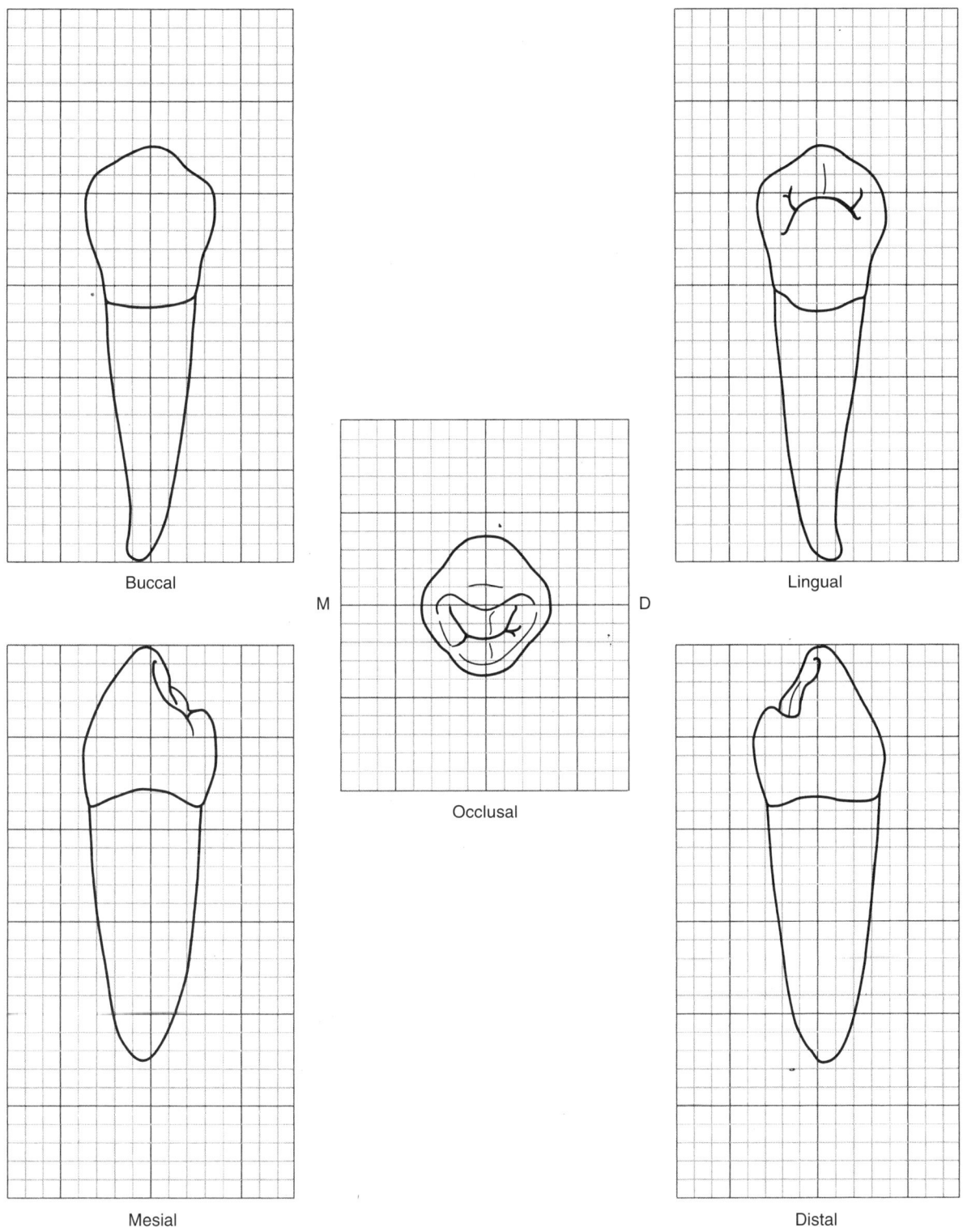

Outline Views of Permanent Maxillary Right First Premolar

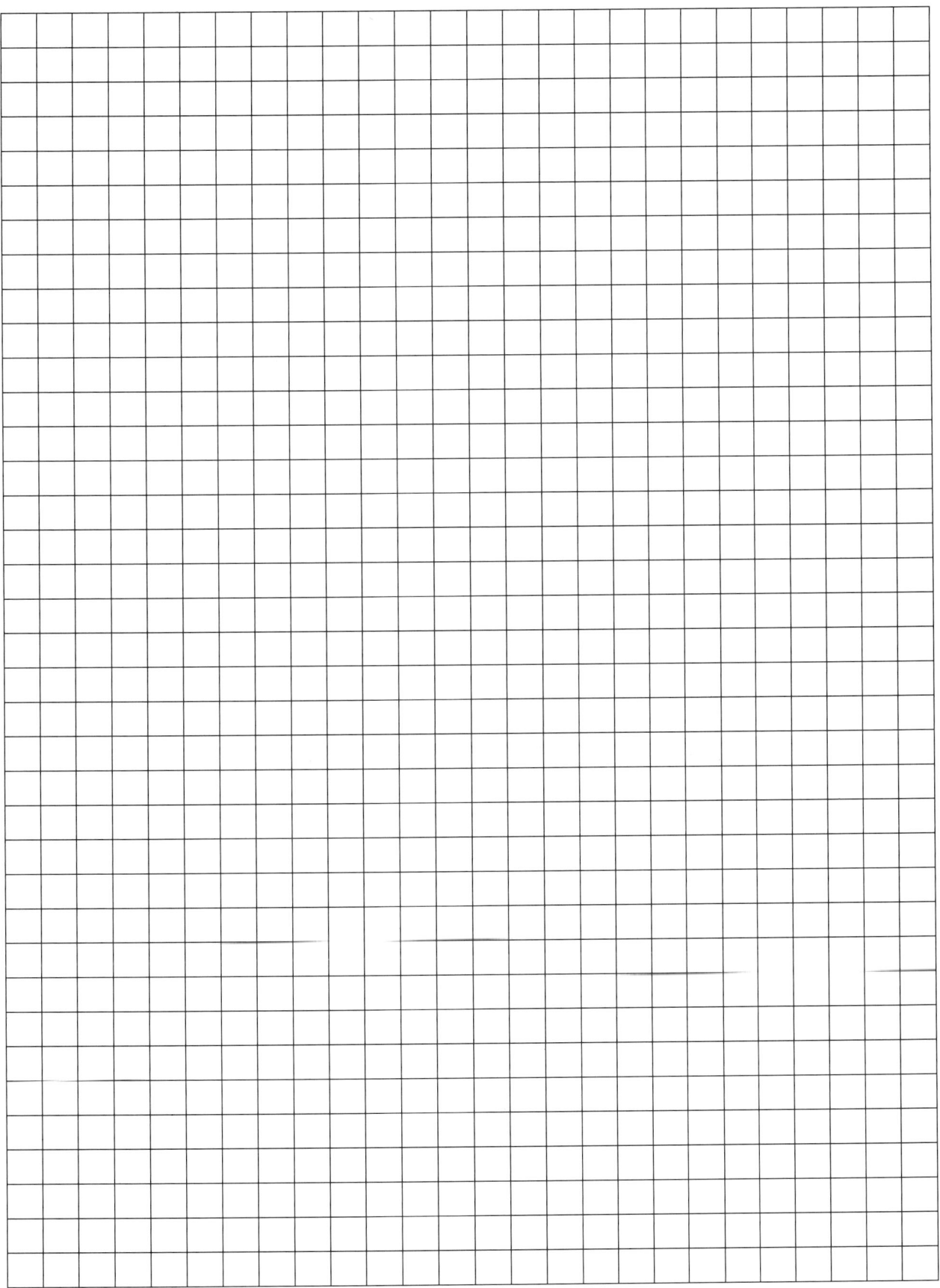

MEASUREMENTS FOR PERMANENT MANDIBULAR FIRST PREMOLAR	
Cervico-occlusal Length of Crown	8.5
Length of Root	14.0
Mesiodistal Diameter of Crown	7.0
Mesiodistal Diameter of CEJ	5.0
Buccolingual Diameter	7.5
Buccolingual Diameter of CEJ	6.5
Curvature of CEJ at Mesial	1.0
Curvature of CEJ at Distal	0.0

CHECKLIST FOR PERMANENT MANDIBULAR FIRST PREMOLAR	
Features Noted	Features Present
Crown Features	
Occlusal table with marginal ridges and cusps with tips, ridges, inclined planes, grooves, fossae, pits	
Smaller lingual cusp of two cusps	
Shorter mesial cusp slope than distal with distinct mesial surface features of deeper mesial CEJ curvature and mesiolingual groove	
Buccal ridge	
Mesial and distal contact just cervical to junction of occlusal and middle thirds with height of contour for buccal in cervical third and lingual in middle third	
Root Features	
Single root	
Proximal root concavities	

Name _____   Tooth Number/Name _____
Date _____   Instructor Rating _____

DRAWING EVALUATION CHECKLIST

RATING SCALE

Completely Correct = 2 points   Major Error = 0 points
Minor Error = 1 point   Note = NA (Not Applicable)

SELF-EVALUATION RATING

Five Views	Clearly Drawn	Accurate Sizing	General Features Included	Specific Features Included
1. Facial View				
2. Lingual View				
3. Mesial View				
4. Distal View				
5. Occlusal View				

Self-Evaluation Rating = $\dfrac{\text{Points received}}{\text{Points possible}}$ = _____ = _____ %

INSTRUCTOR EVALUATION RATING

Five Views	Clearly Drawn	Accurate Sizing	General Features Included	Specific Features Included
1. Facial View				
2. Lingual View				
3. Mesial View				
4. Distal View				
5. Occlusal View				

Instructor Evaluation Rating = $\dfrac{\text{Points received}}{\text{Points possible}}$ = _____ = _____ %

Copyright © 2026 by Elsevier Inc. All rights reserved, including those for text and data mining, AI training, and similar technologies.

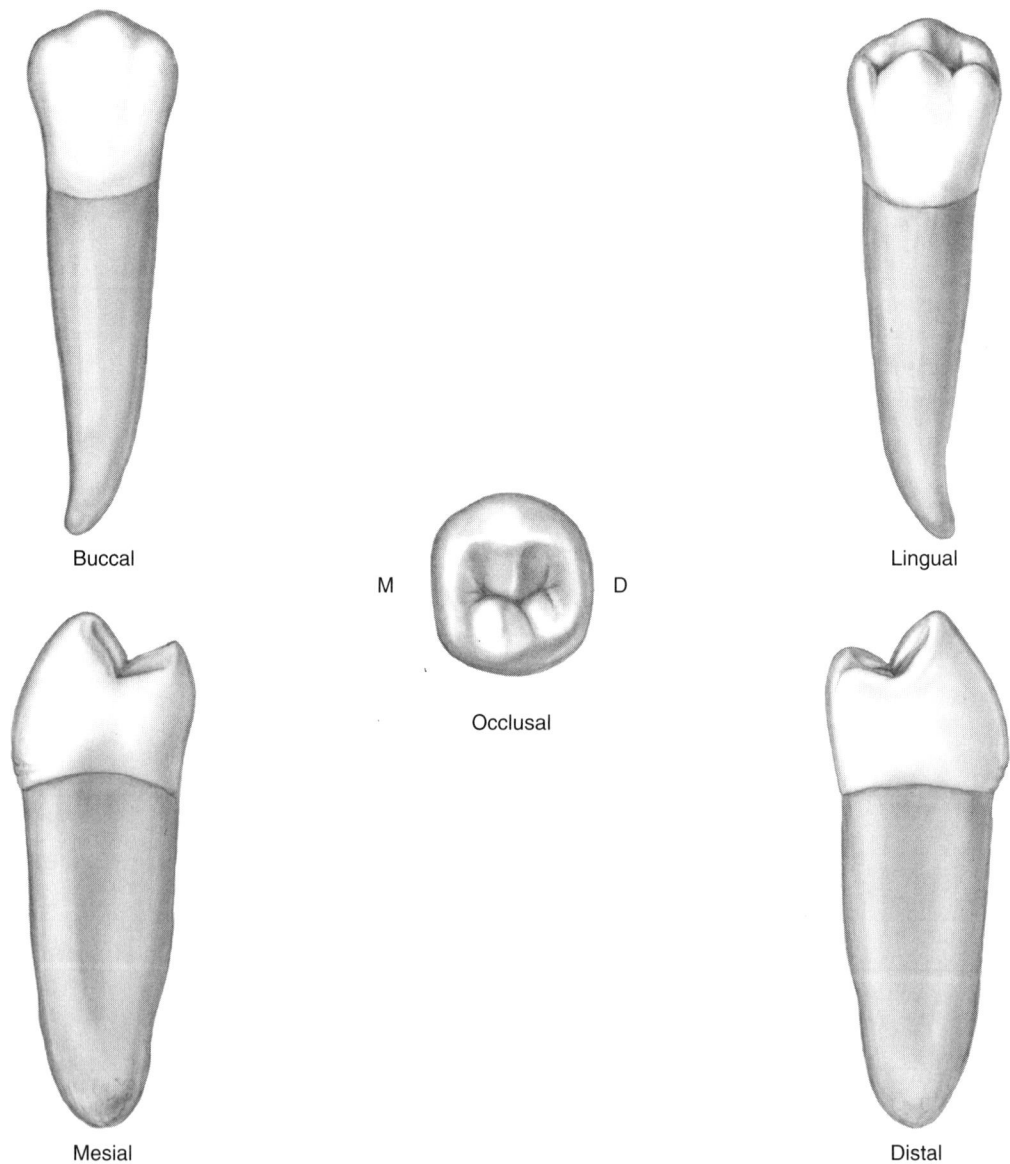

Views of Permanent Mandibular Right Second Premolar (Three-Cusp Type)

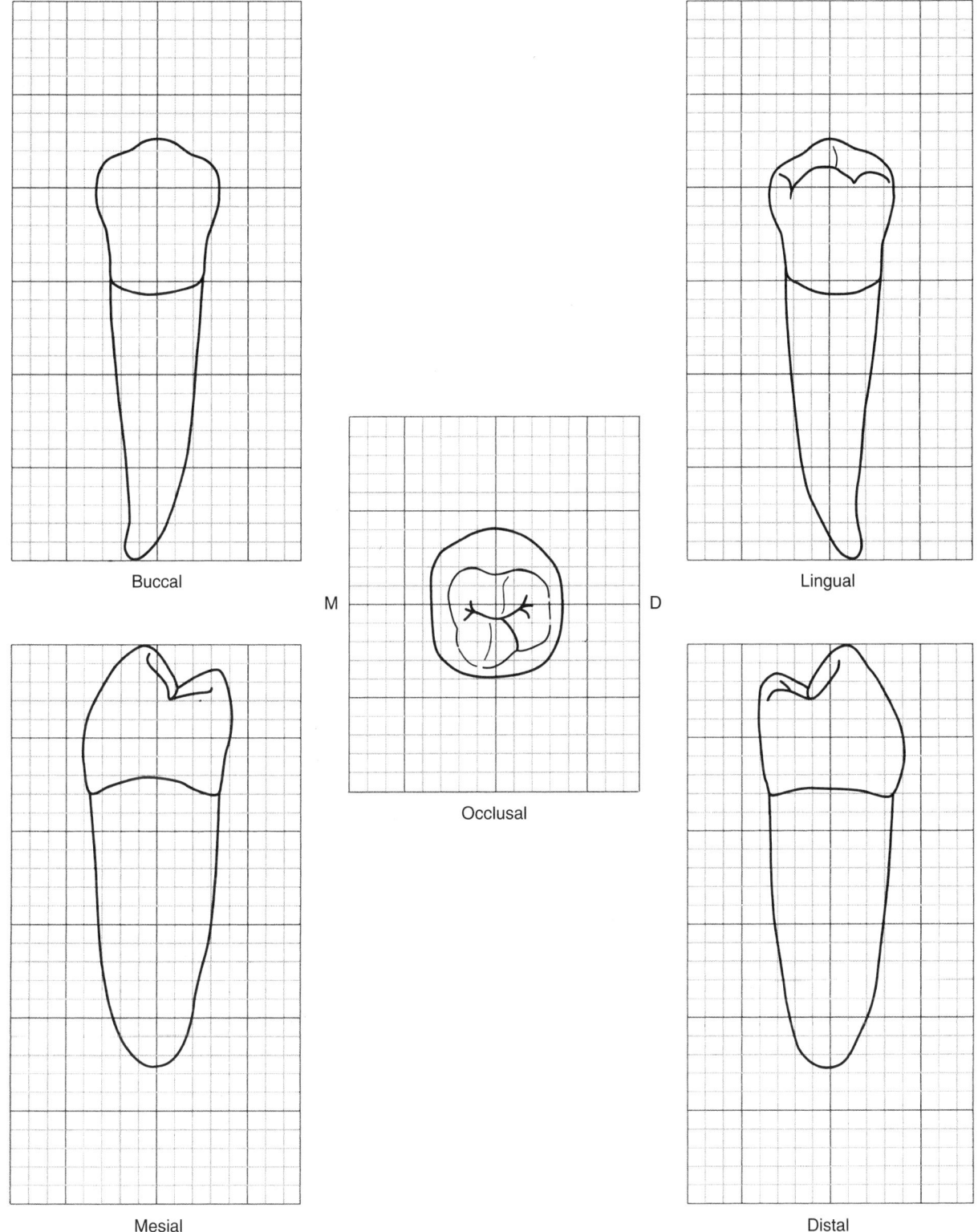

Outline Views of Permanent Mandibular Right Second Premolar (Three-Cusp Type)

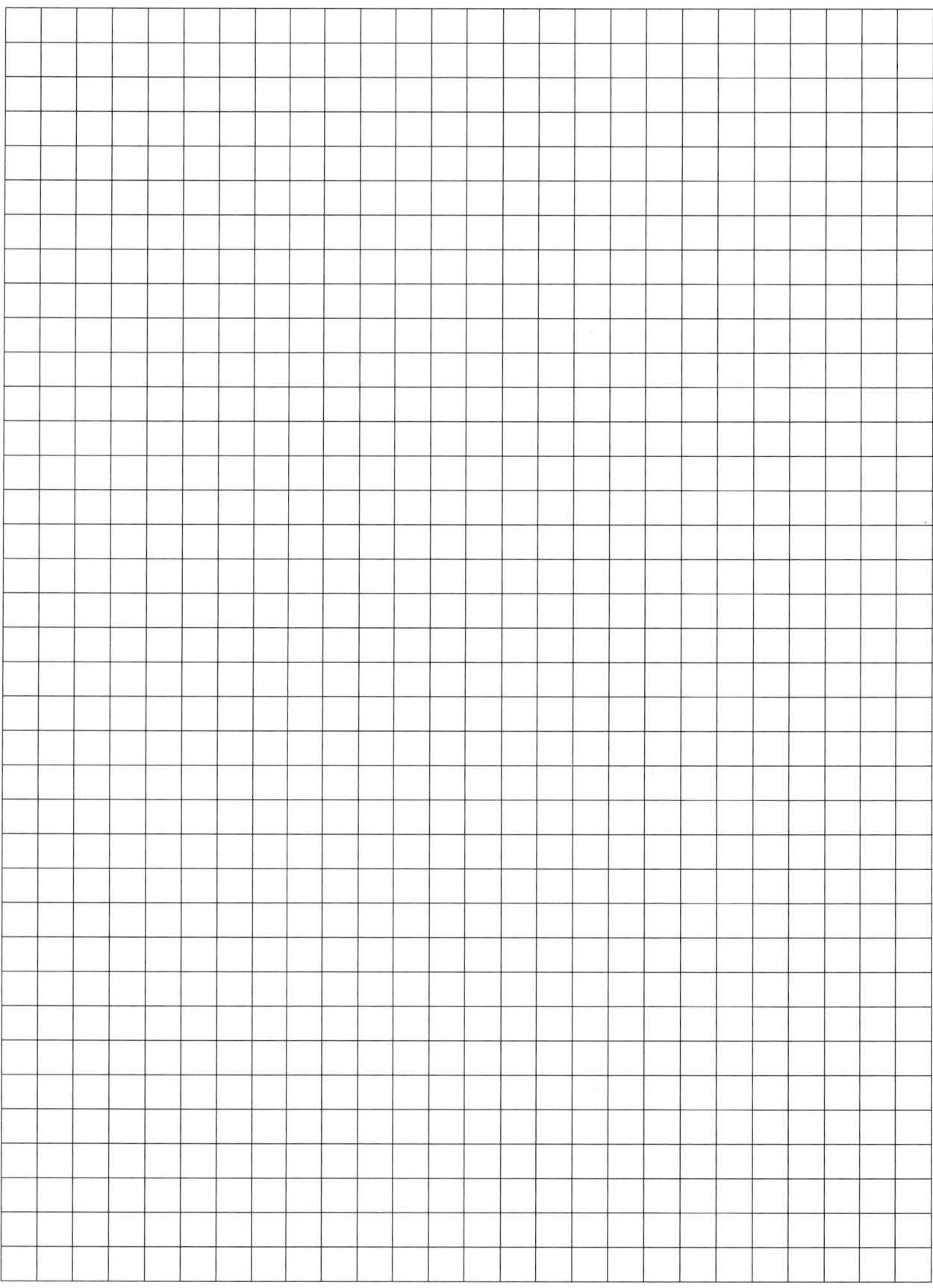

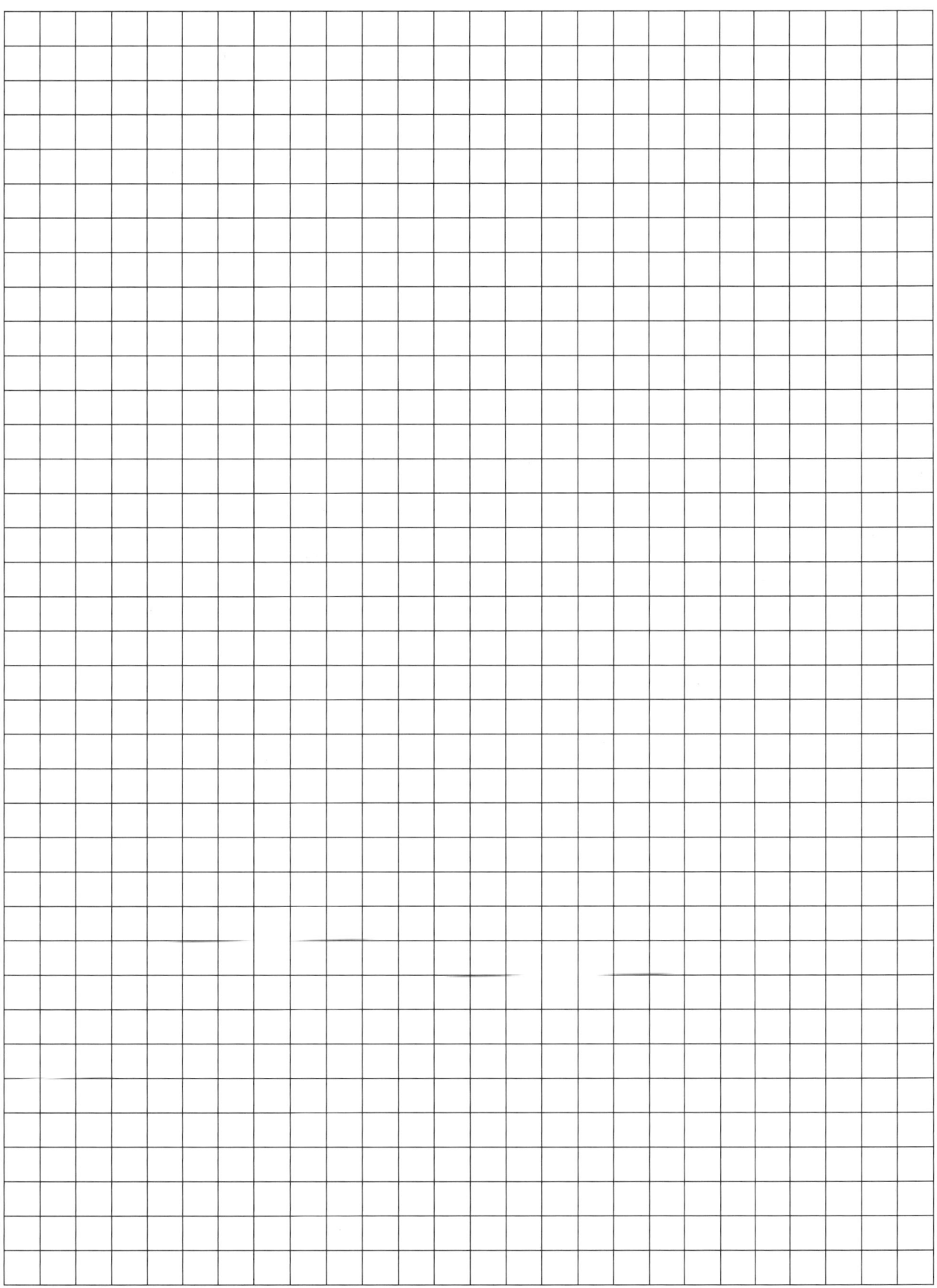

MEASUREMENTS FOR PERMANENT MANDIBULAR SECOND PREMOLAR
(Three-Cusp Type)

Cervico-occlusal Length of Crown	8.0
Length of Root	14.5
Mesiodistal Diameter of Crown	7.0
Mesiodistal Diameter of CEJ	5.0
Buccolingual Diameter	8.0
Buccolingual Diameter of CEJ	7.0
Curvature of CEJ at Mesial	1.0
Curvature of CEJ at Distal	0.0

CHECKLIST FOR PERMANENT MANDIBULAR SECOND PREMOLAR
(Three-Cusp Type)

Features Noted	Features Present
Crown Features	
Occlusal table with marginal ridges and cusps with tips, ridges, inclined planes, grooves, fossae, pits	
Usually three cusps with Y-shaped groove pattern	
Distal marginal ridge more cervically located with more occlusal surface observable from distal	
Buccal ridge	
Mesial and distal contact just cervical to junction of occlusal and middle thirds with height of contour for buccal in cervical third and lingual in middle third	
Root Features	
Single root	
Proximal root concavities	

Name _____   Tooth Number/Name _____
Date _____   Instructor Rating _____

DRAWING EVALUATION CHECKLIST

RATING SCALE

Completely Correct = 2 points   Major Error = 0 points
Minor Error = 1 point   Note = NA (Not Applicable)

SELF-EVALUATION RATING

Five Views	Clearly Drawn	Accurate Sizing	General Features Included	Specific Features Included
1. Facial View				
2. Lingual View				
3. Mesial View				
4. Distal View				
5. Occlusal View				

Self-Evaluation Rating = $\dfrac{\text{Points received}}{\text{Points possible}}$ = _____ = _____ %

INSTRUCTOR EVALUATION RATING

Five Views	Clearly Drawn	Accurate Sizing	General Features Included	Specific Features Included
1. Facial View				
2. Lingual View				
3. Mesial View				
4. Distal View				
5. Occlusal View				

Instructor Evaluation Rating = $\dfrac{\text{Points received}}{\text{Points possible}}$ = _____ = _____ %

Copyright © 2026 by Elsevier Inc. All rights are reserved, including those for text and data mining, AI training, and similar technologies.

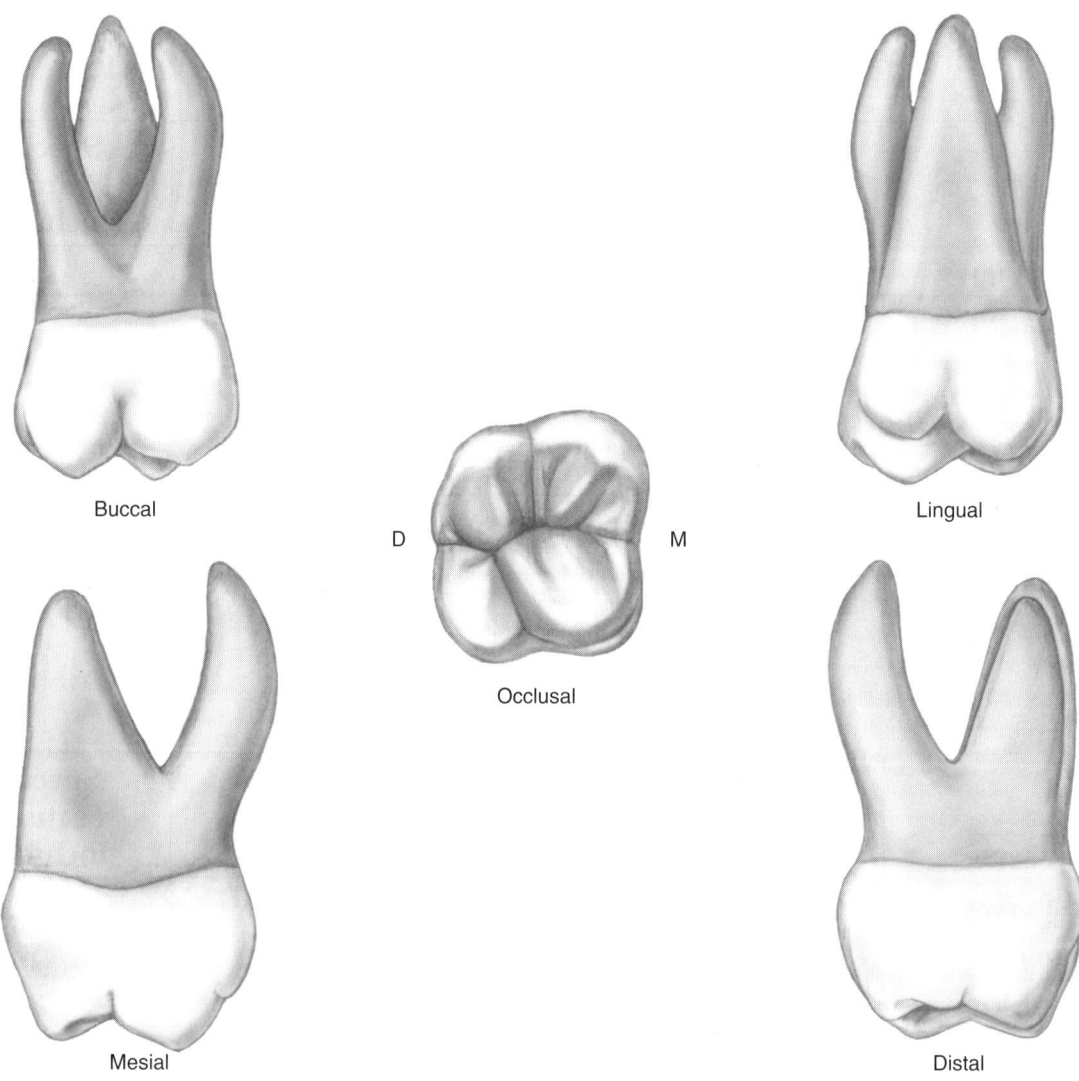

Views of Permanent Maxillary Right First Molar

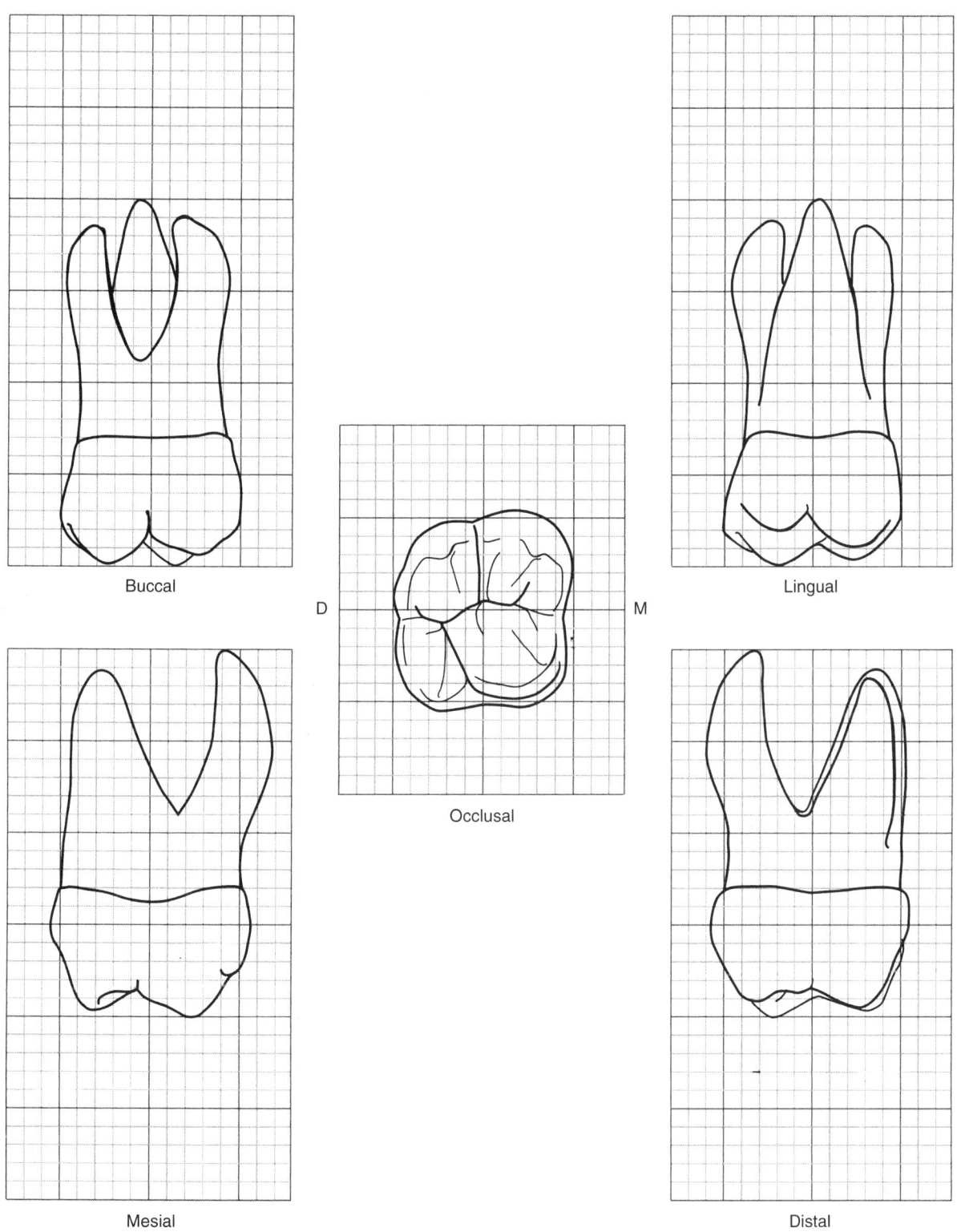

Outline Views of Permanent Maxillary Right First Molar

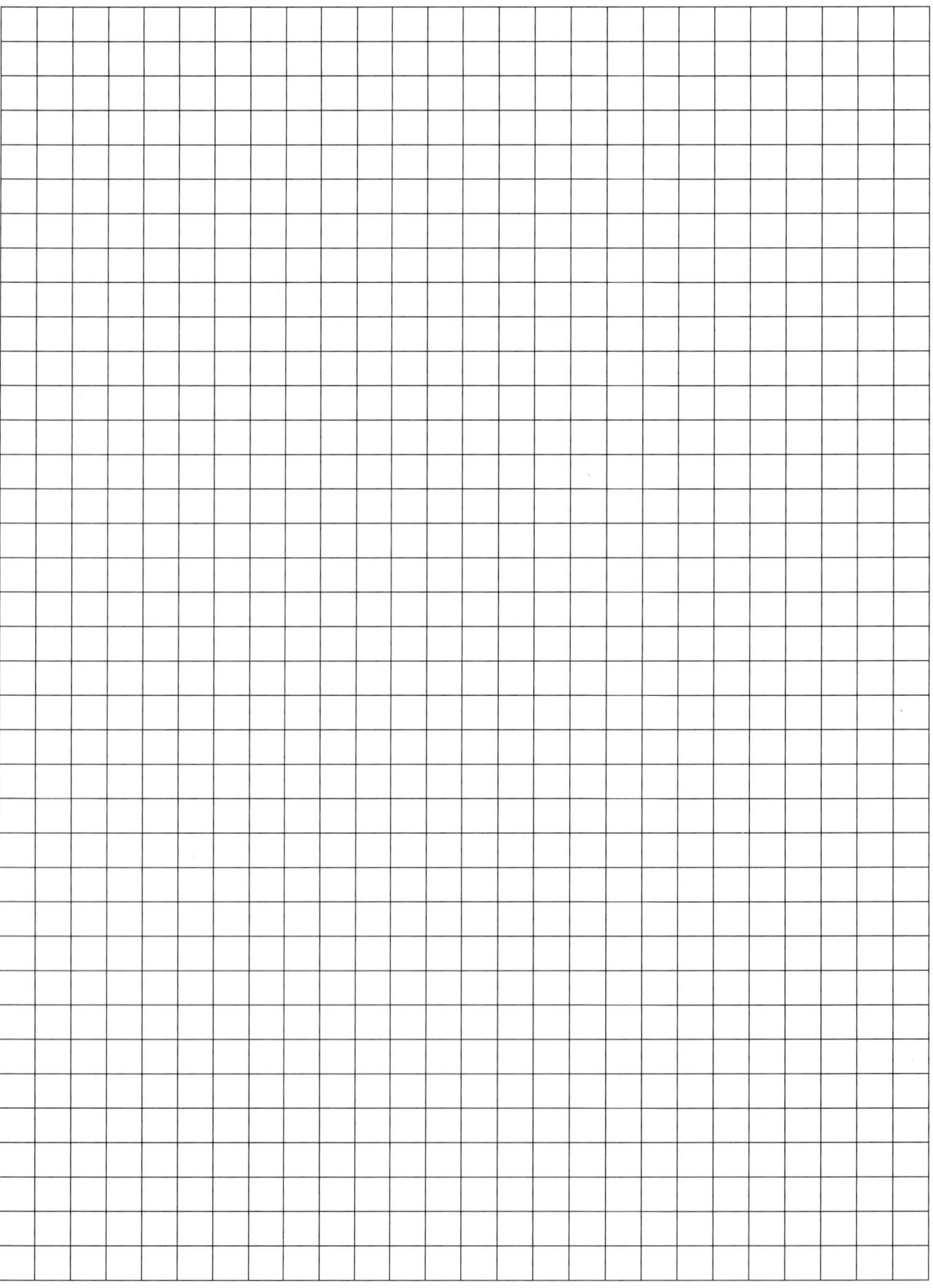

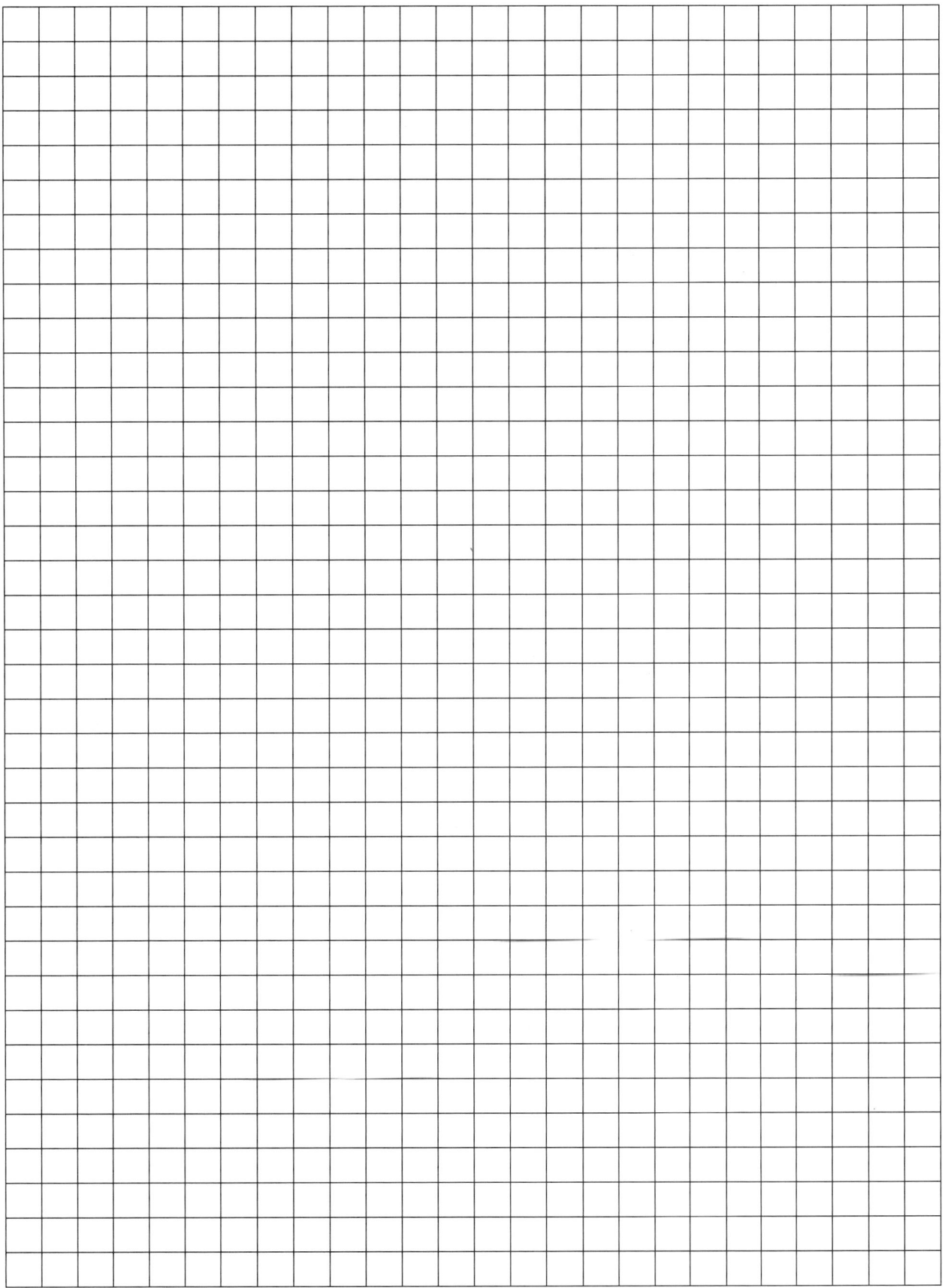

MEASUREMENTS FOR PERMANENT MAXILLARY FIRST MOLAR	
Cervico-occlusal Length of Crown	7.5
Length of Root	Buccal: 12 Lingual: 13
Mesiodistal Diameter of Crown	10.0
Mesiodistal Diameter of CEJ	8.0
Buccolingual Diameter	11.0
Buccolingual Diameter of CEJ	10.0
Curvature of CEJ at Mesial	1.0
Curvature of CEJ at Distal	0.0

CHECKLIST FOR PERMANENT MAXILLARY FIRST MOLAR	
Features Noted	**Features Present**
Crown Features	
Occlusal table with marginal ridges and cusps with tips, ridges, inclined planes, grooves, fossae, pits	
Distinct oblique ridge and distolingual groove	
Four major cusps with buccal cusps almost equal in height	
Fifth minor cusp of Carabelli associated with mesiolingual cusp and groove	
Mesiolingual cusp outline longer and larger but not as sharp as distolingual cusp outline	
Buccal ridge	
Mesial contact at junction of occlusal and middle thirds with height of contour for buccal in cervical third and lingual in middle third	
Distal contact at middle third	
Root Features	
Three roots	
Furcations well removed from CEJ, root trunks, proximal root concavities, divergent roots	

Name _____   Tooth Number/Name _____

Date _____   Instructor Rating _____

DRAWING EVALUATION CHECKLIST

RATING SCALE

Completely Correct = 2 points   Major Error = 0 points
Minor Error = 1 point   Note = NA (Not Applicable)

SELF-EVALUATION RATING

Five Views	Clearly Drawn	Accurate Sizing	General Features Included	Specific Features Included
1. Facial View				
2. Lingual View				
3. Mesial View				
4. Distal View				
5. Occlusal View				

Self-Evaluation Rating = $\frac{\text{Points received}}{\text{Points possible}}$ = _____ = _____ %

INSTRUCTOR EVALUATION RATING

Five Views	Clearly Drawn	Accurate Sizing	General Features Included	Specific Features Included
1. Facial View				
2. Lingual View				
3. Mesial View				
4. Distal View				
5. Occlusal View				

Instructor Evaluation Rating = $\frac{\text{Points received}}{\text{Points possible}}$ = _____ = _____ %

Copyright © 2026 by Elsevier Inc. All rights are reserved, including those for text and data mining, AI training, and similar technologies.

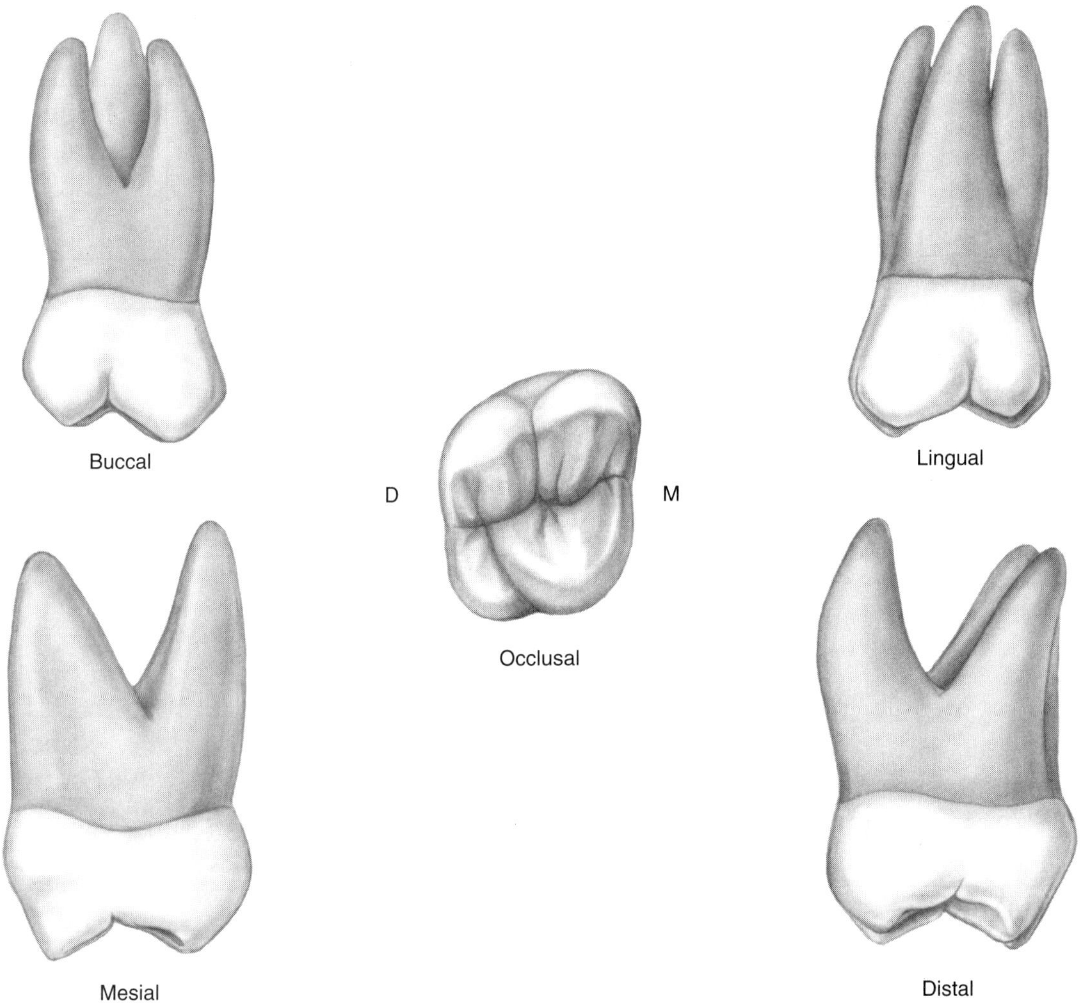

Buccal

D M

Occlusal

Lingual

Mesial

Distal

Views of Permanent Maxillary Right Second Molar (Rhomboidal Crown Outline)

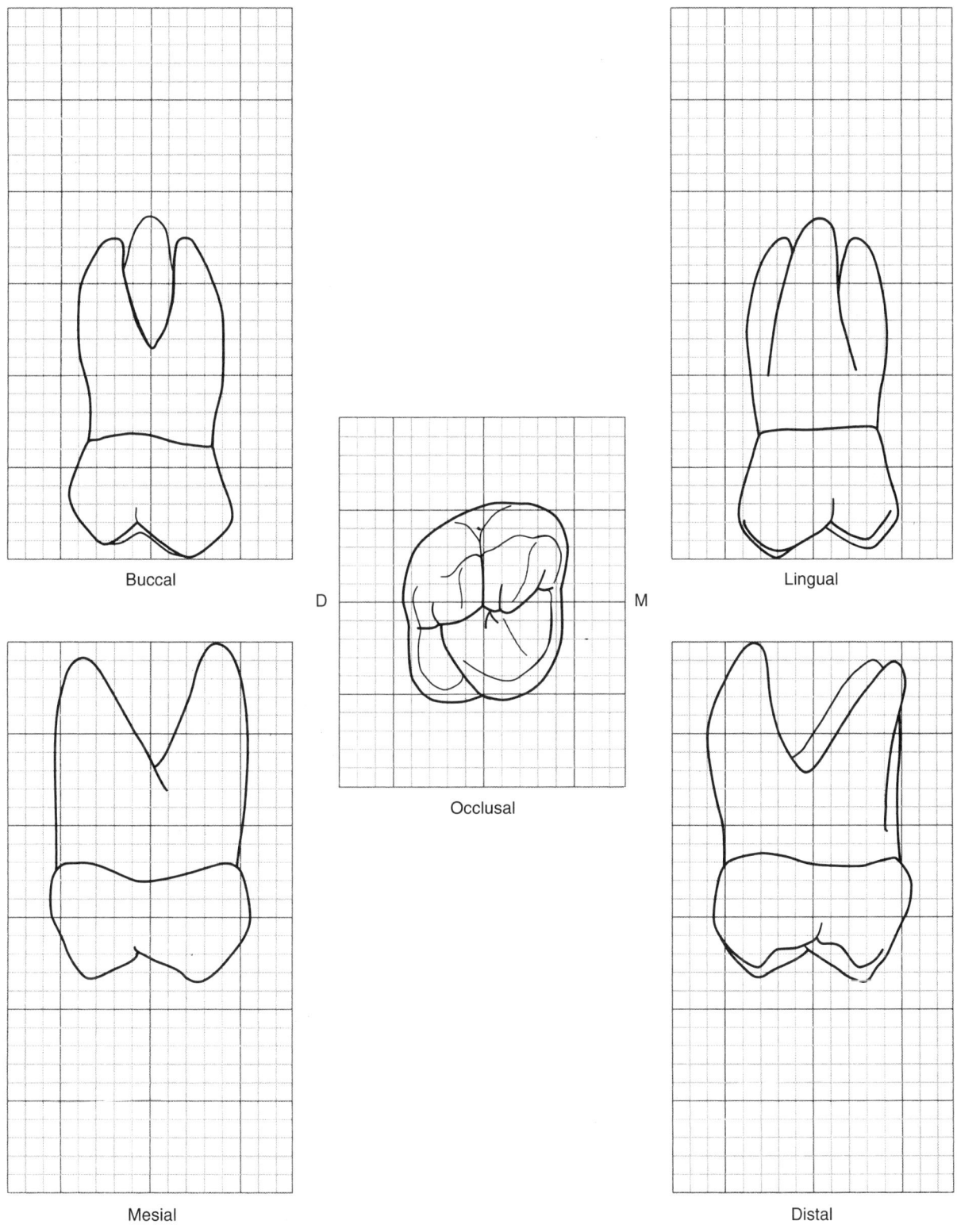

Outline Views of Permanent Maxillary Right Second Molar (Rhomboidal Crown Outline)

190 TOOTH DRAWING EXERCISES

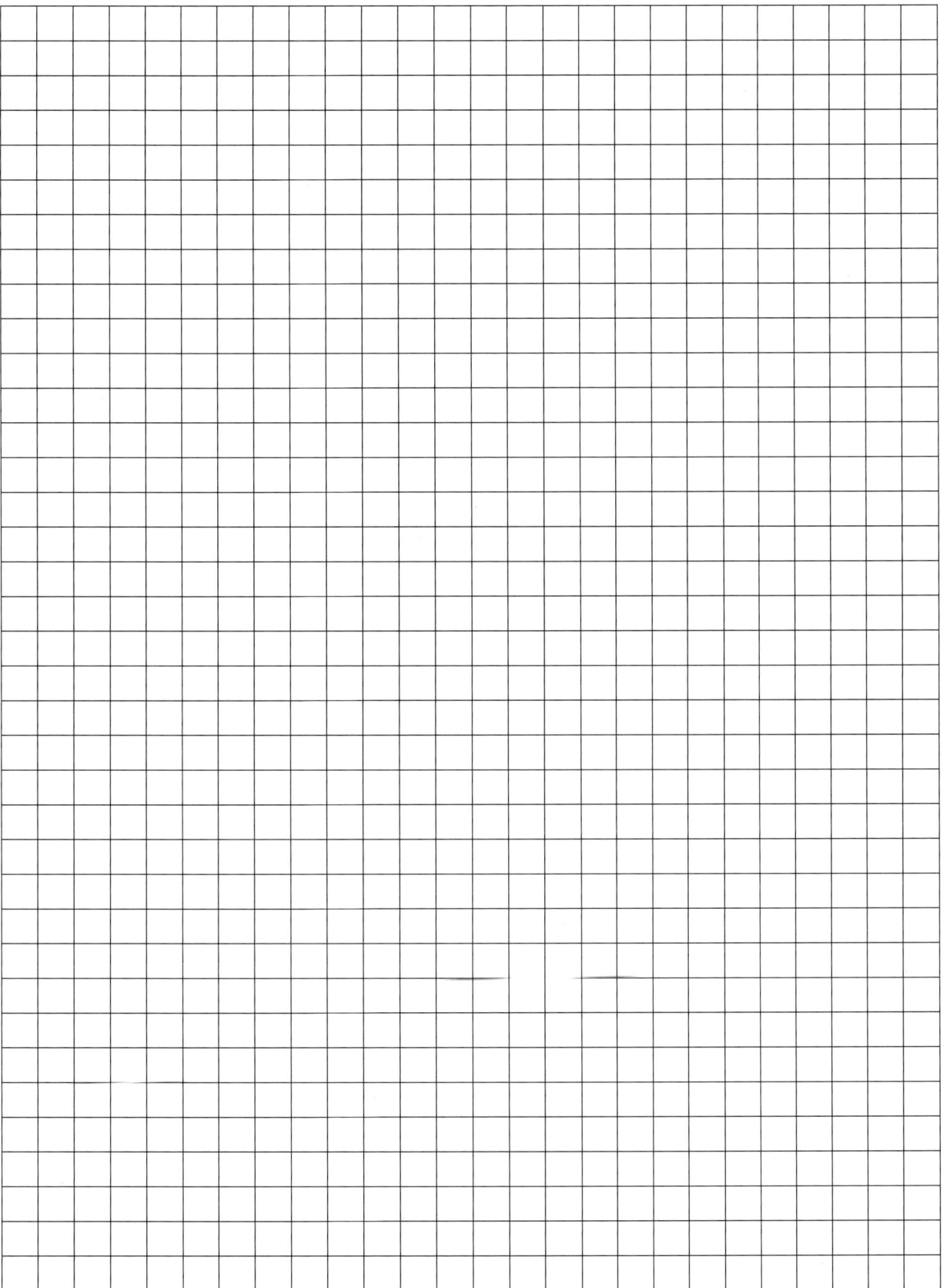

MEASUREMENTS FOR PERMANENT MAXILLARY SECOND MOLAR
(Rhomboidal Crown Outline)

Cervico-occlusal Length of Crown	7.0
Length of Root	Buccal: 11 Lingual: 12
Mesiodistal Diameter of Crown	9.0
Mesiodistal Diameter of CEJ	7.0
Buccolingual Diameter	11.0
Buccolingual Diameter of CEJ	10.0
Curvature of CEJ at Mesial	1.0
Curvature of CEJ at Distal	0.0

CHECKLIST FOR PERMANENT MAXILLARY SECOND MOLAR
(Rhomboidal Crown Outline)

Features Noted	Features Present
Crown Features	
Occlusal table with marginal ridges and cusps with tips, ridges, inclined planes, grooves, fossae, pits	
Less distince oblique ridge	
Four cusps	
Mesiobuccal cusp longer than distobuccal cusp and distolingual cusp smaller with mesiolingual cusp outline longer and larger but not as sharp as distolingual cusp outline	
Buccal ridge	
Mesial contact at middle third	
Distal contact at middle third	
Height of contour for buccal in cervical third and lingual in middle third	
Root Features	
Three roots	
Furcations, root trunks, proximal root concavities, less divergent roots	

Name _____   Tooth Number/Name _____

Date _____   Instructor Rating _____

DRAWING EVALUATION CHECKLIST

RATING SCALE

Completely Correct = 2 points
Minor Error = 1 point

Major Error = 0 points
Note = NA (Not Applicable)

SELF-EVALUATION RATING

Five Views	Clearly Drawn	Accurate Sizing	General Features Included	Specific Features Included
1. Facial View				
2. Lingual View				
3. Mesial View				
4. Distal View				
5. Occlusal View				

Self-Evaluation Rating = $\dfrac{\text{Points received}}{\text{Points possible}}$ = _____ = _____ %

INSTRUCTOR EVALUATION RATING

Five Views	Clearly Drawn	Accurate Sizing	General Features Included	Specific Features Included
1. Facial View				
2. Lingual View				
3. Mesial View				
4. Distal View				
5. Occlusal View				

Instructor Evaluation Rating = $\dfrac{\text{Points received}}{\text{Points possible}}$ = _____ = _____ %

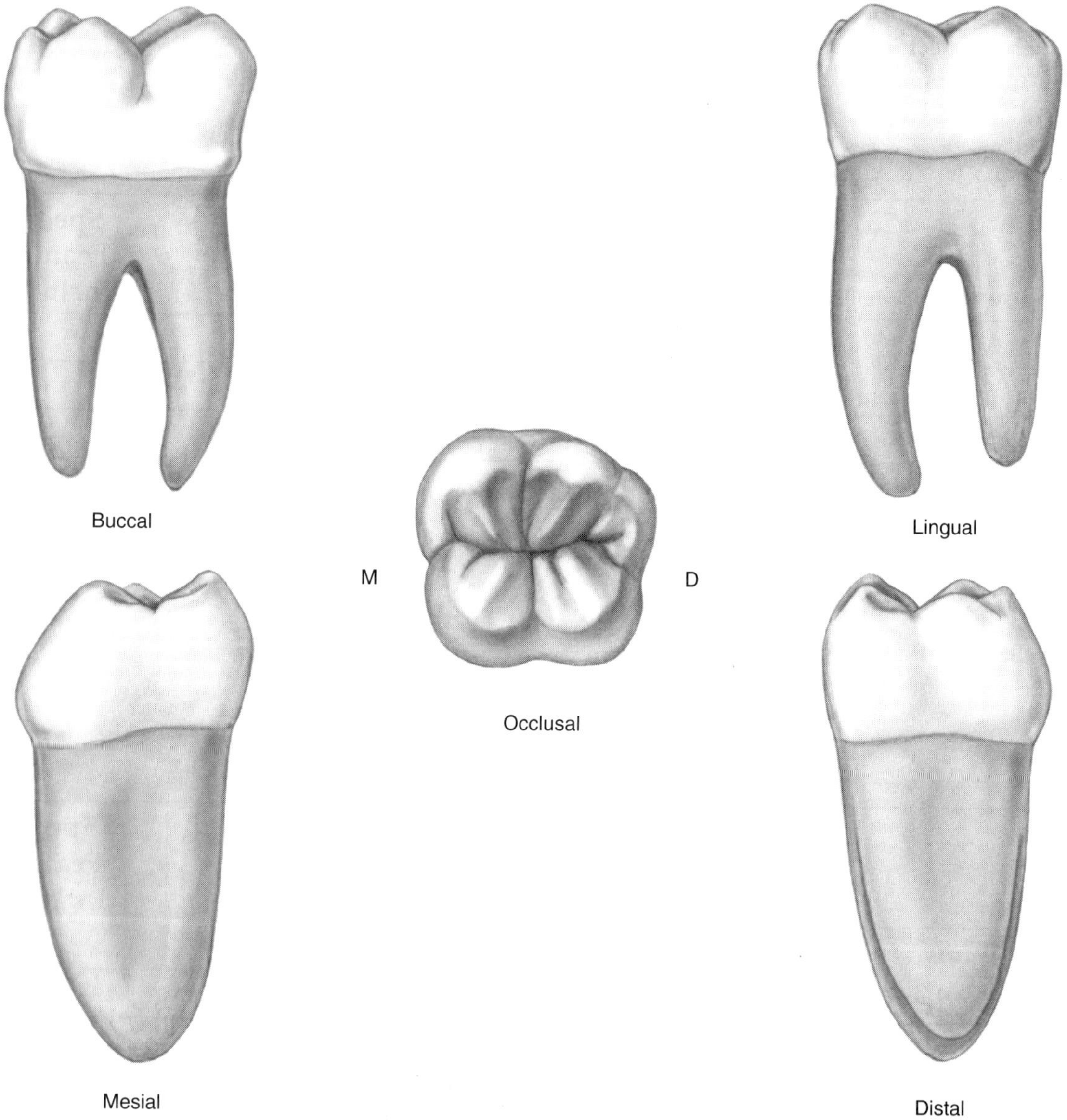

194 TOOTH DRAWING EXERCISES

Buccal

Lingual

M D

Occlusal

Mesial

Distal

Views of Permanent Mandibular Right First Molar

Copyright © 2026 by Elsevier Inc. All rights reserved, including those for text and data mining,
AI training, and similar technologies.

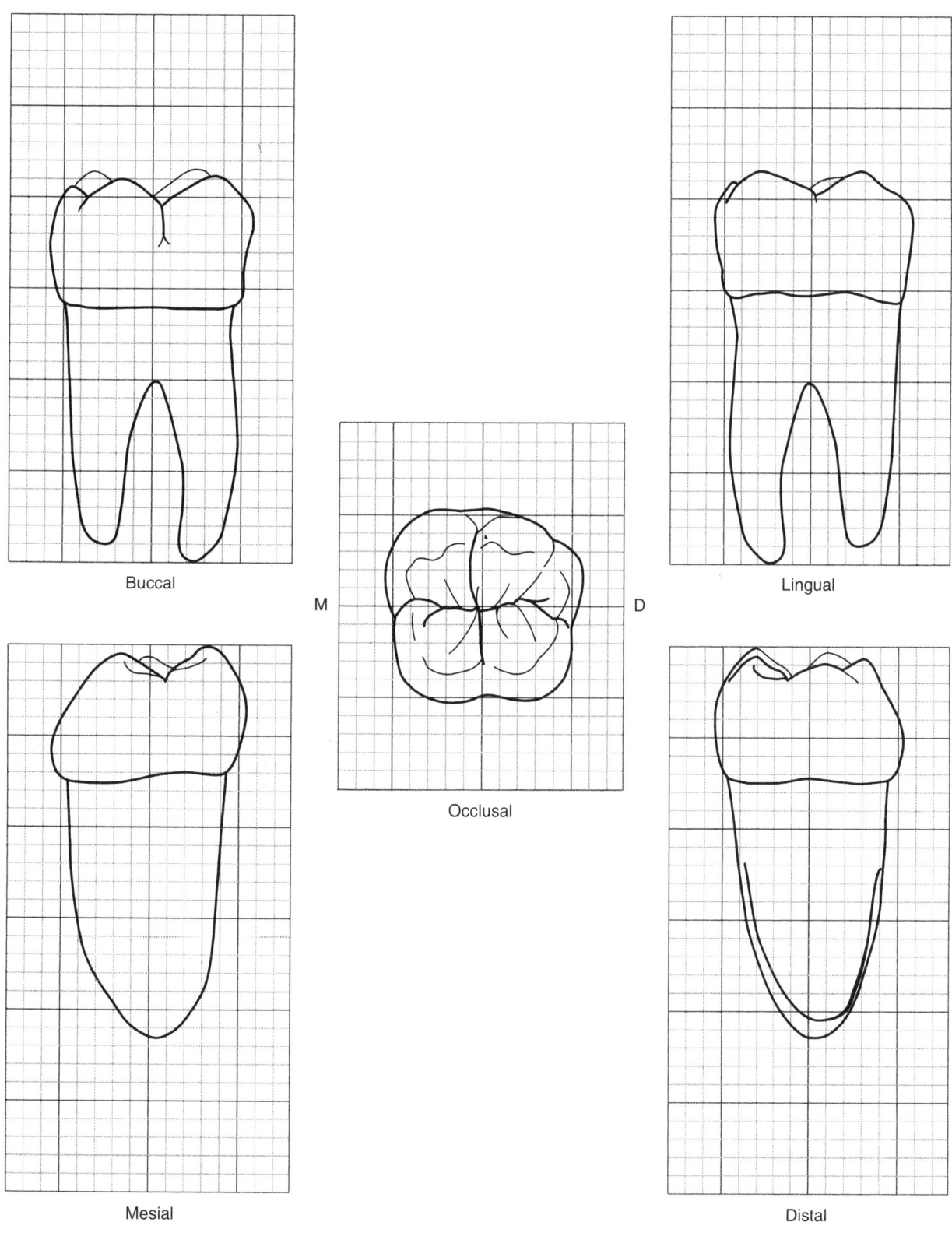

Outline Views of Permanent Mandibular Right First Molar

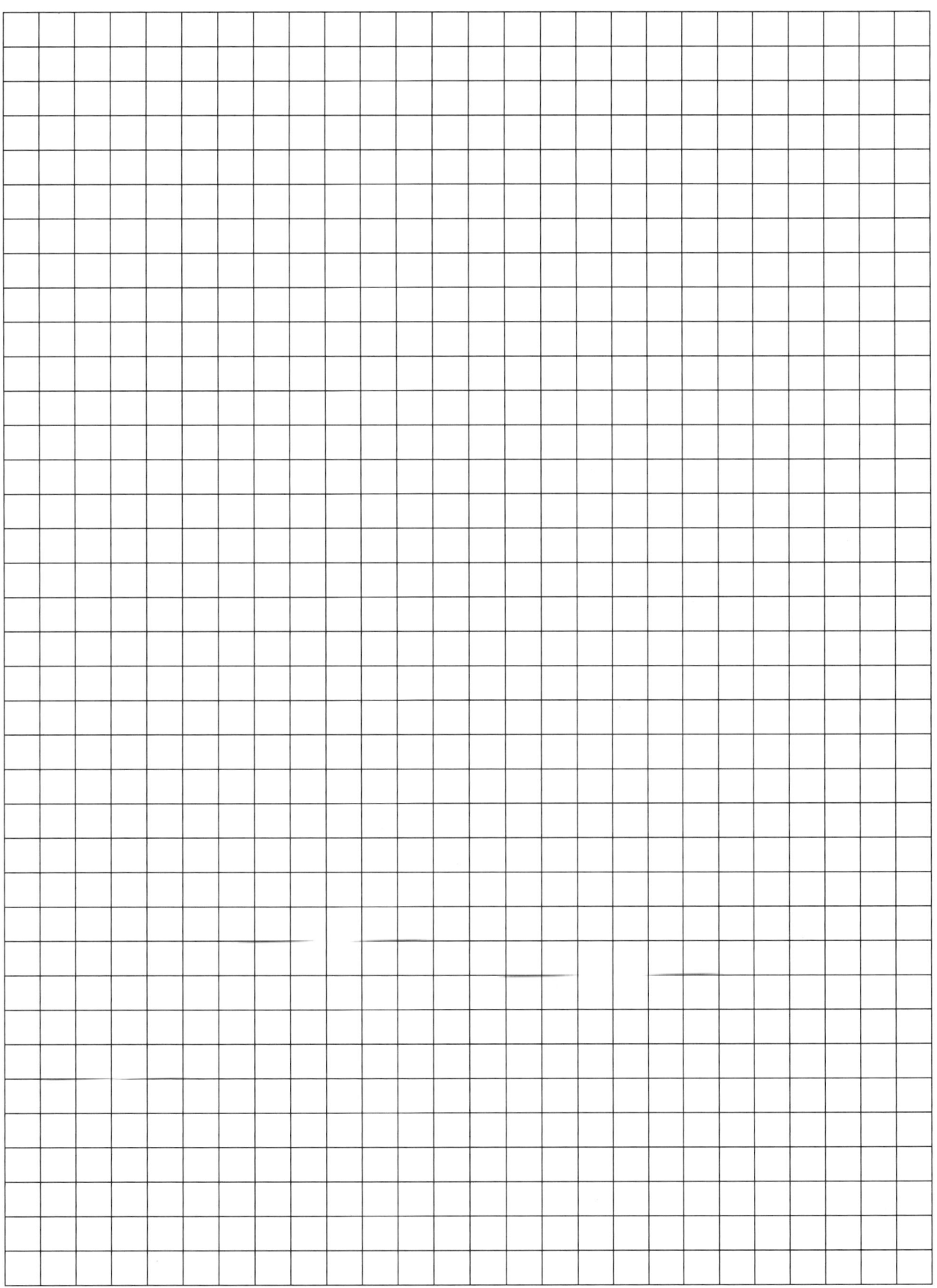

MEASUREMENTS FOR PERMANENT MANDIBULAR FIRST MOLAR	
Cervico-occlusal Length of Crown	7.5
Length of Root	14.0
Mesiodistal Diameter of Crown	11.0
Mesiodistal Diameter of CEJ	9.0
Buccolingual Diameter	10.5
Buccolingual Diameter of CEJ	9.0
Curvature of CEJ at Mesial	1.0
Curvature of CEJ at Distal	0.0

CHECKLIST FOR PERMANENT MANDIBULAR FIRST MOLAR	
Features Noted	Features Present
Crown Features	
Occlusal table with marginal ridges and cusps with tips, ridges, inclined planes, grooves, fossae, pits	
Five cusps with Y-shaped groove pattern and buccal groove	
Distal cusp smallest with sharp cusp	
Buccal ridge	
Mesial and distal contact at junction of occlusal and middle thirds with height of contour for buccal in cervical third and lingual in middle third	
Root Features	
Two roots	
Furcations well removed from CEJ, root trunks, proximal root concavities, more divergent roots	

Name _____   Tooth Number/Name _____
Date _____   Instructor Rating _____

DRAWING EVALUATION CHECKLIST

RATING SCALE

Completely Correct = 2 points   Major Error = 0 points
Minor Error = 1 point   Note = NA (Not Applicable)

SELF-EVALUATION RATING

Five Views	Clearly Drawn	Accurate Sizing	General Features Included	Specific Features Included
1. Facial View				
2. Lingual View				
3. Mesial View				
4. Distal View				
5. Occlusal View				

Self-Evaluation Rating = $\dfrac{\text{Points received}}{\text{Points possible}}$ = _____ = _____ %

INSTRUCTOR EVALUATION RATING

Five Views	Clearly Drawn	Accurate Sizing	General Features Included	Specific Features Included
1. Facial View				
2. Lingual View				
3. Mesial View				
4. Distal View				
5. Occlusal View				

Instructor Evaluation Rating = $\dfrac{\text{Points received}}{\text{Points possible}}$ = _____ = _____ %

Copyright © 2026 by Elsevier Inc. All rights are reserved, including those for text and data mining, AI training, and similar technologies.

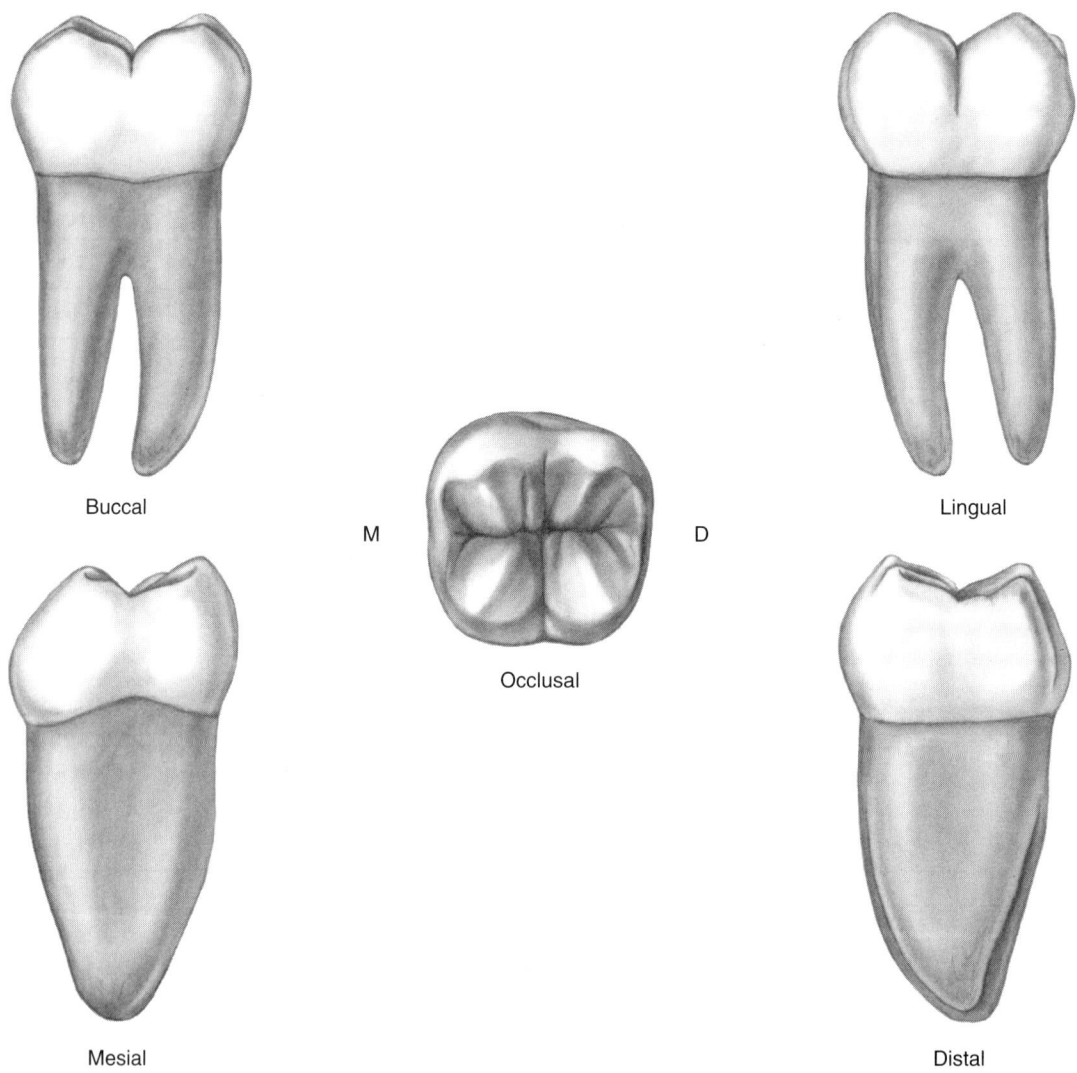

Views of Permanent Mandibular Right Second Molar

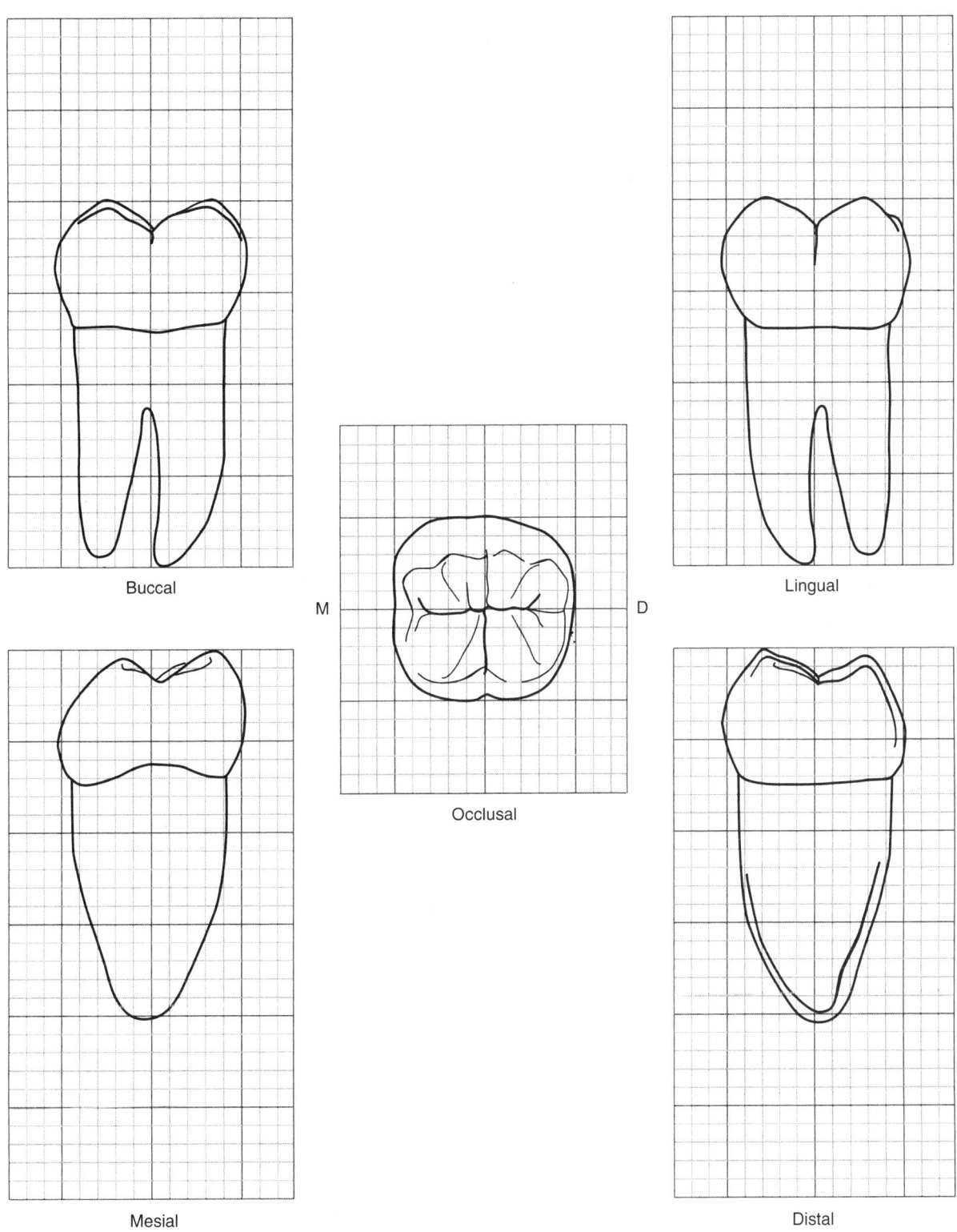

Outline Views of Permanent Mandibular Right Second Molar

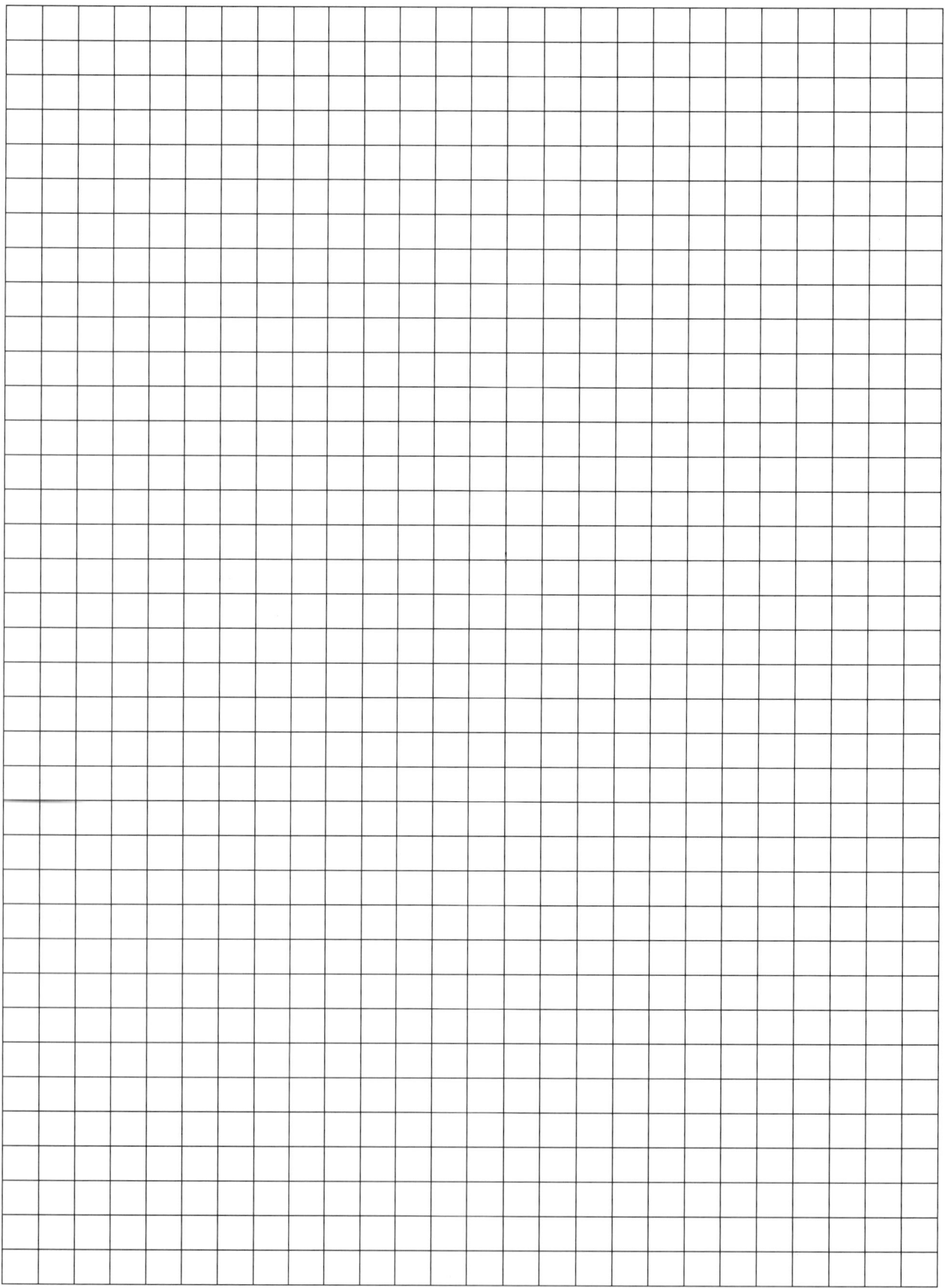

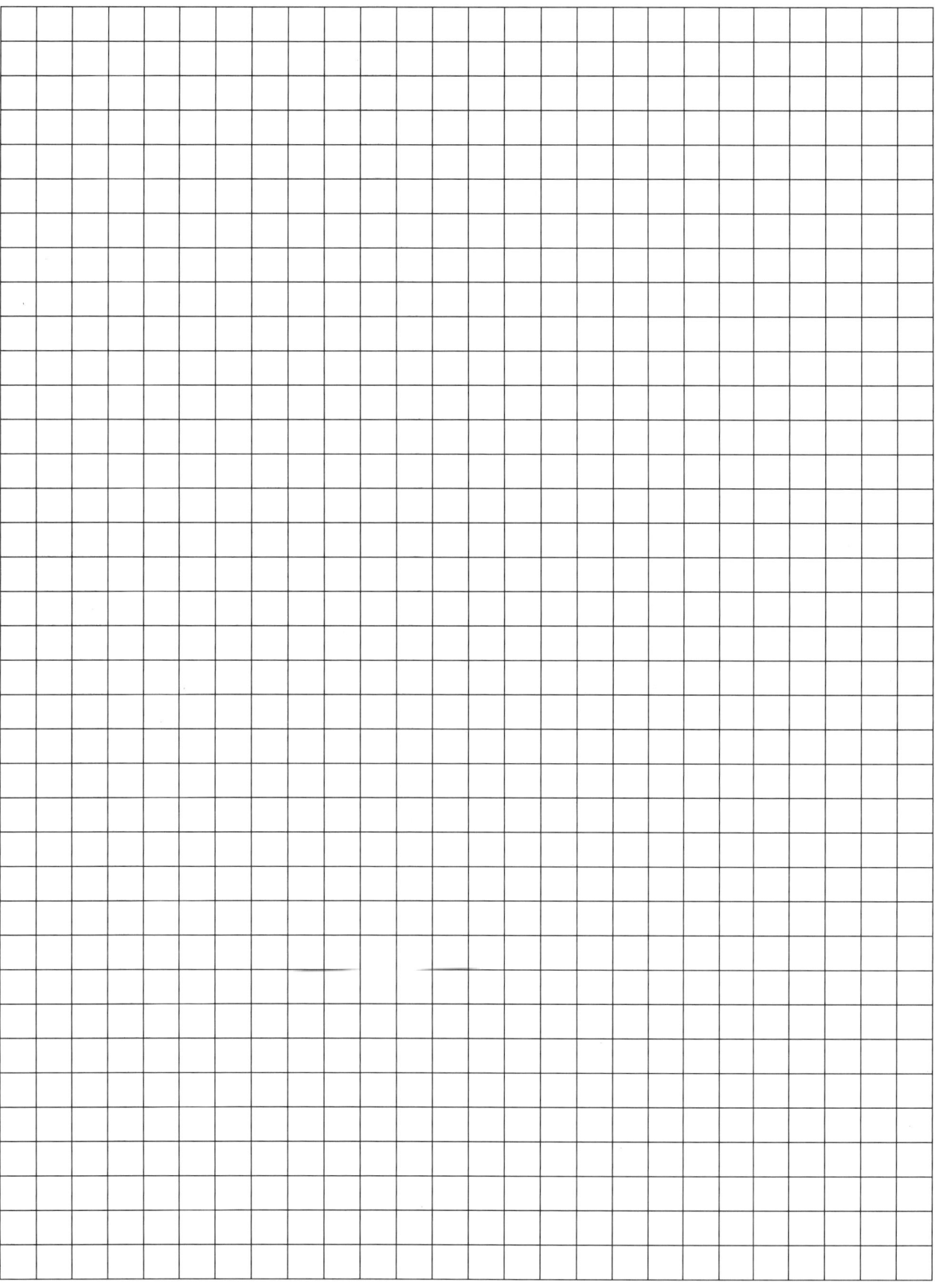

MEASUREMENTS FOR PERMANENT MANDIBULAR SECOND MOLAR	
Cervico-occlusal Length of Crown	7.0
Length of Root	13.0
Mesiodistal Diameter of Crown	10.5
Mesiodistal Diameter of CEJ	8.0
Buccolingual Diameter	10.0
Buccolingual Diameter of CEJ	9.0
Curvature of CEJ at Mesial	1.0
Curvature of CEJ at Distal	0.0

CHECKLIST FOR PERMANENT MANDIBULAR SECOND MOLAR	
Features Noted	**Features Present**
Crown Features	
Occlusal table with marginal ridges and cusps with tips, ridges, inclined planes, grooves, fossae, pits	
Four cusps with cross-shaped groove pattern	
Difference in height of contour for buccal and lingual from each proximal surface and wider on mesial than distal	
Buccal ridge	
Mesial and distal contact at middle third with height of contour for buccal in cervical third and lingual in middle third	
Root Features	
Two roots	
Furcations closer to CEJ, root trunks, proximal root concavities, less divergent roots	

Name _____   Tooth Number/Name _____
Date _____   Instructor Rating _____

DRAWING EVALUATION CHECKLIST

RATING SCALE

Completely Correct = 2 points   Major Error = 0 points
Minor Error = 1 point   Note = NA (Not Applicable)

SELF-EVALUATION RATING

Five Views	Clearly Drawn	Accurate Sizing	General Features Included	Specific Features Included
1. Facial View				
2. Lingual View				
3. Mesial View				
4. Distal View				
5. Occlusal View				

Self-Evaluation Rating = $\dfrac{\text{Points received}}{\text{Points possible}}$ = _____ = _____ %

INSTRUCTOR EVALUATION RATING

Five Views	Clearly Drawn	Accurate Sizing	General Features Included	Specific Features Included
1. Facial View				
2. Lingual View				
3. Mesial View				
4. Distal View				
5. Occlusal View				

Instructor Evaluation Rating = $\dfrac{\text{Points received}}{\text{Points possible}}$ = _____ = _____ %

Copyright © 2026 by Elsevier Inc. All rights are reserved, including those for text and data mining, AI training, and similar technologies.

The following are **concept exercises** that allow the student dental professional to review the ideas presented in the associated textbook *per unit*. This one of the later steps for the student dental professional in understanding dentally related concepts. The first type is **matching exercises** where one matches each term below with its best short description; each single item can only be matched once. And the second type is **true or false exercises** where one designates the statement as either true or false. And finally the third type is **ordering exercises** where one numbers the listed terms in the correct order as desired per description. The **answer key** can be obtained from your instructor and their Evolve Resources.

UNIT 1: OROFACIAL STRUCTURES

Matching Exercises

a.	Lymph nodes	k.	Body	u.	Buccal fat pad
b.	Exostoses	l.	Atypical finding	v.	Alae
c.	Periodontal ligament	m.	Vermilion zone	w.	Maxillary sinus
d.	Vestibules	n.	Mandibular symphysis	x.	Temporomandibular joint
e.	Labial frenum	o.	Fordyce spots	y.	Maxillary tuberosity
f.	Enamel	p.	Mandibular notch	z.	Linea alba
g.	External nose	q.	Anterior teeth		
h.	Parotid papilla	r.	Vertical dimension		
i.	Philtrum	s.	Buccal		
j.	Rami	t.	Tori		

1. Need to be recorded if palpable on a patient _____
2. Main feature of nasal region on face _____
3. Terminates in thicker area of midline of upper lip at tubercle _____
4. Mandibular bony feature between coronoid process and condyle _____
5. Division of face into thirds from forehead to chin _____
6. What most lesions are categorized as by clinicians; *variation from normal* _____
7. Marking midline of mandible of lower face _____
8. Plural of ramus that is present as mandibular bony feature _____
9. Upper and lower horseshoe-shaped spaces in oral cavity _____
10. Disruption of this lip surface feature with solar damage _____
11. Structure orientation that is closest to inner cheek _____
12. Oral feature at midline between labial mucosa and alveolar mucosa on both dental arches _____
13. Small raised tissue area on inner part of buccal mucosa opposite permanent maxillary second molar _____
14. Small yellow bumps within oral mucosa that increase with age _____
15. Heavy horizontal part of maxilla or mandible inferior to roots of teeth _____

16. Attaches tooth to bony surface of alveoli _____
17. Hard outer layer of crown of tooth _____
18. Incisors and canines as group within both dentitions _____
19. Slow-growing bony masses in premolar area noted on radiographs _____
20. Maxillary arch bony growths that may be related to occlusal trauma _____
21. Acts as protective cushion during mastication _____
22. Whiter ridge of calloused tissue extending horizontally where teeth occlude _____
23. Tissue-covered bony elevation just distal to last tooth of maxillary arch _____
24. Nares bounded on each side by winglike cartilaginous structures _____
25. Structure inferior to zygomatic arch and just anterior to external ear _____
26. Structure contained within body of maxilla _____

True or False Exercises

1. An abnormal finding is a discovery of a lesion that is typical but also is a serious pathologic condition. _____
2. On the midline of the upper lip extending downward from the nasal septum is a vertical groove, the philtrum. _____
3. The bone underlying the mental region is the mandible or lower jaw. _____
4. At both sides of the neck are the hyoid bones, which are suspended in the neck. _____
5. Inferior to the hyoid bone is the thyroid cartilage, which is the prominence of the larynx. _____
6. The thyroid gland, an endocrine gland, is located in the midline cervical area. _____
7. The upper and lower lips meet at each corner of the mouth at the labial commissure. _____
8. The bony support for the cheek is the temporomandibular joint. _____
9. The nares are separated by the midline nasal septum. _____
10. The eyeball and all its supporting structures are contained in the orbit of the skull. _____
11. The zygomatic arch extends from just below the lateral margin of the eye toward the middle part of the external nose. _____
12. Those lingual structures closest to the palate are palatal. _____
13. Deep within each vestibule is the vestibular fornix where two tissue types meet at the mucobuccal fold. _____
14. An excess amount of linea alba on either the buccal mucosa or tongue can be associated with certain orofacial parafunctional habits. _____
15. The maxilla is a single bone with a movable articulation with the temporal bones at each temporomandibular joint. _____
16. The etiology of a lesion is its cause. _____
17. The dense pad of tissue located just distal to the last tooth of the mandibular arch is the retromolar pad. _____
18. A similar ridge to the linea alba can sometimes be present on the lateral border of the tongue. _____
19. Each body of the maxilla contains the nasal sinuses. _____
20. The alveolar process is the bony extension for both the maxilla and mandible that contain each alveolus. _____
21. The buccal mucosa covers a dense pad of underlying adipose or fat tissue at the posterior part of each oral vestibule, the retromolar pad. _____
22. Both the labial and buccal mucosa may vary in coloration to include these darker pink tones, especially with darker skin tones. _____

23. The interdental gingiva is the gingival tissue between adjacent teeth adjoining attached gingiva. _____
24. The inner surface of the gingival tissue where each tooth faces a space is the gingival sulcus. _____
25. The region on the inside of the jaws with the teeth is known as the *oral cavity proper*. _____
26. Posteriorly, the opening from the oral cavity proper into the pharynx is the palate. _____
27. The palatine tonsils are located on the lateral side of the tongue. _____
28. A midline ridge of tissue on the hard palate is the retromolar pad. _____
29. The palatine rugae are firm irregular ridges of tissue radiating from the incisive papilla and median palatine raphe. _____
30. The sulcus terminalis separates the base from the body of the tongue. _____
31. If disruption of the vermilion zone and its mucocutaneous junction at the vermilion border has been caused by a traumatic incident, recording it is important, given that the rest of the oral cavity may be affected. _____
32. If considering the diagnosis of cancer, this can be verified only with tissue biopsy and microscopic examination. _____
33. The risk of cancerous changes with the lips can be increased only with chronic alcohol abuse but not with chronic nicotine use. _____
34. The protection of only the lower lip with sunscreen is important because sun exposure increases the risk of cancerous changes. _____
35. Observable surface changes may be caused by underlying associated histologic tissue changes. _____
36. The face can be divided vertically into fourths, and this perspective is considered the vertical dimension of the face. _____
37. A discussion of vertical dimension allows a comparison of the divisions of the face for functional and esthetic purposes using the guidelines of the Golden Proportions. _____
38. Surface changes in the features of the face and neck may be caused by underlying developmental disturbances. _____
39. Knowledge of the surface features of the face and neck additionally allows the dental professionals understand the associated developmental pattern. _____
40. The surface of the tooth is covered by the moderately hard outer enamel layer with an extremely hard inner dentin. _____
41. To examine the area of focus successfully for the dental professional, it is important to know the boundaries, terminology, and divisions of the oral cavity as well as the pharynx. _____
42. The outermost layer of the root(s) is composed of cementum. _____
43. Included within the oral cavity proper are the palate, tongue, and floor of the mouth. _____
44. Exostoses appear on radiographs as radiopaque (light) areas. _____
45. An atypical finding present usually on the facial surface of the alveolar process of the maxillary arch includes a palatal torus. _____
46. Mandibular tori are usually present bilaterally in the area of the premolars and can appear as lobulated or nodular raised areas. _____
47. More serious pathology of the palate, such as a history of cleft palate, needs to be recorded because of its impact on dental care. _____
48. The laryngopharynx is clinically observable in most cases to the dental professional. _____
49. The pharynx has two divisions, the oropharynx and the laryngopharynx. _____
50. The structure of the fauces marks the boundary between the oropharynx and the oral cavity proper. _____

Ordering Exercises

1. In what order should the facial surface features be placed, going from superior to inferior on the face?

    _____ a. Infraorbital region

_____ b. Mental region

_____ c. Orbital region

_____ d. Frontal region

2. In what order should these oral region features be placed, going from the outer part to inner part of the upper lip?

    _____ a. Vermilion zone

    _____ b. Mucocutaneous junction

    _____ c. Tubercle of the upper lip

    _____ d. Philtrum

3. In what order should these facial surface features be placed, going from inner to outer on the face?

    _____ a. Nasal region

    _____ b. External ear

    _____ c. Infraorbital region

    _____ d. Zygomatic region

4. In what order should these facial surface features be placed, going from superior to inferior on the face?

    _____ a. Philtrum

    _____ b. Root of the nose

    _____ c. Nares

    _____ d. Apex of the nose

5. In what order should these neck surface features be placed, going from superior to inferior on the neck?

    _____ a. Thyroid cartilage

    _____ b. Hyoid bone

    _____ c. Mandible

    _____ d. Thyroid gland

6. In what order should these facial surface features be placed, going from inner to outer on the face?

    _____ a. Mandibular condyle

    _____ b. Labial commissures

    _____ c. Mandibular notch

    _____ d. Coronoid process

7. In what order should these oral cavity features be placed, going from superior to inferior on the maxillary arch?

    _____ a. Attached gingiva

    _____ b. Marginal gingiva

    _____ c. Mucogingival junction

    _____ d. Alveolar mucosa

8. In what order should these oral cavity features be placed, going from anterior to posterior on the palate?

    _____ a. Palatal rugae

    _____ b. Incisive papilla

    _____ c. Maxillary incisors

    _____ d. Attached gingiva

9. In what order should these oral cavity features be placed, going from anterior to posterior on the dorsal surface of the tongue?

    _____ a. Body of the tongue

    _____ b. Apex of the tongue

    _____ c. Base of the tongue

    _____ d. Sulcus terminalis

10. In what order should each of these features of both the larynx and pharynx be placed, going from superior to inferior within the neck area?

    _____ a. Nasopharynx

    _____ b. Larynx

    _____ c. Oropharynx

    _____ d. Laryngopharynx

UNIT 2: DENTAL EMBRYOLOGY

Matching Exercises

a.	Cloacal membrane	k.	Mesoderm	u.	Meckel cartilage
b.	Differentiation	l.	Morphogenesis	v.	Secondary palate
c.	Ectoderm	m.	Neural crest cells	w.	Cap stage
d.	Embryonic period	n.	Neuroectoderm	x.	Primary palate
e.	Endoderm	o.	Oropharyngeal membrane	y.	Supernumerary teeth
f.	Fetal period	p.	Placenta	z.	Frontonasal process
g.	Fusion	q.	Preimplantation period		
h.	Induction	r.	Primitive streak		
i.	Maturation	s.	Proliferation		
j.	Mesenchyme	t.	Somites		

1. Period when fertilization and implantation both occur _____
2. Period involving development of embryo _____
3. Second week to eighth week of prenatal development _____
4. Action of one group of cells on another leading establishment of developmental pathway in responding tissue _____
5. Controlled cellular growth and accumulation of by-products _____
6. Change in initially identical embryonic cells to become distinct structurally and functionally _____
7. Development of specific tissue structure or differing form due to embryonic cell migration and inductive interactions _____
8. Adult function and size attainment due to proliferation, differentiation, and morphogenesis _____
9. Originates directly from epiblast layer high columnar cells _____
10. Future layer that involved with dermis, muscle, and bone formation _____
11. Layer of cuboidal cells within embryo involved with respiratory epithelium and gland cell formation _____
12. Considered by many histologists to be fourth embryonic layer _____
13. Prenatal organ that joins pregnant female and developing embryo _____
14. Grooved rod-shaped thickening in midline of embryonic disc _____
15. Differentiates to form most of connective tissue of the head _____
16. Location of future primitive mouth of embryo _____
17. Location of future end of embryo's digestive tract _____
18. Specialized group of cells that differentiates from ectoderm localized to neural plate _____

19. Elimination of groove between two adjacent swellings of tissue or processes on embryo surface _____
20. Mesoderm that additionally differentiates and begins to divide into paired cuboidal condensation of cells _____
21. Most disappear as bony mandible forms by intramembranous ossification _____
22. Forms as bulge of tissue at most cephalic end of embryo _____
23. Initially serves as partial separation between developing oral cavity proper and nasal cavity _____
24. Will develop into posterior two-thirds of hard palate _____
25. Developmental disturbance involving initiation resulting in development of one or more extra teeth _____
26. Stage of unequal growth in different parts of tooth bud to produce different form _____

True or False Exercises

1. The face and its related tissue begin to form during the sixth week of prenatal development. _____
2. All three embryonic layers are involved in facial development. _____
3. Facial development is completed for the most part during the twelfth week of prenatal development. _____
4. The overall growth of the face is in a superior and posterior direction in relationship to the cranial base. _____
5. The stomodeum initially appears as a shallow depression in the embryonic surface ectoderm at the cephalic end. _____
6. Oral epithelium is derived from ectoderm as a result of embryonic folding. _____
7. The paired maxillary processes fuse at the midline to form the mandibular arch. _____
8. The placodes are rounded areas of specialized thickened ectoderm found at the location of developing structures. _____
9. The paired medial nasal processes also fuse internally and grow inferiorly on the inside of the stomodeum, forming the intermaxillary segment. _____
10. The upper lip is formed when each maxillary process fuses with each nearby medial nasal process. _____
11. The beginnings of the embryo's hollow tube are derived from the anterior part of the midgut. _____
12. The stacked bilateral outer swellings of tissue that appear inferior to the stomodeum that include the mandibular arch are the pharyngeal pouches. _____
13. Palatal fusion allows the fusion of swellings or tissue from different surfaces of the embryo. _____
14. The intermaxillary segment develops into the secondary palate. _____
15. The secondary palate will develop into the anterior one-third of the hard palate. _____
16. In the future, the neural crest cells will become involved in the formation of components of the nervous system as well as pigment-producing melanocyte cells. _____
17. The tongue develops during the fourth to eighth weeks of prenatal development. _____
18. Tongue development begins as a triangular median swelling, the tuberculum impar. _____
19. The copula is formed from the fusion of mesenchyme of second, third, and fourth pharyngeal/branchial arches. _____
20. The foramen cecum is the beginning of the thymus gland. _____
21. The oral epithelium grows deeper into the ectomesenchyme and is induced to produce a layer of the dental membrane. _____
22. A depression results in the deepest part of each tooth bud of dental lamina and forms the enamel knot. _____

23. The dental papilla will produce the future dentin and pulp for the inner part of the tooth. _____
24. Three embryologic structures, the enamel organ, dental papilla, and dental sac, are considered together to be the tooth germ. _____
25. After the inner enamel epithelium differentiates into preameloblasts, the outer cells of the dental papilla are induced by the preameloblasts to differentiate into ameloblasts. _____
26. Developmental disturbances can occur within each stage of odontogenesis, affecting the physiologic processes taking place. _____
27. The initial teeth for both dentitions develop in the anterior maxillary region. _____
28. The primary dentition develops during only the embryonic period of prenatal development. _____
29. The second stage of odontogenesis is considered bud stage and occurs at the beginning of the eighth week of prenatal development for the primary dentition. _____
30. The dental sac will produce the periodontium, the supporting tissue types of the tooth. _____
31. Dental professionals need to have a clear understanding of the major events of prenatal development in order to understand the development of the structures of the face, neck, and oral cavity and the underlying relationships among these structures. _____
32. Prenatal development begins with the start of pregnancy and continues and concludes with the formation of the embryo. _____
33. Developmental disturbances can involve the orofacial structures as well as other parts of the body. _____
34. Noninvasive prenatal testing is a cell-free fetal deoxyribonucleic acid testing that involves a simple blood draw from the pregnant female. _____
35. Environmental agents and factors involved in causing developmental disturbances can include infections and radiation but not the use of certain prescription drugs. _____
36. Females of reproductive age should avoid teratogens to protect the developing infant from possible developmental disturbances. _____
37. Down syndrome is developmental disturbance involving an extra chromosome number 12 that remains present after meiotic division. _____
38. The ectomesenchyme is derived from neural crest cells that have migrated to the region of tooth development. _____
39. Ectodermal dysplasia has a hereditary etiology and presents with developmental disturbances of the teeth, skin, hair, nails, eyes, facial structure, and glands. _____
40. If there is failure of migration of the neural crest cells to the neck region, Treacher Collins syndrome develops within the fetus. _____
41. Systemic tetracycline antibiotic therapy of the pregnant female can act as a teratogenic drug during the fetal period. _____
42. A cleft lip results from a failure of the endoderm to grow beneath the mesoderm to obliterate any grooves between these processes or even a deficiency or absence of mesenchyme in the area. _____
43. The structures of the developing palate gradually fuse in a zipper-like manner from a posterior to an anterior direction. _____
44. Most developmental disturbances in the neck originate during transformation of the pharyngeal/branchial apparatus into its mature derivatives. _____
45. The first pharyngeal/branchial grooves occasionally can fail to become obliterated and thus parts remain to form a cervical lymphoepithelial cyst. _____
46. Failure of fusion of the palatal shelves with the primary palate, with each other, or both results in cleft palate. _____
47. Abnormally large teeth result in microdontia; abnormally small teeth result in macrodontia. _____
48. Misplaced ameloblasts can migrate to the surface of the root to produce an enamel pearl. _____

49. Developmental root anatomy variants may involve a linguogingival or palatogingival groove as well as a proximal root groove. _____

50. The primary tooth often starts to erupt before the permanent tooth is fully shed, which may create complications in spacing. _____

Ordering Exercises

1. In what order should these events during prenatal development be noted, going from earlier to later in time span?

   _____ a. Fertilization

   _____ b. Preimplantation period

   _____ c. Fetal period

   _____ d. Embryonic period

2. In what order should these events occurring during prenatal development be noted, going from earlier to later in time span?

   _____ a. Mitosis

   _____ b. Implantation

   _____ c. Meiosis

   _____ d. Sperm and egg union

3. In what order should these structures present during prenatal development be noted, going from earlier to later in time span?

   _____ a. Fetus

   _____ b. Embryo

   _____ c. Blastocyst

   _____ d. Zygote

4. In what order should these prenatal structures be placed, going from closest to farthest in relationship to the endometrium lining the uterus?

   _____ a. Amniotic cavity

   _____ b. Hypoblast layer

   _____ c. Epiblast layer

   _____ d. Yolk sac

5. In what order should these prenatal structures be placed, going from superior to inferior in relationship to the embryo?

   _____ a. Midgut

   _____ b. Hindgut

   _____ c. Foregut

   _____ d. Oropharyngeal membrane

6. In what order should these structures present during prenatal development be noted, going from earlier to later in time span?

   _____ a. Stomodeum

   _____ b. Mandibular processes

   _____ c. Mandibular arch

   _____ d. Primitive mouth

7. In what order should these prenatal structures be placed, going from superior to inferior in relationship to the embryo?

   _____ a. Hyoid arch

   _____ b. Third pharyngeal/branchial arch

   _____ c. Mandibular arch

   _____ d. Fourth pharyngeal/branchial arch

8. In what order should these prenatal structures be placed, going from superior to inferior in relationship to the embryo?

   _____ a. Frontonasal process

   _____ b. Maxillary processes

   _____ c. Mandibular arch

   _____ d. Stomodeum

9. In what order should these structures present during palatal development be noted, going from earlier to later in time span?

   _____ a. Primary palate

   _____ b. Intermaxillary segment

   _____ c. Palatal shelves

   _____ d. Secondary palate

10. In what order should these structures present during tongue development be noted, going from earlier to later in time span?

    _____ a. Hypopharyngeal eminence

    _____ b. Lateral lingual swellings

    _____ c. Epiglottic swelling

    _____ d. Tuberculum impar

11. In what order should these events during odontogenesis be noted, going from earlier to later in time span?

    _____ a. Bud stage

    _____ b. Cap stage

    _____ c. Initiation stage

    _____ d. Bell stage

12. In what order should these layers of the enamel organ be placed, going from the outer part to inner part in relationship to the overall tooth?

    _____ a. Outer enamel epithelium

    _____ b. Stellate reticulum

    _____ c. Inner enamel epithelium

    _____ d. Stratum intermedium

UNIT 3: DENTAL HISTOLOGY

Matching Exercises

a.	Anaphase	k.	Mucoperiosteum	u.	Interglobular dentin
b.	Basement membrane	l.	Nucleoplasm	v.	Lamina dura
c.	Cell	m.	Organ	w.	Sulcular epithelium
d.	Connective tissue	n.	Organelles	x.	Fibroblast
e.	Intercellular fluid	o.	Prophase	y.	Gingival recession
f.	Epithelium	p.	Rete ridges	z.	Attrition
g.	Granulation tissue	q.	System		
h.	Histology	r.	Telophase		
i.	Interphase	s.	Tissue		
j.	Metaphase	t.	von Ebner		

1. Study of microscopic structure and function of cells and tissue _____
2. Smallest living unit of organization _____
3. Collection of similarly specialized cells _____
4. Independent body part formed from tissue _____
5. Organs functioning together _____
6. Semifluid part contained within cell membrane boundary _____
7. Chromatin condenses into chromosomes _____
8. Mitotic spindle forms during cell division _____
9. Migration of chromatids to opposite poles by mitotic spindle _____
10. Reappearance of nuclear membrane _____
11. Cells between divisions involved in this time period _____
12. Specialized metabolically active structures within cell _____
13. Fluid part within nucleus of cell _____
14. Tissue type that covers and lines external and internal body surfaces _____
15. Extensions of epithelium into connective tissue _____
16. Thin acellular structure located between any form of epithelium and its underlying connective tissue _____
17. Most common type of basic tissue by weight _____
18. Immature connective tissue with few fibers and increased amount of blood vessels _____
19. Consisting of mucous membrane combined with periosteum of adjacent bone _____
20. Glands present in submucosa deep to lamina propria of circumvallate lingual papillae _____

21. Wearing of hard tissue as result of tooth-to-tooth contact _____
22. Can cause root dentin to be exposed with thin layer of cementum lost _____
23. Only primary mineralization has occurred within predentin _____
24. Part of alveolar bone proper present on dental imaging _____
25. Most common cell in periodontal ligament _____
26. Stands away from tooth creating gingival sulcus _____

True or False Exercises

1. The interdental gingiva assumes a nonvisible concave form between the facial and lingual gingival surfaces, which is considered the col. _____
2. _____
3. In some cases, a free gingival groove separates the sulcular gingiva from the marginal gingiva. _____
4. The dentogingival junction is the junction between the tooth surface and the periodontal ligament. _____
5. The sulcular epithelium is of an orthokeratinized type, with its cells tightly packed. _____
6. Before the eruption of the tooth and after enamel maturation, the ameloblasts secrete a basal lamina on the surface that serves as a part of the primary epithelial attachment. _____
7. An endocrine gland is a gland having a duct associated with it. _____
8. Saliva supplies the minerals for subgingival calculus formation. _____
9. Mucoserous acini have both a group of mucous cells surrounding the lumen and a serous demilune. _____
10. More than one myoepithelial cell can sometimes be found on a single acinus. _____
11. The submandibular salivary gland is the smallest, most diffuse, and only unencapsulated major salivary gland. _____
12. The parathyroid glands typically consist of two small endocrine glands on each side of the thyroid gland. _____
13. Extracellular fluid drains from the surrounding region into the lymphatic vessels as lymph. _____
14. Each lymphatic follicle has a germinal center containing many immature lymphocytes. _____
15. Intraoral tonsillar tissue consists of nonencapsulated masses of lymphoid tissue located in the lamina propria of the oral mucosa. _____
16. The palatine tonsils are four rounded masses of variable size located between the anterior and posterior faucial pillars. _____
17. The lingual tonsil is an indistinct layer of diffuse lymphoid tissue located on the lateral surface of the tongue. _____
18. Each lateral wall of the nasal cavity has three projecting structures or nasal conchae that extend inward. _____
19. The nasal cavity is lined by a respiratory mucosa like the rest of the respiratory system. _____
20. The moist mucus forms a deep-layered system within the respiratory mucosa near the basement membrane. _____
21. The underlying histologic states of its components provide a clue to the clinical features noted visibly with the periodontium, whether in a healthy or pathologic state. _____
22. The mature cementum consists of mainly calcium hydroxyapatite with the chemical formula of $Ca_{10}(PO4)_6(OH)_2$. _____
23. The trabecular bone appears less uniformly radiopaque and more porous than the uniformly radiopaque lamina dura. _____

24. With the loss of teeth, a patient becomes edentulous, either partially or completely. _____
25. During the chronic advanced type of periodontal disease of periodontitis, the basal bone is the first to be lost. _____
26. The epithelial rests of Malassez are present within the alveolar process but can become cystic. _____
27. The periodontal ligament is wider near the apex and cervix of the tooth. _____
28. During mastication and speech, certain forces are exerted on a tooth, such as rotational, tilting, extrusive, or intrusive. _____
29. The interradicular group of the alveolodental ligament is found only between the alveolar crests of neighboring teeth. _____
30. The dentogingival ligament is the most extensive of the gingival fiber group. _____
31. A type of intercellular junction is formed by a desmosome, which involves an attachment of a cell to an adjacent noncellular surface. _____
32. The turnover time is faster for all types of connective tissue as compared to epithelium. _____
33. The details of the basement membrane are not noted with lower-power magnification. _____
34. The amount of scar tissue varies, depending on the type and size of the injury, amount of granulation tissue, and movement of tissue after injury. _____
35. By age 10, the skin begins to deteriorate and by the age of 20 is in a rapid state of degradation because of the aging process. _____
36. Microscopically a cross-section of bone demonstrates layers related to its development that look like growth rings in a tree. _____
37. Changes such as hyperkeratinization are reversible if the source of the injury is removed, but it takes time for the keratin to be shed by the tissue. _____
38. The two types of taste bud cells are the supporting cells and the taste cells. _____
39. The lesion of geographic tongue shows the sensitivity of the fungiform lingual papillae to changes in their environment. _____
40. The pigmentation of both the oral mucosa and skin may increase with certain endocrine pathologic conditions. _____
41. All regions of the oral cavity have a faster turnover time than the skin. _____
42. The formation of increased scar tissue in the oral mucosa is useful both esthetically and functionally when oral or periodontal surgery is performed. _____
43. The biologic width describes the heights of the suprabony soft tissue. _____
44. The gingival phenotype is the width of the gingiva within the mesiodistal dimension. _____
45. The junctional epithelium is attached on the other side to the laminal propria of nearby gingiva, as is the sulcular epithelium. _____
46. The junctional epithelium has only one basal lamina and it faces the tooth. _____
47. The amount of gingival overgrowth through drug-influenced gingival hyperplasia is related to the drug dosage. _____
48. The increased production of saliva is considered xerostomia and can result in overall moist mouth or hypersalivation. _____
49. A common developmental disturbance is the deepened pit and groove patterns on the facial surface of anterior teeth and on the root surface of posterior teeth. _____
50. An unwanted side effect of rapid orthodontic therapy can be root apex resorption, reducing the overall length of the tooth. _____

Ordering Exercises

1. In what order should these cellular structures be placed, going from outer part to inner part of the cell?

    _____ a. Cell membrane

    _____ b. Nucleolus

    _____ c. Nucleus

    _____ d. Nuclear membrane

2. In what order should these components of the body be noted, going from a simple to a more complex type of organization?

   _____ a. Cell

   _____ b. Organ

   _____ c. Tissue

   _____ d. System

3. In what order should these phases present during mitosis be noted, going from earlier to later in time span?

   _____ a. Anaphase

   _____ b. Prophase

   _____ c. Metaphase

   _____ d. Telophase

4. In what order should these bone layers be placed, going from superficial to deeper layers in the tissue?

   _____ a. Compact bone

   _____ b. Endosteum

   _____ c. Periosteum

   _____ d. Cancellous bone

5. In what order should these steps present during endochondral ossification be noted, going from earlier to later in time span?

   _____ a. Formation of primary ossification centers

   _____ b. Osteoblasts penetrate cartilage

   _____ c. Production of osteoid in layers

   _____ d. Cartilage disintegrates

6. In what order should these components of skeletal muscle be placed, going from superficial to deeper layers in relationship to the muscle bundle?

   _____ a. Myofilaments

   _____ b. Myofibers

   _____ c. Myofibrils

   _____ d. Muscle fascicles

7. In what order should these layers of orthokeratinized stratified squamous epithelium be placed, going from superficial to deeper layers in the tissue?

   _____ a. Keratin layer

   _____ b. Basal layer

   _____ c. Prickle layer

   _____ d. Granular layer

8. In what order should these salivary glands be noted, going from largest to smallest as related to individual size?

   _____ a. von Ebner gland

   _____ b. Submandibular gland

   _____ c. Parotid gland

   _____ d. Sublingual gland

9. In what order should these components of salivary glands be placed, going from larger to smaller in size as well as superficial to deeper within the gland?

   _____ a. Lobes

   _____ b. Acini

   _____ c. Capsule

   _____ d. Lobules

10. In what order should these components of salivary glands be placed, going from superficial to deeper in the gland?

    _____ a. Intercalated duct

    _____ b. Acinus

    _____ c. Striated duct

    _____ d. Excretory duct

11. In what order should these components of the thyroid gland be placed, going from larger to smaller in size as well as superficial to deeper within the gland?

    _____ a. Lobes

    _____ b. Follicles

    _____ c. Capsule

    _____ d. Lobules

12. In what order should these components of a lymph node be noted, going the same way as the flow of lymph first entering and then exiting the node?

    _____ a. Efferent vessel

    _____ b. Lymphatic vessel

    _____ c. Afferent vessel

    _____ d. Hilus

13. In what order should these components of a lymph node be placed, going from larger to smaller in size as well as superficial to deeper within the node?

    _____ a. Lymphatic follicle

    _____ b. Trabeculae

    _____ c. Capsule

    _____ d. Germinal center

14. In what order should these events involving the ameloblasts during odontogenesis be placed, going from earlier to later in time span?

    _____ a. Forming enamel matrix from Tomes process

    _____ b. Actively transporting materials for mineralization

    _____ c. Becoming part of reduced enamel epithelium

    _____ d. Removing water and organic material from enamel

15. In what order should these zones in pulp be placed, going from the outer pulpal wall near the dentin to the inner part of the pulp?

    _____ a. Pulpal core

    _____ b. Cell-rich zone

    _____ c. Cell-free zone

    _____ d. Odontoblastic layer

16. In what order should these fiber groups of the alveolodental ligament of the periodontal ligament be placed, going from the cementoenamel junction to the tooth apex?

    _____ a. Horizontal group

    _____ b. Oblique group

    _____ c. Alveolar crest group

    _____ d. Apical group

UNIT 4: DENTAL ANATOMY

Matching Exercises

a.	Anatomic root	k.	Furcation	u.	Occlusal table
b.	Bicuspid	l.	Mamelons	v.	Transverse ridge
c.	Bifurcated	m.	Occlusion	w.	Trifurcated
d.	Bruxism	n.	Overjet	x.	Curve of Wilson
e.	Centric relationship	o.	Palmer Notation Method	y.	Wisdom teeth
f.	Cervical ridge	p.	Primate spaces	z.	Articular fossa
g.	Cingulum	q.	Sextant		
h.	Contact	r.	Adult teeth		
i.	Cuspids	s.	Supplemental grooves		
j.	Diastema	t.	Supporting cusps		

1. Other name for permanent dentition that is more commonly used by patients _____

2. Tooth numbering system commonly used during orthodontic therapy _____

3. Used to describe anatomic alignment of teeth and relationship to rest of masticatory system _____

4. Division of each dental arch into three parts based on relationship to midline _____

5. Part of root covered by layer of cementum _____

6. Raised rounded area on cervical third of lingual surface of anterior teeth _____

7. Rounded enamel extensions on incisal ridge from either labial or lingual views _____

8. Mainly considered as open contact between permanent maxillary central incisors _____

9. Another term for canines that is still commonly used by patients _____

10. Occlusal surface is bordered by marginal ridges to create inner surface _____

11. Joining of two triangular ridges crossing occlusal surface from labial to lingual outline _____

12. Secondary grooves on occlusal surface that appear as shallow and more irregular linear depressions _____

13. Another term for premolar that is still commonly used by patients _____

14. Maxillary first premolars having two root branches _____

15. Common name used by patients for third molars _____

16. Area between two or more of the root branches before division from root trunk _____

17. Maxillary molars with three root branches _____

18. Spaces between primary maxillary lateral incisor and canine and also between primary mandibular canine and first molar _____

19. Ridge more prominent on primary molars than any similar structure on permanent molar _____

20. Cause of extensive wear of incisal edge of primary incisor _____

21. End point of closure of mandible _____

22. Maxillary dental arch horizontally overlaps mandibular arch _____

23. Area on proximal surfaces of teeth with same-arch neighbors _____

24. Concave curve that results when sectioning through each set of molars _____

25. Cusps that function during centric occlusion _____

26. Depression on inferior aspect of temporal bone _____

True or False Exercises

1. The curve of Wilson is produced by the curved alignment of all the teeth and is especially evident when viewing the posterior teeth from the buccal. _____

2. Phase three of arch development begins when the canines wedge themselves between the lateral incisors and the first premolars. _____

3. Open contacts allow areas of food impaction from opposing cusps resulting in trauma to the gingivosulcular area; these opposing cusps are considered. _____

4. Overbite is measured in millimeters with the tip of a periodontal probe. _____

5. If a tooth is lost for a longer period, the neighboring teeth usually become more upright in an effort to fill the edentulous space. _____

6. Triangular grooves separate a marginal ridge from the triangular ridge of a cusp and at their terminations form the triangular fossae. _____

7. The contact areas of posterior teeth are wider than anterior teeth and usually located to the lingual of center as well as nearer the same level on each proximal surface. _____

8. Some inclined cuspal planes are functional and thus involved in the occlusion of the teeth. _____

9. The crown of each posterior tooth has an occlusal surface as its masticatory surface, bordered by the raised marginal ridges, which are located on both the facial surface and lingual surface. _____

10. Most permanent maxillary first premolars are trifurcated, having two root branches in the apical third, with a buccal root and a lingual root. _____

11. Permanent maxillary second premolars erupt between 10 and 12 years of age. _____

12. There is one form of permanent mandibular first premolars, the tricuspidate form, which is a three-cusp type. _____

13. The permanent dentition is also sometimes considered the nonsuccedaneous dentition because all of these permanent teeth succeed primary predecessors. _____

14. The molars, because of their tapered shape and their prominent single cusp, function to pierce or tear food during mastication. _____

15. A tooth numbering system that is commonly used in orthodontic therapy is the Palmer Notation Method. _____

16. The joint capsule outer layer is a synovial membrane, which consists of a thin connective tissue with nerves and blood vessels. _____

17. The central area of the temporomandibular joint disc is vascularized and has innervation. _____

18. Lateral deviation of the mandible, or lateral excursion, which involves shifting the lower jaw to one side, occurs during mastication. _____

19. Not all patients with temporomandibular disorders have abnormalities in the joint disc or even in the joint itself; most symptoms seem to originate from the muscles. _____

20. The Palmer Notation Method is recorded using an easy to view graphic system. _____

21. The permanent dentition period begins with the eruption of the primary mandibular central incisors. _____

22. The mixed dentition period occurs between 6 and 12 years of age. _____
23. A growth center is located in the head of each mandibular condyle before an individual can reach maturity. _____
24. Lateral deviation involves only gliding movements of contralateral temporomandibular joints in their respective joint cavities. _____
25. When the teeth of the occlusion are in the position of centric occlusion, each tooth of one arch is in occlusion with two others in the opposing arch, except for a few teeth. _____
26. Premature contacts are where one or two teeth contact after the other teeth. _____
27. The permanent canine on each side should usually be the only tooth in function during lateral occlusion. _____
28. The permanent central incisors are closest to the midline, and the permanent lateral incisors are the second teeth from the midline. _____
29. The pulp chamber of the permanent maxillary central incisor has two sharp elongations: the mesial and distal pulp horns. _____
30. The lingual surface of the crown of a permanent maxillary lateral incisor is narrower overall than the labial surface. _____
31. The crown of a permanent mandibular central incisor is quite asymmetrical from the labial view. _____
32. Because of their tapered shape and prominent single cusp, the permanent canines function to pierce or tear food during mastication. _____
33. The mesial half of the crown of a permanent maxillary canine resembles a part of a premolar, and the distal half resembles a part of a permanent incisor. _____
34. Like anterior teeth, multirooted permanent premolars and molars originate as a single root on the base of the crown. _____
35. Because the permanent maxillary first molar has both a buccal and lingual root, it also has two furcations. _____
36. The lingual cusp is slightly displaced to the distal, which helps distinguish the permanent maxillary right second premolar from the left. _____
37. Both types of permanent mandibular premolars can present difficulties during periodontal instrumentation due to narrow lingual surfaces combined with the lingual inclination of the crown. _____
38. The permanent mandibular first molar has the most complex developmental groove pattern of all the permanent mandibular molars. _____
39. The two roots of a permanent mandibular first molar are smaller, shorter, and less divergent than those of a second molar. _____
40. The pulp cavity of a permanent mandibular first molar is more likely to have three pulp canals, distal, mesiobuccal, and mesiolingual with and five pulp horns. _____
41. Permanent maxillary third molars, along with the mandibular third molars, commonly are involved with partial anodontia, being developmentally missing. _____
42. The distinct oblique ridge is less pronounced on the permanent maxillary second molar than on the first molar. _____
43. From the mesial, the mesial contact area of a permanent maxillary second molar is larger, and the cervical flattening or concavity is never as pronounced as in a first molar. _____
44. The two roots on permanent maxillary second molars are smaller than the first molars. _____
45. Loss of the tooth is followed by mesial inclination and drift of the maxillary second molar into the open arch space, and the mandibular first molar, if present, also supererupts. _____
46. On the permanent maxillary first molar, the two marginal ridges and two cusp ridges of the four major cusps are found bordering the occlusal table on the buccal and lingual margins. _____
47. The crown of any primary tooth is short in relation to its total length. _____
48. Overall, the dentin of the primary dentition is thicker than that of the permanent counterparts. _____

49. From the labial aspect, the crown of the primary maxillary central incisor appears wider mesiodistally than incisocervically, the opposite of its permanent successor. _____

50. The crown of the primary maxillary first molar does not resemble any other crown of either dentition. _____

Ordering Exercises

1. In what order should the following general dental terms be placed when giving the name of a tooth, going from the largest number of teeth included in an adult to the smallest number of teeth?

    _____ a. Dentition

    _____ b. Quadrant

    _____ c. Arch

    _____ d. Sextant

2. In what order should the following line angles of an anterior tooth be placed, going from mesial to distal for the front surface of the tooth and then in the same direction for the back surface of the tooth?

    _____ a. Mesiolabial

    _____ b. Distolabial

    _____ c. Mesiolingual

    _____ d. Distolingual

3. In what order should the following permanent incisors be placed, going from largest in overall size to smallest?

    _____ a. Mandibular lateral

    _____ b. Mandibular central

    _____ c. Maxillary central

    _____ d. Maxillary lateral

4. In what order should the following permanent teeth be placed according to their approximate eruption dates, going from earlier to later in time span?

    _____ a. Mandibular central incisors

    _____ b. Maxillary canines

    _____ c. Maxillary first premolars

    _____ d. Mandibular first molars

5. In what order should the following cusps of the permanent mandibular first molar be placed, going from largest in overall size to smallest?

    _____ a. Mesiolingual

    _____ b. Distolingual

    _____ c. Distobuccal

    _____ d. Mesiobuccal

6. In what order should the following cusps of the permanent maxillary first molar be placed, going from largest in overall size to smallest?

    _____ a. Mesiolingual

    _____ b. Distolingual

    _____ c. Distobuccal

    _____ d. Mesiobuccal

7. In what order should the following events during formation of the primary dentition be placed, going from earlier to later in time span?

    _____ a. All teeth have started mineralization

    _____ b. Beginning of tooth mineralization

    _____ c. Completion of full dentition

    _____ d. Eruption of first tooth into oral cavity

8. In what order should these skull features be placed, going from anterior to posterior on the skull?

    _____ a. Postglenoid process

    _____ b. Articular eminence

    _____ c. Zygomatic arch

    _____ d. Articular fossa

9. In what order should the following permanent premolars be placed, going from largest in overall size to smallest?

    _____ a. Mandibular first

    _____ b. Mandibular second

    _____ c. Maxillary first

    _____ d. Maxillary second

10. In what order should the following permanent teeth be placed according to their approximate eruption dates, going from earlier to later in time span?

    _____ a. Maxillary lateral incisors

    _____ b. Mandibular canines

    _____ c. Maxillary second premolars

    _____ d. Mandibular second molars

The following are **case studies exercises** with questions *per unit* that are based on the National Board Examination Format as determined by the Joint Commission on National Dental Examinations of the American Dental Association. In addition, parts of this exercise are similar those scenarios presented by the National Dental Examining Board of Canada as well as other dental professional examinations worldwide.

Thus these case studies help prepare the student dental professional for competency examinations as well as future clinical situations. Contained within each **patient box** is information available to the dental professional at the time of the dental visit. The clinician should closely consider this information when answering the follow-up questions. If no information is presented in each area of the patient box, then the clinician shoulld assume the information is either unknown or is not available. Figures courtesy M.J. Fehrenbach, RDH, MS, unless otherwise noted.

UNIT 2: DENTAL EMBRYOLOGY CASE STUDY 1

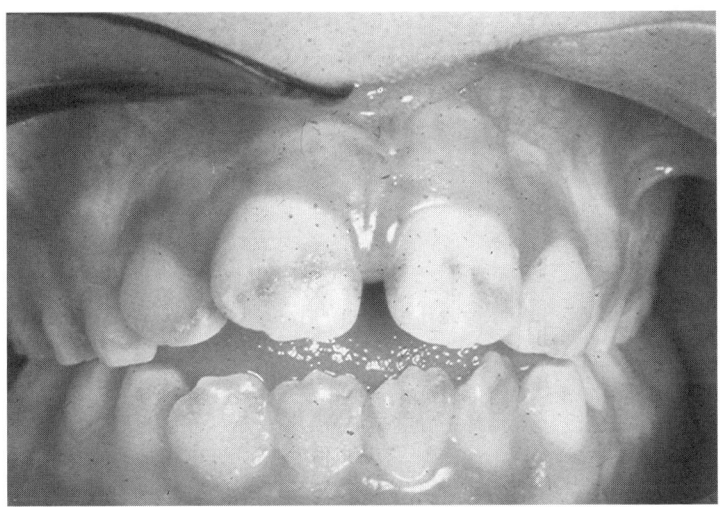

Patient	23 years old
Chief Complaint	"Can we whiten my front teeth as soon as possible?"
Background and/or Patient History	First-grade teacher getting ready for family pictures Regular 6-month dental care until recent move States teeth always appeared stained with past dental office with recommendation of full-coverage crowns when fully erupted High level of fluoride in well water used for drinking as child Digit sucking as child
Current Findings	New patient appointment with previous records including photographs of dentition No fluoridated drinking water or toothpaste used now Regularly chews sugared gum

1. Which of the following developmental disturbances is present involving the patient's anterior teeth of both dental arches?
   A. Concrescence
   B. Enamel dysplasia
   C. Dentin dysplasia
   D. Anodontia

2. Which of the following cell types were mostly disturbed during tooth development so as to cause the chief complaint by the patient?
   A. Odontoblasts
   B. Fibroblasts
   C. Ameloblasts
   D. Cementoblasts

3. During which of the following stage(s) of odontogenesis does this developmental disturbance of the anterior teeth occur?
   A. Bud stage
   B. Initiation stage
   C. Cap or bell stages
   D. Apposition and maturation stages

4. What is the exact type of staining present involving the patient's anterior teeth from the developmental disturbance?
   A. Extrinsic
   B. Intrinsic
   C. Transient
   D. Temporary

5. Because of the bite pattern noted after an evaluation of the occlusion, what is also present on the masticatory surface of the mandibular anterior teeth?
   A. Attrition
   B. Perikymata
   C. Mamelons
   D. Occlusal tables

UNIT 2: DENTAL EMBRYOLOGY CASE STUDY 2

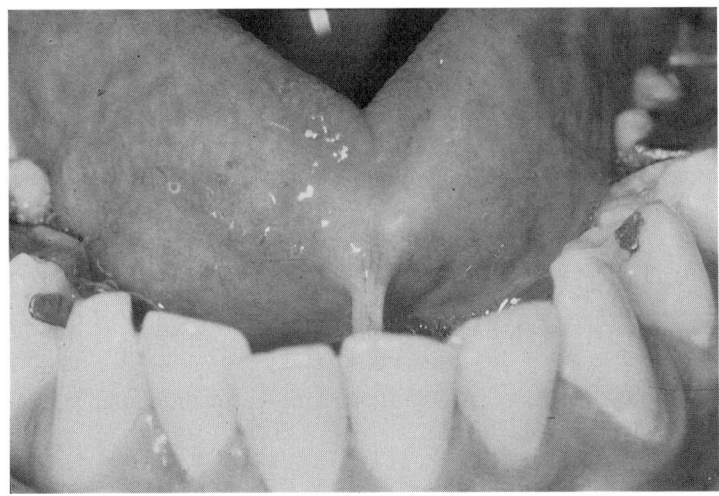

Patient	52 years old
Chief Complaint	"My lower teeth are getting more crowded."
Background and/or Patient History	Historian at local university Stated no history of orofacial surgery or speech therapy
Current Findings	New patient appointment without previous records Mandibular anterior teeth crowded with moderate lingual supragingival calculus Moderate speech impediment Photograph of developmental disturbance taken

1. Which of the following developmental disturbances is present with the patient?
   A. Gemination
   B. Fusion
   C. Ankyloglossia
   D. Mesial drift

2. The developmental disturbance present mostly involves what part of the oral cavity?
   A. Lingual frenum
   B. Soft tissue of floor of the mouth
   C. Mandibular anterior teeth
   D. Mandibular alveolar process

3. In what week of prenatal development does the associated structure involved in the developmental disturbance begin its specific development?
   A. First week
   B. Second week
   C. Third week
   D. Fourth week

4. Which of the following is one of the superficial demarcations for the usual manner of fusion noted in the associated structure(s) involved in this developmental disturbance?
   A. Labial developmental lobes
   B. Sublingual fold
   C. Median lingual sulcus
   D. Cementoenamel junction

5. During which prenatal developmental time span does the associated structure involved in the developmental disturbance complete its fusion?
   A. Fetal period
   B. Embryonic period
   C. Initiation stage
   D. Maturation stage

UNIT 2: DENTAL EMBRYOLOGY CASE STUDY 3

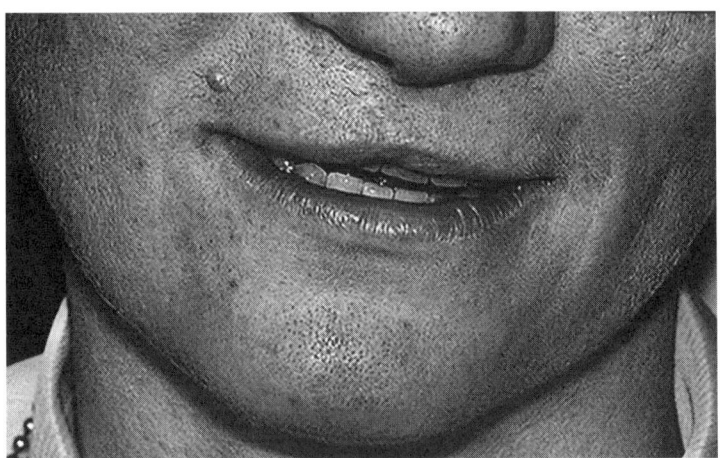

Patient	45 years old
Chief Complaint	"Why do I have so much tartar on my teeth?"
Background and/or Patient History	Surgery as child for "birth defect" left with scar on skin Speech therapy as child but still slight speech impediment Former smoker Allergy to pollens Premenopausal Medications: OTC decongestant spray, short-term hormone replacement therapy
Current Findings	New patient appointment No functional defects noted during occlusal evaluation Mouth breather Maxillary anterior sextant with moderate BOP Generalized moderate supragingival calculus Slight to moderate xerostomia with hyposalivation Photograph of developmental disturbance taken

1. Which of the following developmental disturbances was present at birth as observed on an extraoral examination of the patient?
   A. Tubercle of upper lip
   B. Cleft palate
   C. Cleft lip
   D. Actinic cheilitis

2. Which of the following processes is mostly involved in the developmental disturbance?
   A. Maxillary process
   B. Lateral nasal process
   C. Mandibular process
   D. Frontonasal process

3. Which of the following tissue types shows a failure to grow as well as possibly a deficiency or absence with this distubance?
   A. Mesenchyme
   B. Endoderm
   C. Dermis
   D. Hypodermis

4. Which of the following statements is correct concerning this developmental disturbance?
   A. Only hereditary etiologic factors noted
   B. May be associated with other disturbances
   C. Only occurs unilaterally
   D. Occurs mainly on right side

5. During which prenatal developmental time span does this developmental disturbance usually occur?
   A. Preimplantation period
   B. Embryonic period
   C. Initiation stage
   D. Apposition stage

UNIT 2: DENTAL EMBRYOLOGY CASE STUDY 4

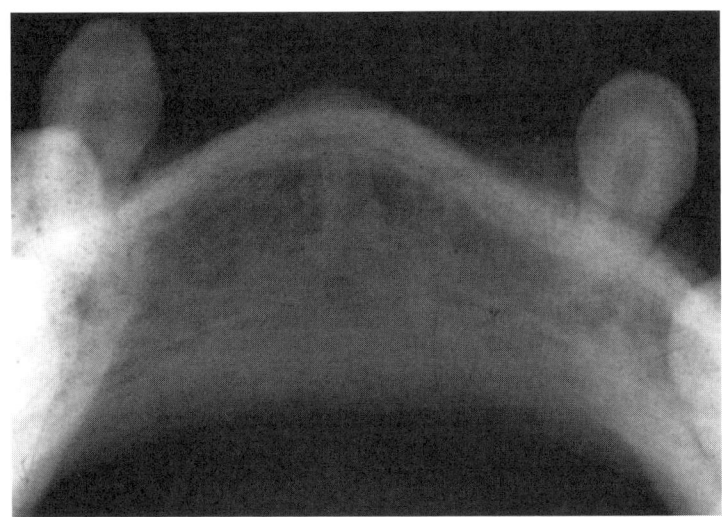

Patient	23 years old
Chief Complaint	"I need to know if I can have those implant teeth put in and when it can happen."
Background and/or Patient History	Aspiring actor after finishing high school drama with honors Needs special measures to keep body temperature regulated Hearing difficulty due to genetic defect States periodic partial dentures replaced over time since preschool
Current Findings	New patient at community dental clinic referred by university nurse Looks older because of sparse hair but has typical orofacial features Missing many teeth and wears ill-fitting upper and lower partial dentures States saving for dental implants placed through reduced-fee program at local dental school Occlusal radiograph taken of mandibular anterior sextant

1. Which of the following developmental disturbances is present with the patient?
   A. Fetal alcohol syndrome
   B. Down syndrome
   C. Ectodermal dysplasia
   D. Treacher Collins syndrome

2. Which of the following can be noted with this developmental disturbance case?
   A. Various levels of intellectual disability
   B. Indistinct philtrum and thin upper lip
   C. Abnormalities of skin, hair, and nails
   D. Epicanthic folds near orbital region

3. The noted developmental disturbance involves which of the following etiologic factors?
   A. Teratogenic
   B. Hereditary
   C. Radiation
   D. Drug usage

4. Which of the following was recommended for the patient in the past and temporarily served both a cosmetic and functional purpose?
   A. Orthodontic therapy
   B. Replacement partial dentures
   C. Surgical removal of many teeth
   D. Monitored speech therapy

5. The structures involved with this developmental disturbance are formed during which prenatal developmental time span?
   A. Fetal period
   B. Embryonic period
   C. Initiation stage
   D. Maturation stage

UNIT 2: DENTAL EMBRYOLOGY CASE STUDY 5

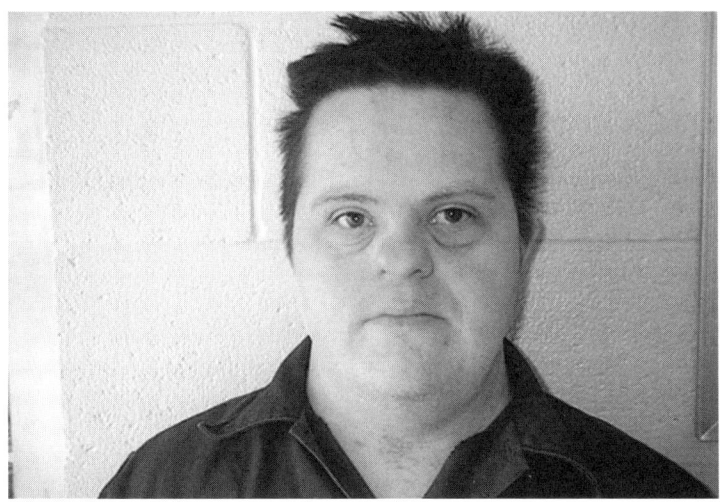

Patient	26 years old
Chief Complaint	"I need teeth done."
Background and/or Patient History	Group home after being home schooled Works part time at library Hypothyroidism related to developmental disturbance Treated for sleep apnea Past speech therapy Medications: Thyroid hormone, antiseizure medication
Current Findings	Patient of record 6-month appointment with identification photograph noted Microdontia Chronic periodontitis with moderate early horizontal bone loss Xerostomia with mouth breathing

1. Which of the following developmental disturbances is present with the patient?
   A. Fetal alcohol syndrome
   B. Down syndrome
   C. Ectodermal dysplasia
   D. Treacher Collins syndrome

2. During which prenatal developmental event does this disturbance occur?
   A. Meiosis
   B. Mitosis
   C. Maturation stage
   D. Mesoderm formation

3. What situation was mostly involved to cause this developmental disturbance?
   A. Toxic teratogen
   B. Hereditary factors
   C. Chromosomal abnormality
   D. Cell migration failure

4. Which of the following may also be present and observed on clinical examination of the patient?
   A. Fissured tongue
   B. Enlarged tongue
   C. Lingual papillae hyperplasia
   D. Grooved upper lip

5. Which of the following is the correct number of chromosomes present after the joining of the sperm and ovum?
   A. 12
   B. 23
   C. 46
   D. 92

UNIT 2: DENTAL EMBRYOLOGY CASE STUDY 6

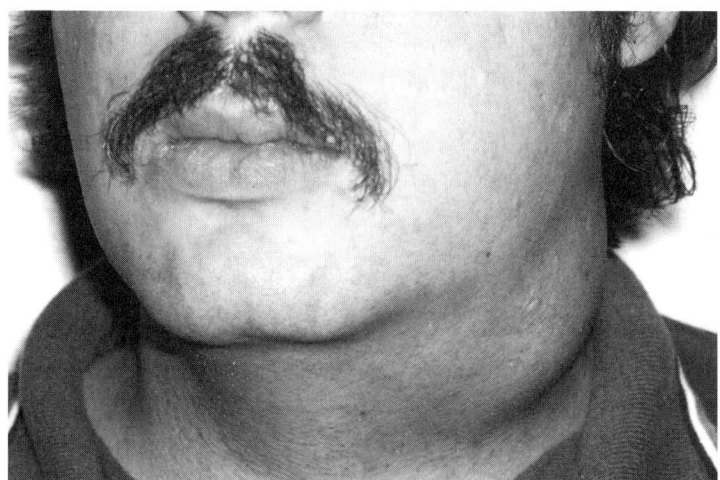

From Neville BW: *Oral and Maxillofacial Pathology*, ed. 5, Elsevier, 2024.

Patient	32 years old
Chief Complaint	"What is the swelling here on my neck?"
Background and/or Patient History	Business administrator who wants diagnosis before taking new job position without insurance Referred by outpatient medical clinic Allergy to pollen No history of night sweats, unexplained weight loss, or chronic fatigue when asked at clinic Medications: OTC allergy pills
Current Findings	New patient appointment with limited examination Large soft swelling on left side of neck near angle of mandible States that lesion present for over 2 years and slowly growing larger No skin discoloration noted over lesion No fever or soreness noted upon palpation of neck lesion Wave effect felt upon palpation of neck lesion No caries or endodontic involvement of any permanent mandibular left posterior teeth noted upon full mouth dental imaging Photograph of cervical region also taken

1. Which of the following is the most likely cause for the patient's neck swelling?
   A. Lymph node infection
   B. Thyroid gland goiter
   C. Temporomandibular disorder
   D. Cervical lymphoepithelial cyst

2. Why does this lesion occur in this region of the neck?
   A. Transformation of pharyngeal/branchial apparatus
   B. Serious infection of regional primary lymph nodes
   C. Secondary pain impulses from nearby joint
   D. Growth from surge in specific hormones

3. Which of the following events usually occurs during the development of the thyroid gland?
   A. Foramen cecum shows origin of thyroid gland
   B. Migration of gland into the jaw region
   C. Foramen cecum opens up to become persistent
   D. Cystic formation near pharyngeal/branchial apparatus

4. Which of the following events usually occurs during the development of pharyngeal/branchial apparatus?
   A. Tuberculum impar remains after further formation
   B. Area pharyngeal/branchial grooves are not obliterated
   C. First two arch pairs develop to greatest extent
   D. Migration pathway of thyroid gland into region

5. Which of the following is present within the tissue of healthy lymph nodes?
   A. Germinal centers containing only mature lymphocytes
   B. Budding of nearby blood vessels into follicle
   C. Hilus at depression on one side of node
   D. Presence of many more efferent than afferent vessels

UNIT 3: DENTAL HISTOLOGY CASE STUDY 1

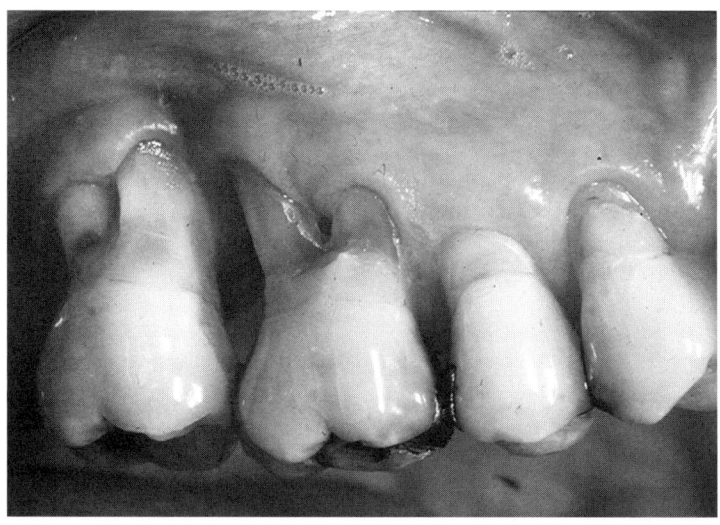

Patient	57 years old
Chief Complaint	"Why do my teeth look so long lately and are also so loose?"
Background and/or Patient History	Retired tennis player Skin cancer history States regular dental care including diagnosis and treatment of "gum disease" until 15 years ago when dentist retired
Current Findings	New patient appointment without previous records Generalized slight BOP, moderate mobility, generalized moderate to severe gingival recession Bilateral photographs of dentition taken along with full mouth dental imaging

1. What part of the patient's alveolar process has undergone resorption between the roots of the molars?
   A. Basal bone
   B. Alveolar crest bone
   C. Interdental bone
   D. Interradicular bone

2. What fiber group of the periodontal ligament is the last group to be affected by periodontal disease?
   A. Alveolar crest group
   B. Horizontal group
   C. Oblique group
   D. Interdental group

3. Both the patient's lost alveolar process levels and altered associated periodontal ligament are considered part of which of the following orofacial structures?
   A. Periodontium
   B. Alveolodental ligament
   C. Principal fiber groups
   D. Temporomandibular joint

4. What type of hard tissue of the teeth was first lost as a result of the root exposure?
   A. Predentin
   B. Secondary dentin
   C. Cellular cementum
   D. Coronal enamel

5. Which cell population has been the most active in removing the alveolar process because of the patient's periodontal diagnosis?
   A. Ameloblast
   B. Osteoclast
   C. Odontoblast
   D. Odontoclast

UNIT 3: DENTAL HISTOLOGY CASE STUDY 2

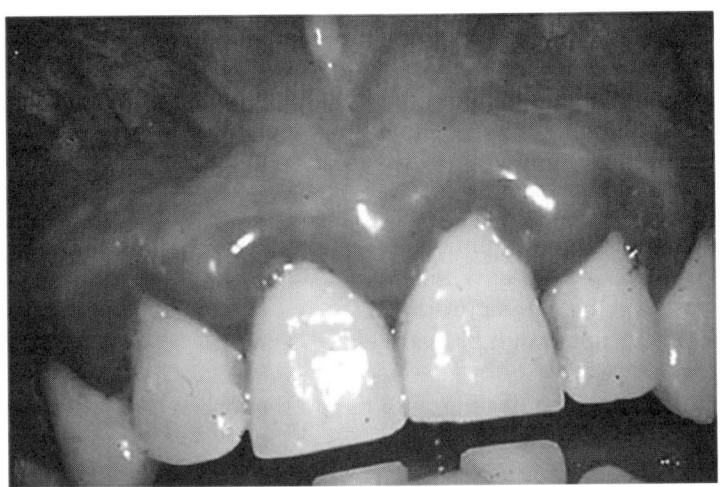

Patient	32 years old
Chief Complaint	"Why do my teeth keep bleeding now when I eat?"
Background and/or Patient History	Real estate agent with four children Diabetes mellitus type 2 diagnosed at age 30 Medications: Oral diabetes pill States does not routinely take medication or test blood levels since recent job loss 2 weeks ago
Current Findings	New patient appointment without previous records Estimated height: 5 feet, 11 inches (1.80 meters) Estimated weight: 280 pounds (127 kilograms) BP: 110/85 Blood glucose: 240 mg/dL Angry manner when asked to take blood glucose reading Generalized slight to moderate gingival BOP No bone loss on present full mouth dental imaging States does not regularly brush or floss since recent job loss Photograph of oral cavity also taken for homecare discussion

1. What type of mucosa is involved in the patient's chief complaint noted?
   A. Lining mucosa
   B. Specialized mucosa
   C. Masticatory mucosa
   D. Paranasal mucosa

2. Which fiber group of the periodontal ligament could be the first group to be affected with this patient in the future without any changes to patient history or current findings?
   A. Gingival group
   B. Alveolar crest group
   C. Horizontal group
   D. Oblique group

3. What is the main underlying cause of the patient's chief complaint?
   A. Thickening of the junctional epithelium
   B. Repair of the lamina propria's blood vessels
   C. Increased blood vessels in the lamina propria
   D. Increased collagen production around blood vessels

4. What is the classification used when dealing with the present orofacial condition of the patient?
   A. Acute gingivitis
   B. Chronic gingivitis
   C. Acute periodontitis
   D. Chronic periodontitis

5. What histologic situation can be noted in this case with both the epithelium and lamina propria at the mucogingival junction?
   A. Smooth interface at basement membrane between tissue types
   B. Decreased numbers of migrating white blood cells
   C. Presence of rete pegs and connective tissue papillae
   D. All signs of hyperplasia throughout

UNIT 3: DENTAL HISTOLOGY CASE STUDY 3

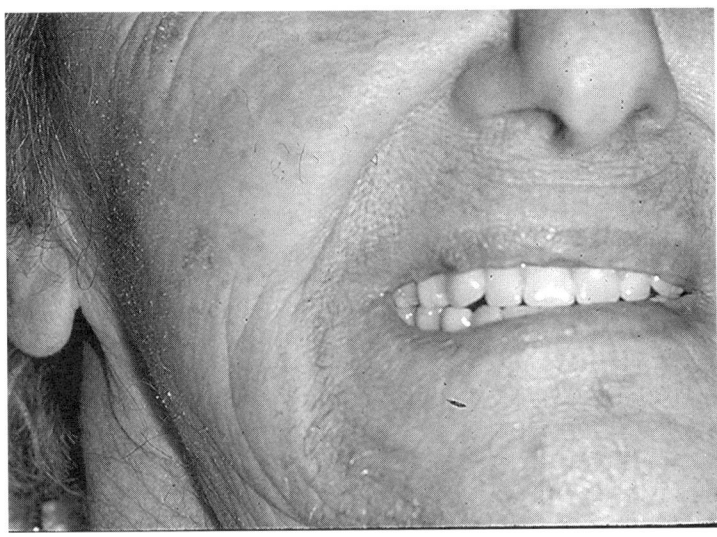

Patient	82 years old
Chief Complaint	"My mouth feels like sandpaper."
Background and/or Patient History	Extended care facility resident Alzheimer disease in early stages Former smoker (cigarettes) Medications: Antidepressant
Current Findings	New patient appointment at limited facility dental clinic States that complete dentures do not fit comfortably Photograph taken of patient wearing dentures

1. What is the correct term used to describe the oral condition present with the patient?
   A. Attrition
   B. Abfraction
   C. Hypersalivation
   D. Xerostomia

2. Which is the largest salivary gland present in the body?
   A. Parotid
   B. Submandibular
   C. Sublingual
   D. von Ebner

3. What salivary gland usually produces the most saliva in the oral cavity?
   A. Parotid
   B. Submandibular
   C. Sublingual
   D. von Ebner

4. What part of each of the patient's jaws is mostly still present in this case?
   A. Basal bone
   B. Alveolar process
   C. Interdental bone
   D. Interradicular bone

5. What is the change in the height of the lower third of the patient's face correctly termed?
   A. Increase of Golden Proportions
   B. Loss of vertical dimension
   C. Partially edentulous state
   D. Mesial drift with supereruption

UNIT 3: DENTAL HISTOLOGY CASE STUDY 4

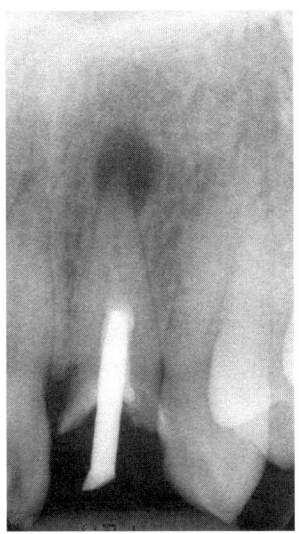

Patient	45 years old
Chief Complaint	"Can you fix my painful broken tooth?"
Background and/or Patient History	High school basketball coach No longer chews spit tobacco States involved tooth had endodontic therapy 20 years ago by referred specialist due to "tooth anomaly"
Current Findings	New patient appointment with limited examination States has bad taste in mouth Periapical radiograph taken of involved tooth Pain on percussion on involved tooth

1. What is the developmental disturbance that was present upon eruption of the patient's involved tooth?
   A. Microdontia
   B. Gemination
   C. Dens in dente
   D. Peg lateral

2. Why is there presence of pain for the patient with the involved tooth?
   A. Secondary dentin filling pulp chamber
   B. Inflammatory edema pressing on nerves
   C. Inert material extruding from the pulp
   D. Apical bone forming at the apex

3. What is the best explanation for the present state of the patient's involved tooth?
   A. Hyperplasia of pulpal tissue
   B. Failure during lobular division
   C. Loss of tooth vitality
   D. Placement of gutta-percha

4. What is the main path by which pulpal infection travels to the surrounding periodontium to cause a collection of purulent exudate?
   A. Apical foramen
   B. Pulp horns
   C. Accessory canals
   D. Dentinal tubules

5. Which of the following cell populations can produce additional pulp tissue?
   A. Lined up odontoblasts
   B. Red blood cell clotting
   C. White blood cell migration
   D. Undifferentiated mesenchymal cells

UNIT 3: DENTAL HISTOLOGY CASE STUDY 5

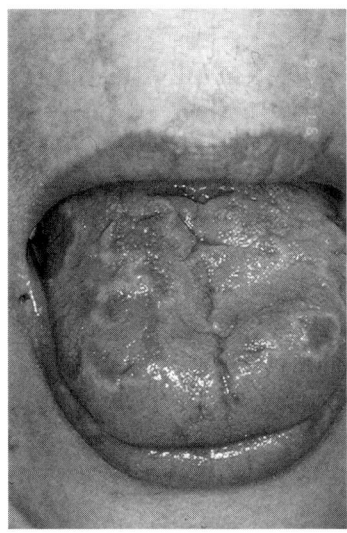

Patient	32 years old
Chief Complaint	"Why does the top of my tongue always look so different?"
Background and/or Patient History	Chef in restaurant Osteoporosis diagnosed recently Medications: Bone-building pills
Current Findings	Second visit at dental school clinic after screening examination Uses electric toothbrush since recommended at last visit States tongue has always looked this way Brushes dorsal surface of tongue regularly

1. What is the lesion noted on the patient's dorsal surface of the tongue?
   A. Fissured tongue
   B. Mucocele or ranula
   C. Geographic tongue
   D. Black hairy tongue

2. What type of oral structure is mostly involved in this tongue lesion?
   A. Filiform lingual papilla
   B. Floor of mouth
   C. Circumvallate lingual papilla
   D. Lingual tonsil

3. What type of oral mucosa is mostly associated with this lesion?
   A. Masticatory
   B. Lining
   C. Specialized
   D. Paranasal

4. Which of the following is directly associated with sensory neuron processes when the patient is checking their career work in progress?
   A. Taste pore
   B. Taste cells
   C. Supporting cells
   D. Surrounding tongue epithelium

5. Fungiform lingual papillae are present in all areas noted below EXCEPT one area. Which of the following areas is the EXCEPTION?
   A. Sulcus terminalis
   B. Tip of tongue
   C. Body of tongue
   D. Median lingual sulcus

UNIT 3: DENTAL HISTOLOGY CASE STUDY 6

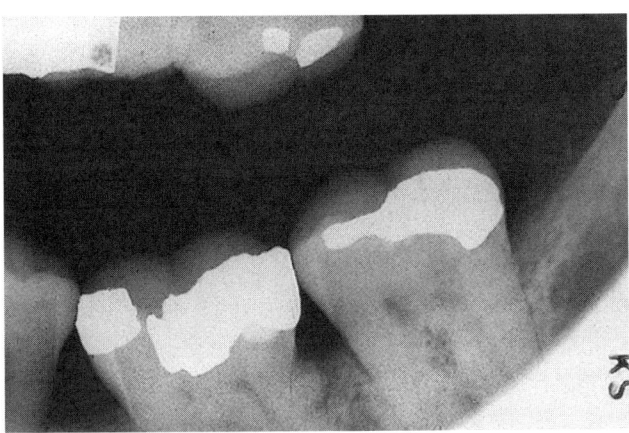

Patient	34 years old
Chief Complaint	"I can feel hard bumps on the sides of my lower molars when I floss."
Background and/or Patient History	Student nurse professional States has dental phobia Diabetes mellitus type 1 diagnosed at age 7 Medications: Insulin injections twice daily
Current Findings	New patient appointment Bitewing radiograph taken of area of concern Very nervous during dental imaging Generalized slight BOP in area of concern but no calculus noted Noncavitated lesion on occlusal surface of #13 (#25) States just started flossing teeth

1. What could be causing the situation with the molars noted by the patient?
   A. Denticles
   B. Enamel pearls
   C. Calculus
   D. Cementicles

2. What does this noted situation with the molars involve on a histologic level?
   A. Deposition by misplaced ameloblasts
   B. Irregular deposition by cementocytes
   C. Mineralization around microorganism debris
   D. Calcified masses of dentin

3. What is the main histologic tissue associated with this situation with the molars?
   A. Cementoblasts
   B. Dentinal tubules
   C. Enamel rods
   D. Collagen

4. Which of the following is most important to stress to this patient to maintain oral health?
   A. Avoidance of flossing
   B. Taking medication as prescribed
   C. Avoiding dental imaging
   D. Rinsing with salt water

5. Which of the following dental procedures need to be completed for tooth #13 (#25)?
   A. Amalgam restoration
   B. Monitoring lesion
   C. Resin restoration
   D. Dental sealant

UNIT 4: DENTAL ANATOMY CASE STUDY 1

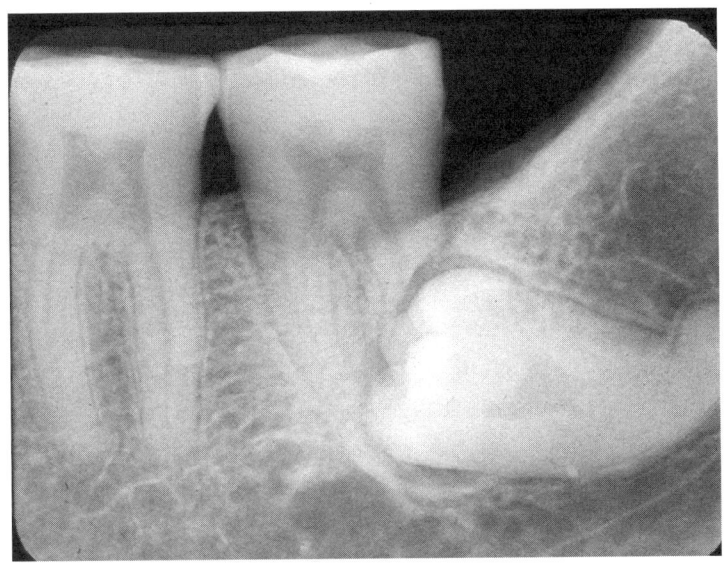

Patient	25 years old
Chief Complaint	"Why does my lower jaw hurt even when using my guard?"
Background and/or Patient History	Chemistry postgraduate student Orthodontic therapy 10 years ago at referred orthodontic office Low caries risk Moderate level of bruxism Generalized moderate attrition
Current Findings	Patient of record annual appointment Early symptoms of bilateral jaw joint disorder States uses nightguard regularly Painful area in lower left jaw but no dental or intraoral lesions present upon examination Periapical radiograph of area of concern

1. What is the condition noted on the radiograph that is probably causing the patient's oral pain?
   A. Eruption cyst
   B. Supernumerary tooth
   C. Dilaceration
   D. Impacted third molar

2. Which of the following are features of the involved tooth that is causing the discomfort?
   A. Three roots
   B. Four pulp horns
   C. Consistent crown form
   D. Square crown outline

3. When does this involved tooth usually complete its roots?
   A. 10 to 14 years old
   B. 13 to 17 years old
   C. 17 to 21 years old
   D. 18 to 25 years old

4. What are the radiopaque structures noted in the pulp chambers of some of the mandibular posterior teeth?
   A. Denticles
   B. Pulp stones
   C. Sialoliths
   D. Enamel pearls

5. Which structure is located on the temporal bone anterior to the articular fossa of the jaw joint?
   A. Joint capsule
   B. Articular eminence
   C. Synovial membrane
   D. Articulating surface of the condyle

UNIT 4: DENTAL ANATOMY CASE STUDY 2

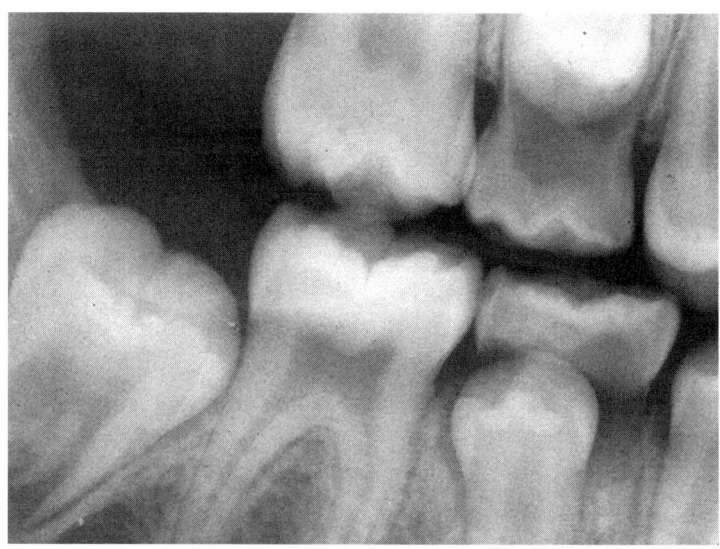

Patient	13 years old
Chief Complaint	"Why do my back teeth feel really loose when I wiggle them?"
Background and/or Patient History	Likes to play basketball Sips sports drinks regularly
Current Findings	Patient of record annual appointment Dental sealants placed last appointment Four posterior teeth have slight mobility with nearby teeth partially erupted with tissue inflamed Bilateral bitewing radiographs taken

252 CASE STUDY EXERCISES

1. On which of the patient's teeth were dental sealants placed at last dental appointment?
   A. First premolars
   B. Second premolars
   C. First molars
   D. Second molars

2. Which partially erupted teeth may require placement of dental sealants at the patient's next dental appointment because of caries risk profile?
   A. First premolars
   B. Second premolars
   C. First molars
   D. Second molars

3. Which of the following teeth may show signs of mobility and ready to be exfoliated?
   A. S (#84)
   B. T (#85)
   C. #2 (#17)
   D. #30 (#46)

4. The crown of which of the following appears similar to the crown anatomy of one of the nearby mobile teeth?
   A. S (#84)
   B. T (#85)
   C. #2 (#17)
   D. #30 (#46)

5. Which of the following teeth may be considered to be exfoliated?
   A. S (#84)
   B. T (#85)
   C. #2 (#17)
   D. #30 (#46)

UNIT 4: DENTAL ANATOMY CASE STUDY 3

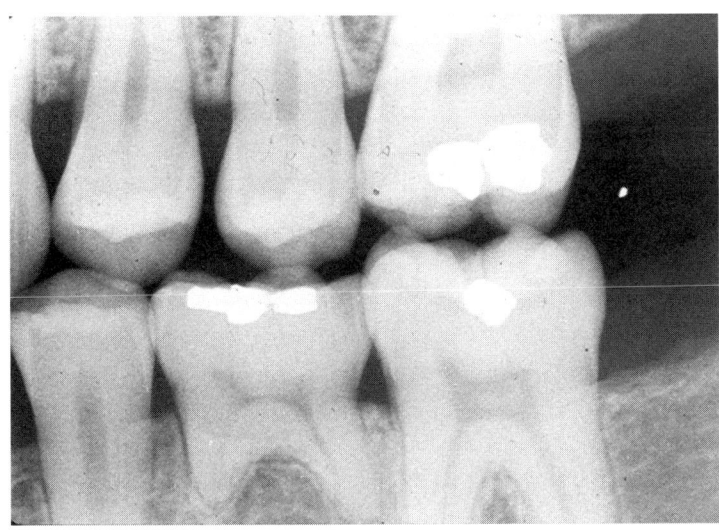

Patient	25 years old
Chief Complaint	"Why is one of my back teeth on each side smaller than the rest?"
Background and/ or Patient History	Dental sealants placed at age 6 but later restored due to margin failure Four permanent posterior teeth extracted at age 13 because of extensive caries Four permanent teeth extracted at age 18 because of impaction Stated that childhood dentist said some "adult teeth" were never going to erupt Does not have fluoridated drinking water
Current Findings	New patient appointment with previous records Regularly sucks on sugared mints Bilateral bitewing radiographs taken

1. Which of the patient's permanent posterior teeth exhibit partial anodontia?
   A. Second premolars
   B. First molars
   C. Second molars
   D. Third molars

2. Which of the patient's permanent posterior teeth were extracted as an adolescent?
   A. Second premolars
   B. First molars
   C. Second molars
   D. Third molars

3. Which of the patient's permanent posterior teeth were extracted as a young adult?
   A. Second premolars
   B. First molars
   C. Second molars
   D. Third molars

4. Which of the patient's permanent posterior teeth have been restored because of failure of the dental sealants?
   A. Second premolars
   B. First molars
   C. Second molars
   D. Third molars

5. Which of the following permanent mandibular teeth in the patient's dentition have two roots?
   A. Second premolars
   B. First molars
   C. Second molars
   D. Third molars

UNIT 4: DENTAL ANATOMY CASE STUDY 4

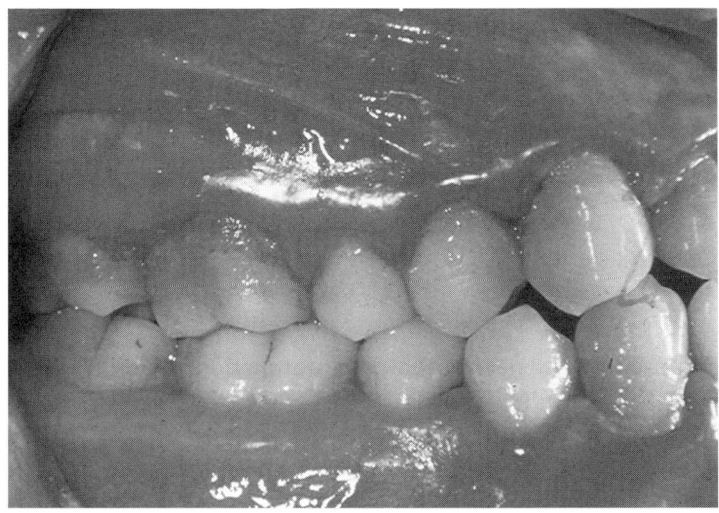

Patient	42 years old
Chief Complaint	"Why are my bottom eyeteeth so sensitive at gumline when I drink anything cold?"
Background and/or Patient History	Long-haul truck driver High blood pressure controlled with medication Former smoker (cigars) Orthodontic therapy 25 years ago but does not use any form of retention Extracted permanent third molars at age 20 with infection present Not been to dental office for 12 years States grinding teeth at night when working Medications: Diuretic
Current Findings	New patient appointment Estimated height: 5 feet, 10 inches (1.78 meters) Estimated weight: 180 pounds (81.6 kilograms) BP: 115/95 No caries noted after full mouth dental imaging and clinical examination Generalized moderate gingival inflammation with generalized soft deposits Uses soft toothbrush Gargles with OTC medicated mouthrinse

1. What is the Angle classification of malocclusion noted on the patient's right side?
   A. Class I
   B. Class II, Division I
   C. Class II, Division II
   D. Class III

2. What other occlusal evaluation notes can be made regarding the right side of the dentition?
   A. Severe crossbite
   B. Open bite
   C. Severe overjet
   D. End-to-end bite

3. What may be occurring on the mandibular teeth to make them sensitive to cold drinks?
   A. Erosion
   B. Abfraction
   C. Pulpitis
   D. Toothbrush abrasion

4. What is the correct term used for the noted orofacial parafunctional habit concerning the teeth?
   A. Clenching
   B. Xerostomia
   C. Bruxism
   D. Passive eruption

5. What part of the anatomy of the sensitive teeth is first to be lost due to the orofacial parafunctional habit?
   A. Fossae
   B. Pits
   C. Grooves
   D. Cusps

UNIT 4: DENTAL ANATOMY CASE STUDY 5

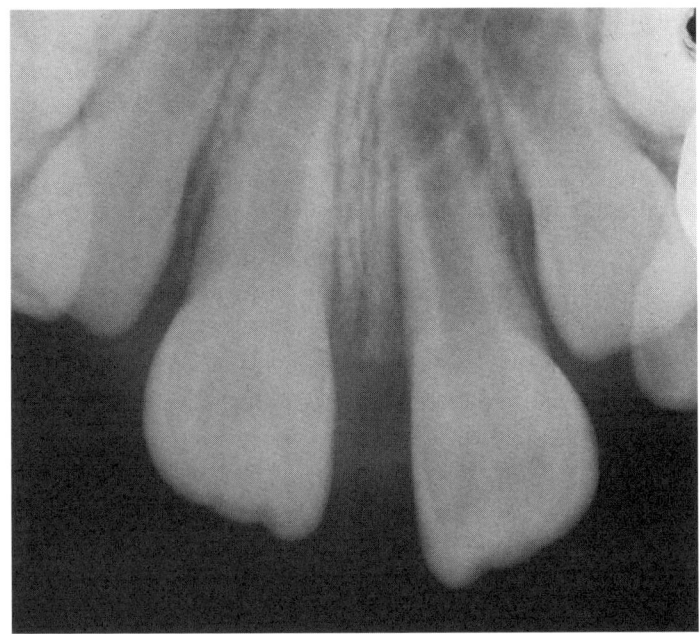

From Dean JA: *McDonald and Avery's Dentistry for the Child and Adolescent*, 10th ed., Elsevier, 2016.

Patient	8 years old
Chief Complaint	Supervising adult: "The front tooth looks different now!"
Background and/or Patient History	Supervising adult states child slipped in tub and hit upper front tooth 60 minutes earlier with EMT called No past medical concerns
Current Findings	Patient of record emergency appointment Generalized slight BOP in maxillary anterior sextant with swollen upper lip No other trauma noted and negative for concussion by EMT Periapical radiograph taken of maxillary anterior sextant

1. What is the correct term for the dentition period that is present for the patient and how many teeth could be involved within the dentition?
   A. Deciduous dentition period, 10 teeth
   B. Primary dentition period, 20 teeth
   C. Mixed dentition period, 24 teeth
   D. Transitional dentition period, 30 teeth

2. Which of the following teeth in the patient should be expected to be fully erupted?
   A. Incisors, canines, first molars
   B. Incisors, canines, molars
   C. Incisors, canines, premolars
   D. Incisors, canines, premolars, molars

3. What effect might this accident have on the future development of the involved tooth?
   A. Pulpal involvement
   B. Slight crown shortening
   C. Additional primary dentin layers
   D. None anticipated

4. When does the root commonly complete its development for the involved tooth?
   A. 6 years old
   B. 7 years old
   C. 10 years old
   D. 12 years old

5. Which of the following is considered a distinct feature of the involved tooth?
   A. Nonsuccedaneous tooth
   B. Distal contact at middle third
   C. Wider labiolingually than mesiodistally
   D. Labial and lingual height of contour in cervical third

Notes

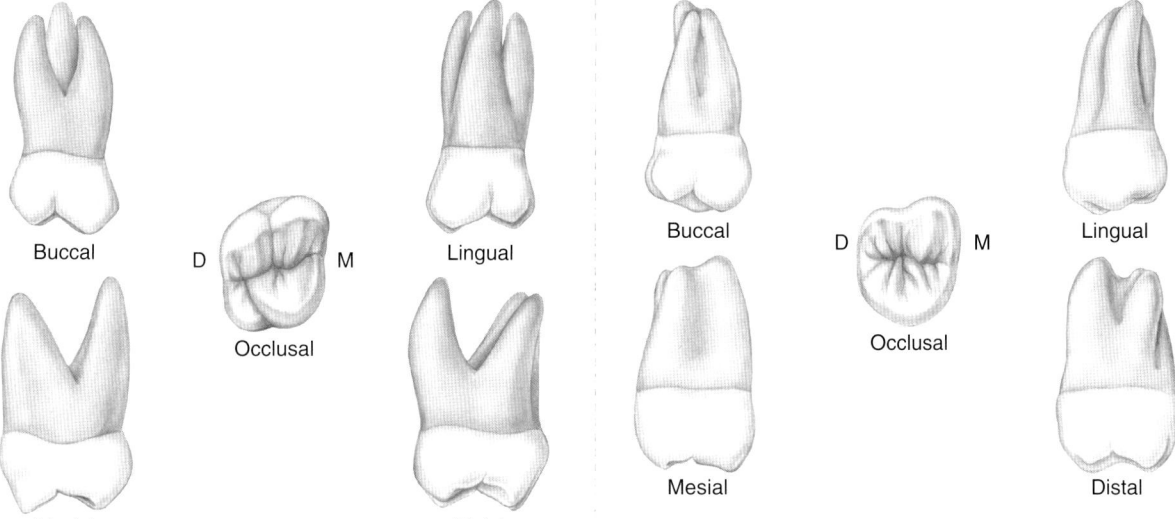

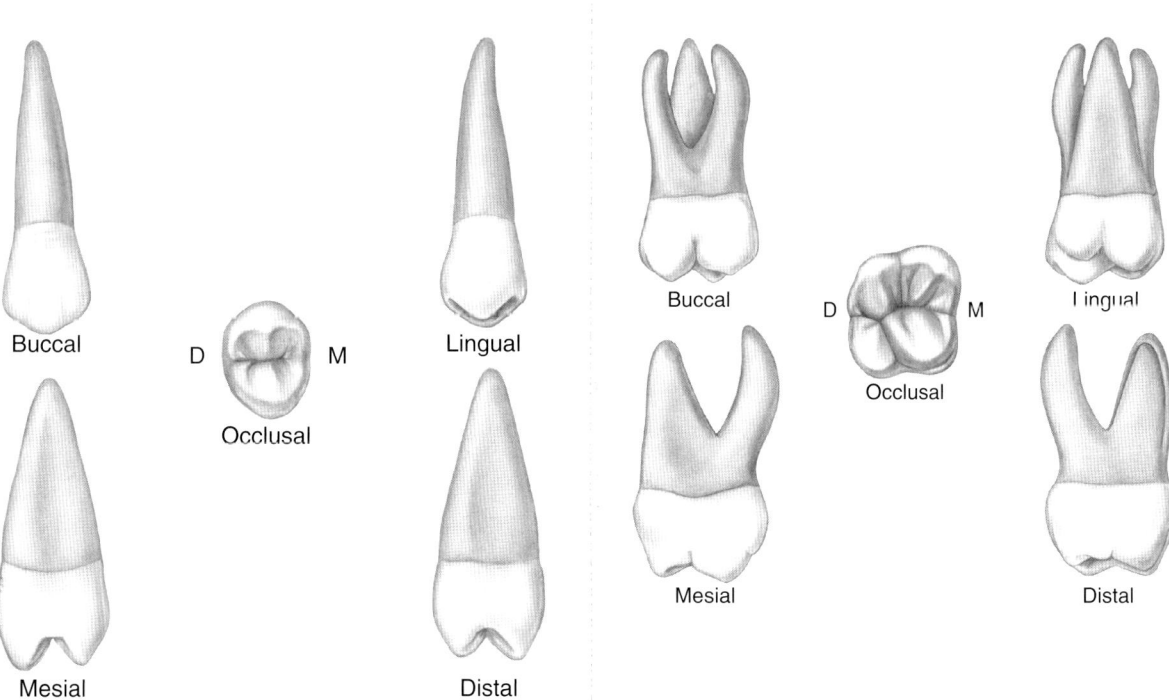

Maxillary Right Third Molar (Heart-Shaped Occlusal Crown Outline)

Universal Number: #1 **International Number:** #18
Eruption: 17-21 **Root completion:** 18-25
General crown features: Occlusal table with marginal ridges and cusps with tips, inclined planes, ridges, grooves, fossae, pits
Specific crown features: Smaller crown than second and variable in form. Heart-shaped or rhomboidal occlusal crown outline (in order) with three or four cusps. Trapezoidal proximal crown outline. Buccal ridge
Height of contour: Buccal: cervical third; Lingual: middle third
Mesial contact: Middle third **Distal contact:** None
Distinguishing right from left: Distobuccal cusp shorter than mesiobuccal cusp
Root features: Three less divergent roots usually fused curving distally

Maxillary Right Second Molar (Rhomboidal Occlusal Crown Outline)

Universal Number: #2 **International Number:** #17
Eruption: 12-13 **Root completion:** 14-16
General crown features: Occlusal table with marginal ridges and cusps with tips, inclined planes, ridges, grooves, fossae, pits
Specific crown features: Smaller crown than first. Rhomboidal or heart-shaped occlusal crown outline (in order) with three or four cusps. Less distinct oblique ridge and more supplemental grooves. Mesiobuccal cusp longer than distobuccal cusp. Distolingual cusp smaller than on first or absent. No fifth cusp. Less distinct oblique ridge and more supplemental grooves. Trapezoidal proximal crown outline. Buccal ridge.
Height of contour: Buccal: cervical third; Lingual: middle third
Mesial and distal contact: Middle third
Distinguishing right from left: Mesiolingual cusp outline longer and larger but not as sharp as distolingual cusp outline
Root features: Three less divergent roots. Root trunks, furcations, proximal root concavities

Maxillary Right First Molar

Universal Number: #3 **International Number:** #16
Eruption: 6-7 **Root completion:** 9-10
General crown features: Occlusal table with marginal ridges and cusps with tips, inclined planes, ridges, grooves, fossae, pits
Specific crown features: Largest tooth in arch and largest crown in dentition. Four major cusps with buccal cusps almost equal in height. Fifth minor cusp and groove of Carabelli with mesiolingual cusp and distinct oblique ridge. Rhomboidal occlusal and trapezoidal proximal crown outline. Distolingual groove possibly ending in lingual pit. Buccal ridge
Height of contour: Buccal: cervical third; Lingual: middle third
Mesial contact: Junction of occlusal and middle thirds **Distal contact:** Middle third
Distinguishing right from left: Mesiolingual cusp outline longer and larger but not as sharp as distolingual
Root features: Three divergent roots: lingual largest and longest extending beyond crown outline, mesiobuccal second largest, and distobuccal third largest; latter two with extreme curvature. Root trunks, furcations, proximal root concavities

Maxillary Right Second Premolar

Universal Number: #4 **International Number:** #15
Eruption: 10-12 **Root completion:** 12-14
General crown features: Occlusal table with marginal ridges and cusps with tips, ridges, inclined planes, grooves, fossae, pits
Specific crown features: Smaller than first. Hexagonal but rounder occlusal crown outline. Two cusps same length with short central groove and increased supplemental grooves. No distinct mesial surface features like first. Trapezoidal proximal crown outline. Buccal ridge
Height of contour: Buccal: cervical third; Lingual: middle third
Mesial and distal contact: Just cervical to junction of occlusal and middle thirds
Distinguishing right from left: Lingual cusp to offset to mesial
Root features: Single root. Elliptical on cervical cross section. Proximal root concavities

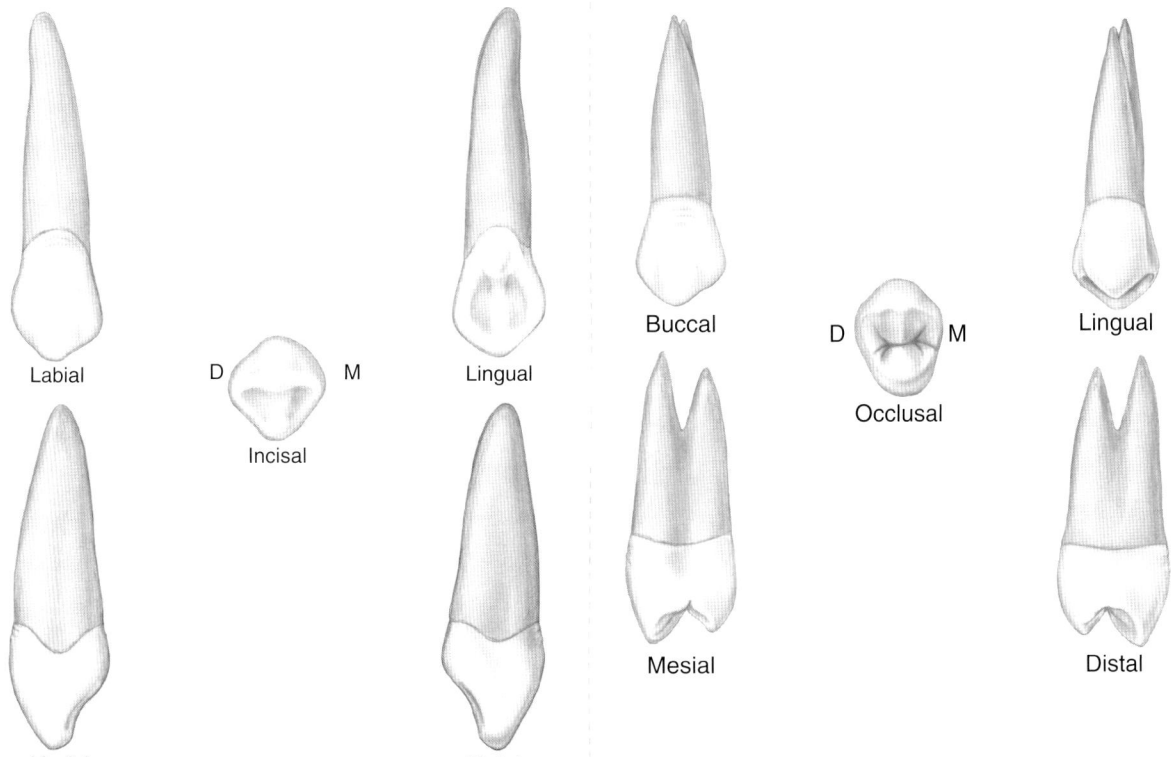

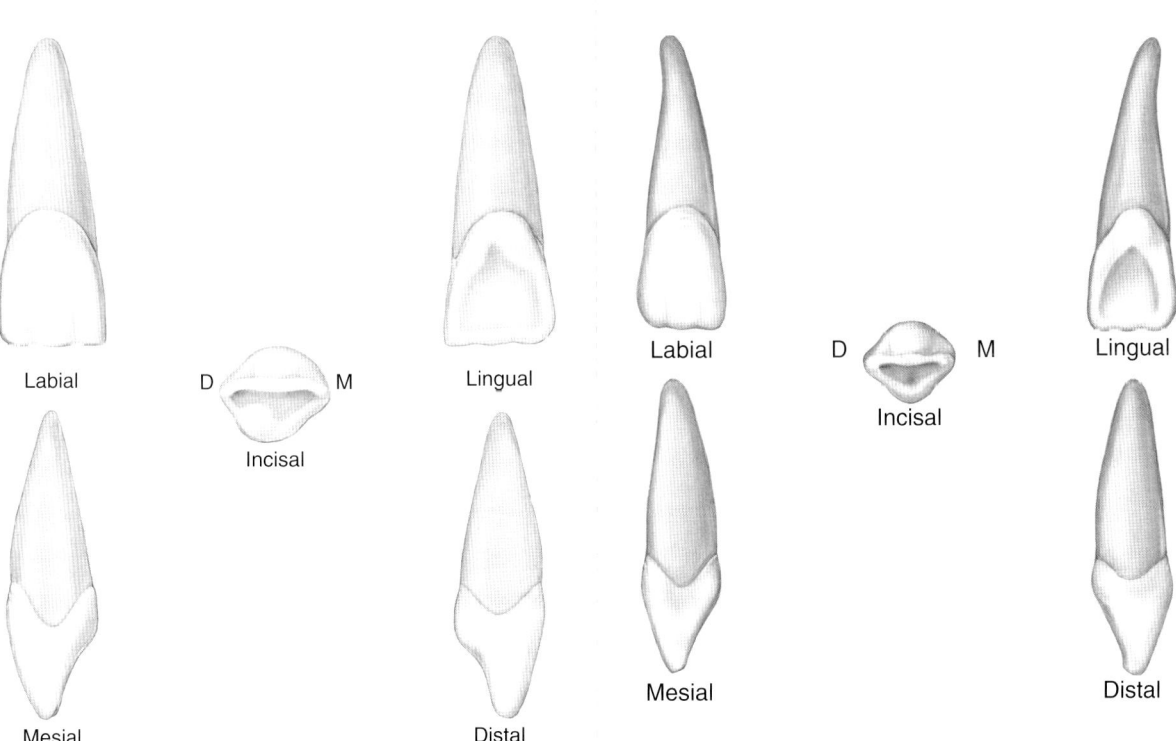

Maxillary Right First Premolar

Universal Number: #5 **International Number:** #14
Eruption 10-11 **Root completion:** 12-13
General crown features: Occlusal table with marginal ridges and cusps with tips, ridges, inclined planes, grooves, fossae, pits
Specific crown features: Larger than second. Hexagonal occlusal crown outline. Buccal cusp longer of two cusps. Long central groove. Distinct mesial surface features unlike second. Trapezoidal proximal crown outline. Buccal ridge
Height of contour: Buccal: cervical third; Lingual: middle third
Mesial and distal contact: Just cervical to junction of occlusal and middle thirds
Distinguishing right from left: Longer mesial cusp slope than distal and with distinct mesial features: deeper CEJ curvature, marginal groove, developmental depression, especially deep mesial root concavity
Root features: Two roots with root trunk. Elliptical on cervical cross section. Proximal root concavities

Maxillary Right Canine

Universal Number: #6 **International Number:** #13
Eruption: 11-12 **Root completion:** 13-15
General crown features: Single cusp with tip, slopes, labial ridge, cingulum, lingual ridge, marginal ridges, lingual fossae
Specific crown features: Longest tooth in arch. More pronounced lingual surface with sharp cusp tip
Height of contour: Labial: cervical third; Lingual: middle third
Mesial contact: Junction of incisal third and middle thirds **Distal contact:** Middle third
Distinguishing right from left: Shorter mesial cusp slope than distal with more pronounced mesial CEJ curvature. More cervical contact on distal. Shorter distal outline than mesial on labial and with depression between distal contact and CEJ
Root features: Long, thick single root. Oval on cervical cross section. Proximal root concavities. Blunt root apex

Maxillary Right Lateral Incisor

Universal Number: #7 **International Number:** #12
Eruption: 8-9 **Root completion:** 11
General crown features: Incisal ridge, incisal angles, cingulum, marginal ridges, lingual fossa
Specific crown features: Greatest crown variation. Like smaller central. Pronounced lingual surface with centered narrower cingulum and more pronounced marginal ridges with deeper lingual fossa
Height of contour: Cervical third
Mesial contact: Incisal third **Distal contact:** Middle third
Distinguishing right from left: Sharper mesio-incisal angle and rounder disto-incisal angle. More pronounced mesial CEJ curvature
Root features: Single root. Oval on cervical cross section. Same or longer than central but thinner. Overall conical shape. No proximal root concavities. Root curves distally with sharp apex

Maxillary Right Central Incisor

Universal Number: #8 **International Number:** #11
Eruption: 7-8 **Root completion:** 10
General crown features: Incisal ridge, incisal angles, cingulum, marginal ridges, lingual fossa
Specific crown features: Widest crown mesiodistally. Greatest CEJ curve and height of contour. Pronounced distal offset wide cingulum and marginal ridges with wide and deep lingual fossa of various depths
Height of contour: Cervical third
Mesial contact: Incisal third **Distal contact:** Junction of incisal and middle thirds
Distinguishing right from left: Sharper mesio-incisal angle and rounder disto-incisal angle. More pronounced mesial CEJ curvature
Root features: Single root. Triangular on cervical cross section. Overall conical shape. No proximal root concavities. Rounded apex

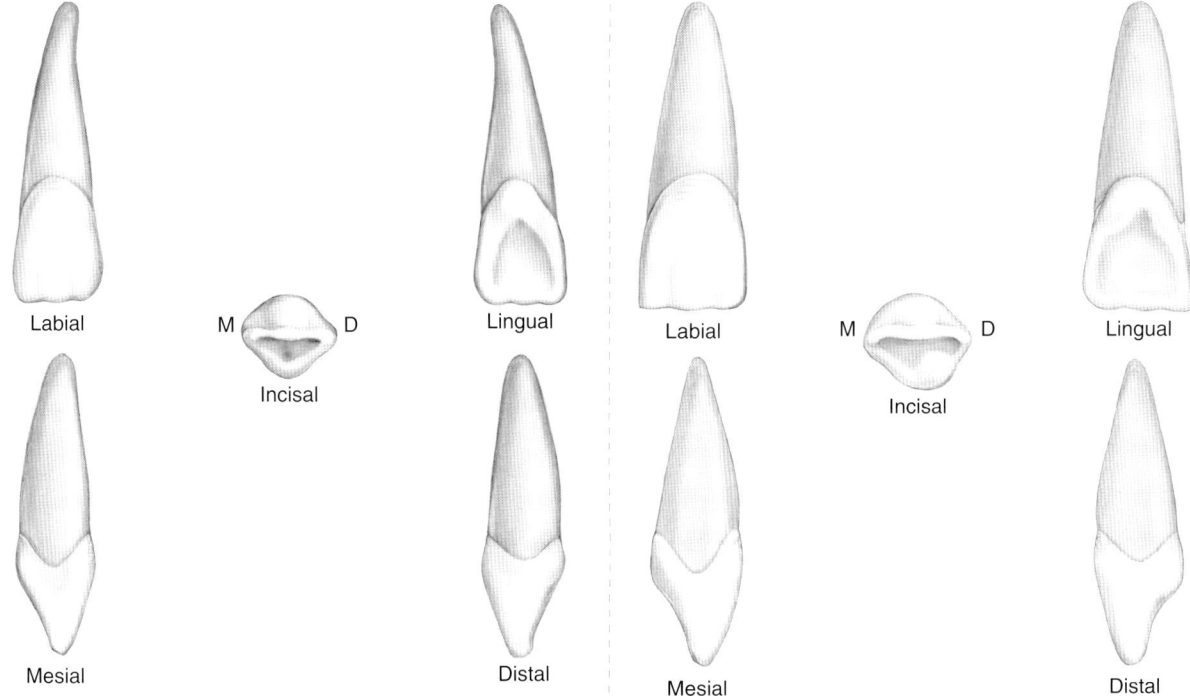
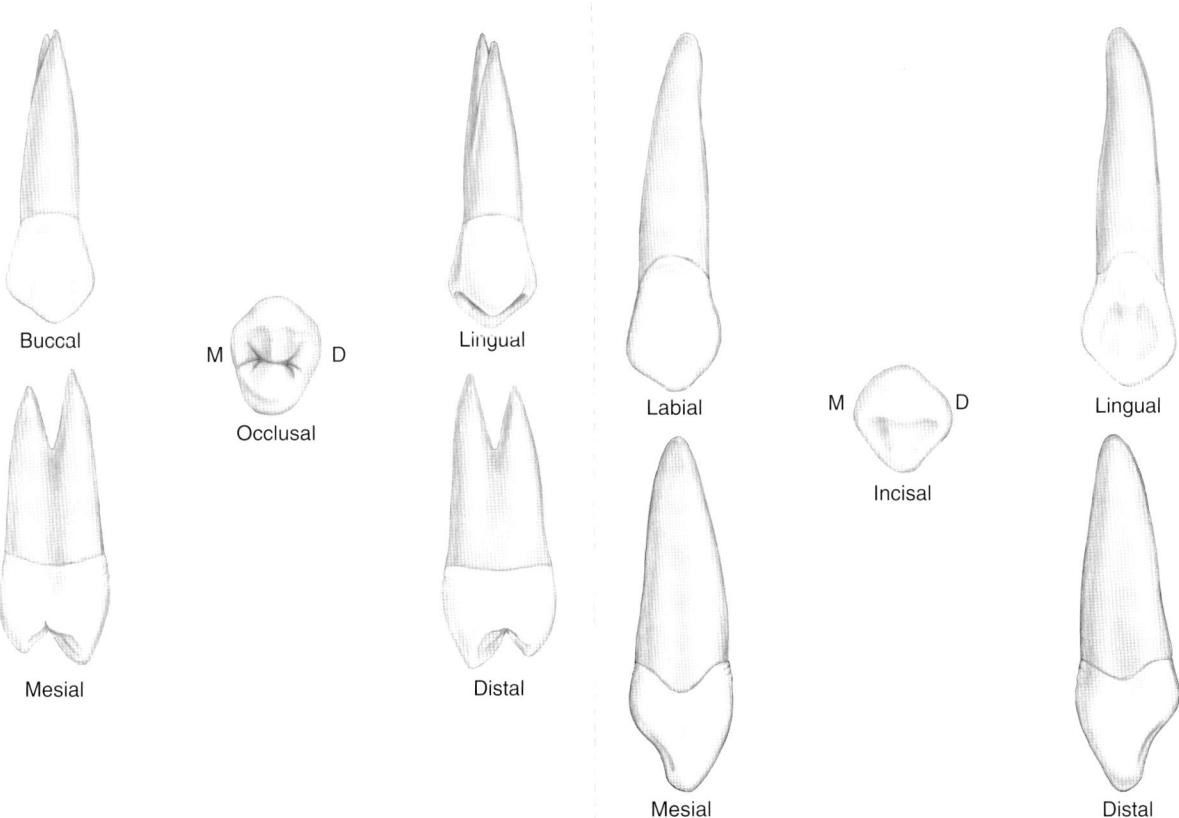

Maxillary Left Central Incisor

Universal Number: #9 **International Number:** #21
Eruption: 7-8 **Root completion:** 10
General crown features: Incisal ridge, incisal angles, cingulum, marginal ridges, lingual fossa
Specific crown features: Widest crown mesiodistally. Greatest CEJ curve and height of contour. Pronounced distal offset wide cingulum and marginal ridges with wide and deep lingual fossa of various depths
Height of contour: Cervical third
Mesial contact: Incisal third **Distal contact:** Junction of incisal and middle thirds
Distinguishing right from left: Sharper mesio-incisal angle and rounder disto-incisal angle. More pronounced mesial CEJ curvature
Root features: Single root. Triangular on cervical cross section. Overall conical shape. No proximal root concavities. Rounded apex

Maxillary Left Lateral Incisor

Universal Number: #10 **International Number:** #22
Eruption: 8-9 **Root completion:** 11
General crown features: Incisal ridge, incisal angles, cingulum, marginal ridges, lingual fossa
Specific crown features: Greatest crown variation. Like smaller central. Pronounced lingual surface with centered narrower cingulum and more pronounced marginal ridges with deeper lingual fossa
Height of contour: Cervical third
Mesial contact: Incisal third **Distal contact:** Middle third
Distinguishing right from left: Sharper mesio-incisal angle and rounder disto-incisal angle. More pronounced mesial CEJ curvature
Root features: Single root. Oval on cervical cross section. Same or longer than central but thinner. Overall conical shape. No proximal root concavities. Root curves distally with sharp apex

Maxillary Left Canine

Universal Number: #11 **International Number:** #23
Eruption: 11-12 **Root completion:** 13-15
General crown features: Single cusp with tip, slopes, labial ridge, cingulum, lingual ridge, marginal ridges, lingual fossae
Specific crown features: Longest tooth in arch. More pronounced lingual surface with sharp cusp tip
Height of contour: Labial: cervical third; Lingual: middle third
Mesial contact: Junction of incisal third and middle thirds **Distal contact:** Middle third
Distinguishing right from left: Shorter mesial cusp slope than distal with more pronounced mesial CEJ curvature. More cervical contact on distal. Shorter distal outline than mesial on labial and with depression between distal contact and CEJ
Root features: Long, thick single root. Oval on cervical cross section. Proximal root concavities. Blunt root apex

Maxillary Left First Premolar

Universal Number: #12 **International Number:** #24
Eruption: 10-11 **Root completion:** 12-13
General crown features: Occlusal table with marginal ridges and cusps and with tips, ridges, inclined planes, grooves, fossae, pits
Specific crown features: Larger than second. Hexagonal occlusal crown outline. Buccal cusp longer of two cusps. Long central groove. Distinct mesial surface features unlike second. Trapezoidal proximal crown outline. Buccal ridge
Height of contour: Buccal: cervical third; Lingual: middle third
Mesial and distal contact: Just cervical to junction of occlusal and middle thirds
Distinguishing right from left: Longer mesial cusp slope than distal with distinct mesial **features:** deeper CEJ curvature, marginal groove, developmental depression, especially deep mesial root concavity
Root features: Two roots with root trunk. Elliptical on cervical cross section. Proximal root concavities

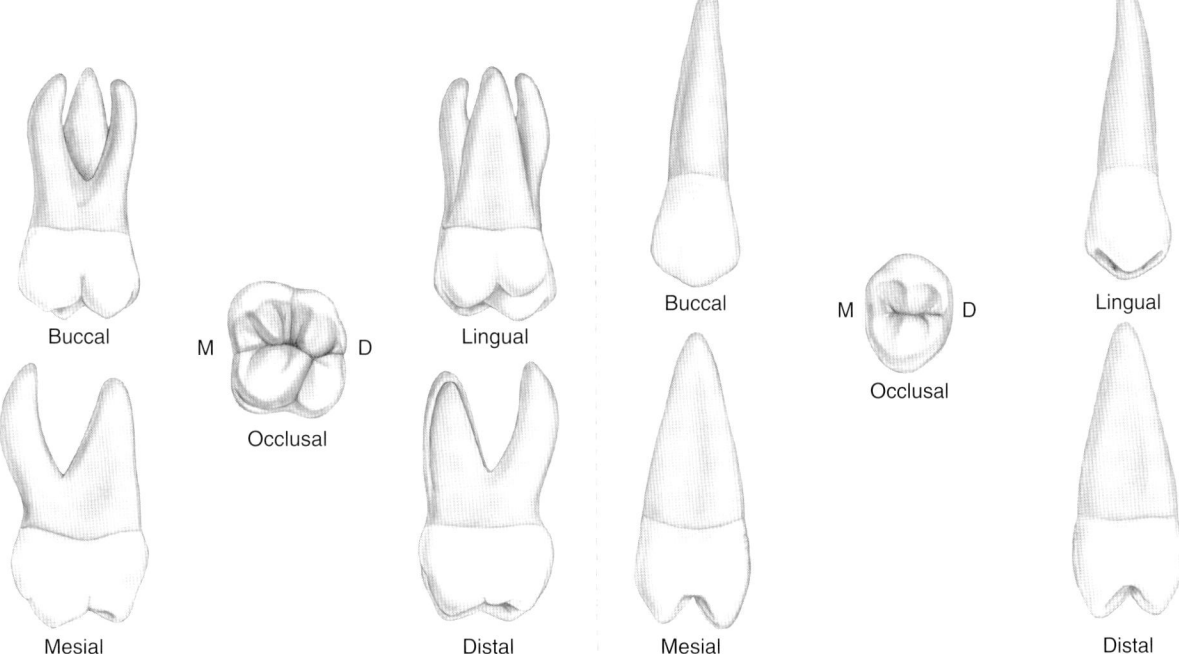

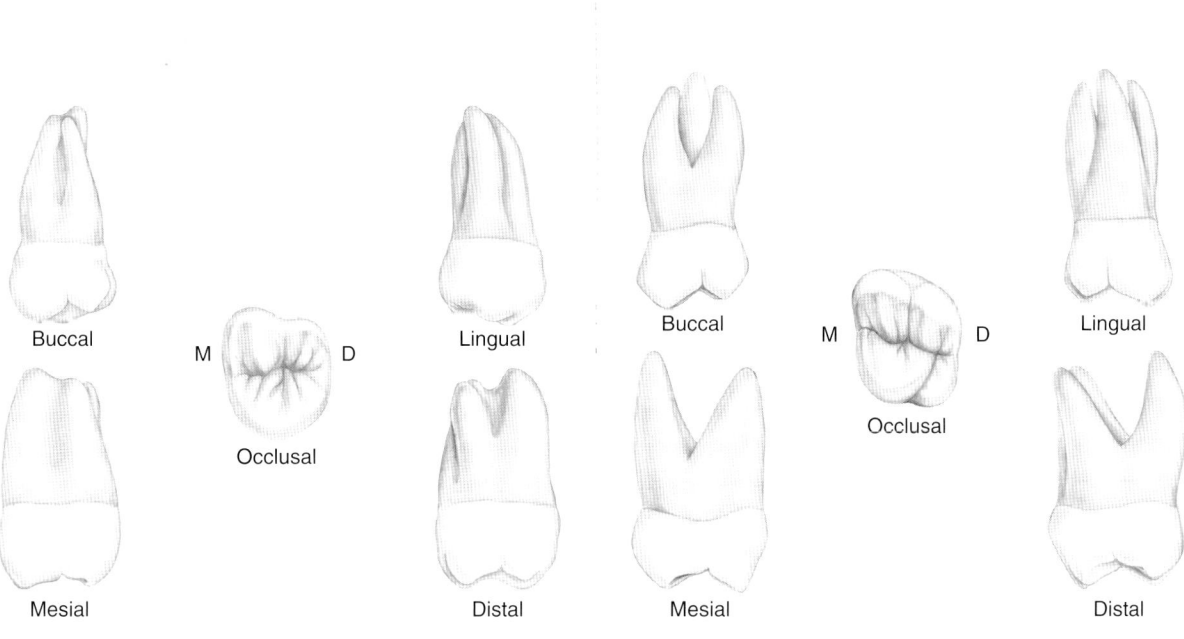

Maxillary Left Second Premolar

Universal Number: #13 **International Number:** #25
Eruption: 10-12 **Root completion:** 12-14
General crown features: Occlusal table with marginal ridges and cusps with tips, ridges, inclined planes, grooves, fossae, pits
Specific crown features: Smaller than first. Hexagonal but rounder occlusal crown outline. Two cusps same length with short central groove with increased supplemental grooves. No distinct mesial surface features like first. Trapezoidal proximal crown outline. Buccal ridge
Height of contour: Buccal: cervical third; Lingual: middle third
Mesial and distal contact: Just cervical to junction of occlusal and middle thirds
Distinguishing right from left: Lingual cusp to offset to mesial
Root features: Single root. Elliptical on cervical cross section. Proximal root concavities

Maxillary Left First Molar

Universal Number: #14 **International Number:** #26
Eruption: 6-7 **Root completion:** 9-10
General crown features: Occlusal table with marginal ridges and cusps with tips, inclined planes, ridges, grooves, fossae, pits
Specific crown features: Largest tooth in arch and largest crown in dentition. Four major cusps with buccal cusps almost equal in height. Fifth minor cusp and groove of Carabelli with mesiolingual cusp and distinct oblique ridge. Rhomboidal occlusal and trapezoidal proximal crown outline. Distolingual groove possibly ending in lingual pit. Buccal ridge
Height of contour: Buccal: cervical third; Lingual: middle third
Mesial contact: Junction of occlusal and middle thirds **Distal contact:** Middle third
Distinguishing right from left: Mesiolingual cusp outline longer and larger but not as sharp as distolingual
Root features: Three divergent roots: lingual largest and longest extending beyond crown outline, mesiobuccal second largest, and distobuccal third largest; latter two with extreme curvature. Root trunks, furcations, proximal root concavities

Maxillary Left Second Molar (Rhomboidal Occlusal Crown Outline)

Universal Number: #15 **International Number:** #27
Eruption: 12-13 **Root completion:** 14-16
General crown features: Occlusal table with marginal ridges and cusps with tips, inclined planes, ridges, grooves, fossae, pits
Specific crown features: Smaller crown than first. Rhomboidal or heart-shaped occlusal crown outline (in order) with three or four cusps. Mesiobuccal cusp longer than distobuccal cusp. Distolingual cusp smaller than on first or absent. No fifth cusp. Less distinct oblique ridge and more supplemental grooves. Trapezoidal proximal crown outline. Buccal ridge
Height of contour: Buccal: cervical third; Lingual: middle third
Mesial and distal contact: Middle third
Distinguishing right from left: Mesiolingual cusp outline longer and larger but not as sharp as distolingual cusp outline
Root features: Three roots less divergent roots. Root trunks, furcations, and proximal root concavities

Maxillary Left Third Molar (Heart-Shaped Occlusal Crown Outline)

Universal Number: #16 **International Number:** #28
Eruption: 17-21 **Root completion:** 18-25
General crown features: Occlusal table with marginal ridges and cusps with tips, inclined planes, ridges, grooves, fossae, pits
Specific crown features: Smaller crown than second and variable in form. Heart-shaped or rhomboidal occlusal crown outline (in order) with three or four cusps. Trapezoidal proximal crown outline. Buccal ridge
Height of contour: Buccal: cervical third; Lingual: middle third
Mesial contact: Middle third **Distal contact:** None
Distinguishing right from left: Distobuccal cusp shorter than mesiobuccal cusp
Root features: Three roots less divergent roots usually fused curving distally

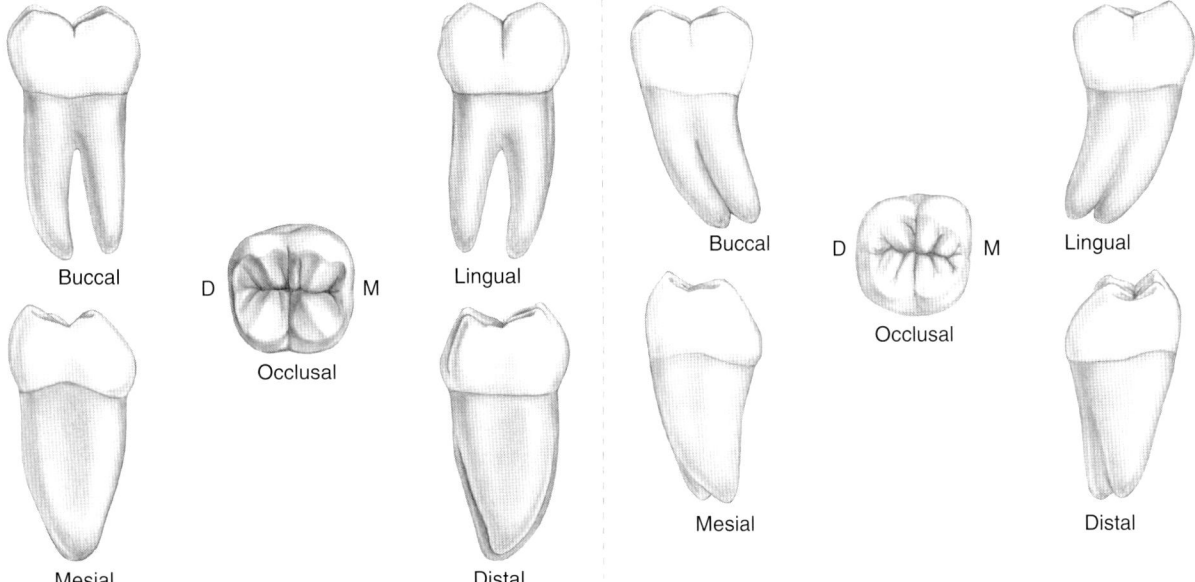
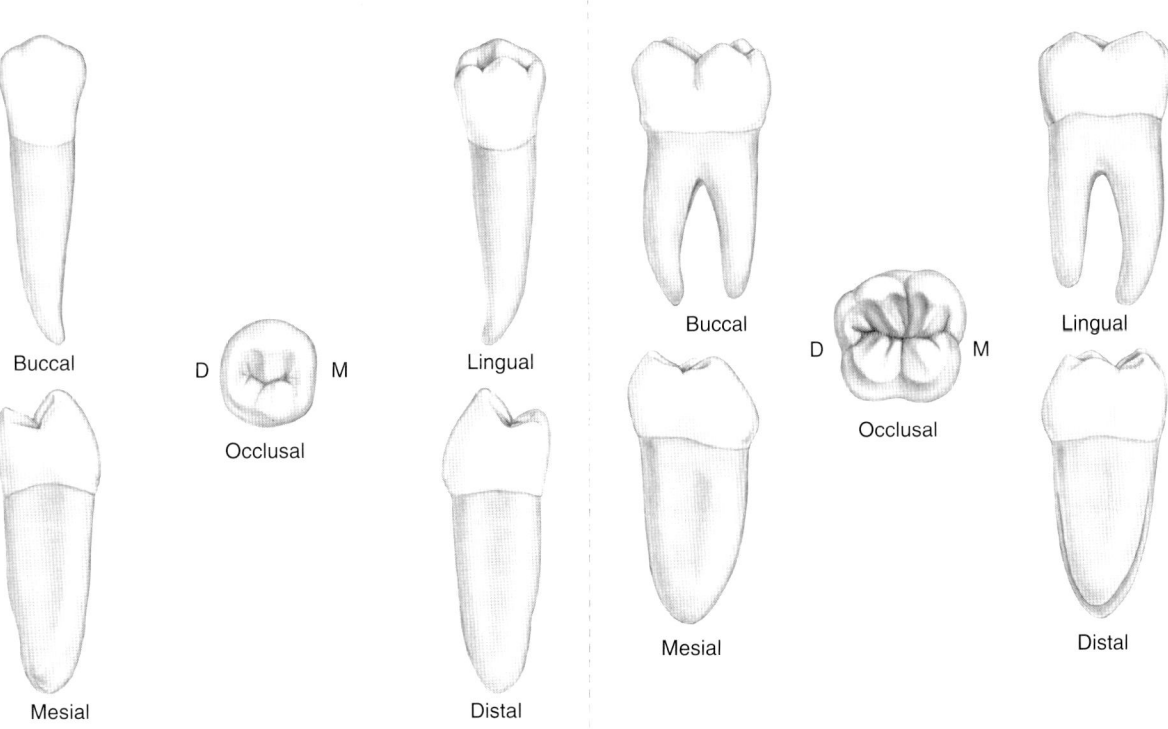

Mandibular Left Third Molar

Universal Number: #17 **International Number:** #38
Eruption: 17-21 **Root completion:** 18-25
General crown features: Occlusal table with marginal ridges and cusps with tips, inclined planes, ridges, grooves, fossae, pits
Specific crown features: Smaller crown than second. More oval occlusal crown outline. Rhomboidal proximal crown outline. Buccal ridge
Height of contour: Buccal: cervical third; Lingual: middle third
Mesial contact: Cervical third **Distal contact:** None
Distinguishing right from left: Wider buccolingually on mesial than on distal
Root features: Two roots fused, irregularly curved, with sharp apices

Mandibular Left Second Molar

Universal Number: #18 **International Number:** #37
Eruption: 11-13 **Root completion:** 14-15
General crown features: Occlusal table with marginal ridges and cusps with tips, inclined planes, ridges, grooves, fossae, pits
Specific crown features: Smaller crown than first. Rectangular occlusal crown outline. Four cusps with cross-shaped groove pattern. Rhomboidal proximal crown outline.
Height of contour: Buccal: cervical third; Lingual: middle third
Mesial and distal contact: Middle third
Distinguishing right from left: Difference in height of contour for buccal and lingual from each proximal surface and wider on mesial than distal
Root features: Two roots less divergent and smaller than first. Root trunks, furcations, and proximal root concavities

Mandibular Left First Molar

Universal Number: #19 **International Number:** #36
Eruption: 6-7 **Root completion:** 9-10
General crown features: Occlusal table with marginal ridges and cusps with tips, inclined planes, ridges, grooves, fossae, pits
Specific crown features: First permanent tooth to erupt. Widest crown mesiodistally of dentition. Pentagonal occlusal crown outline. Five cusps with Y-shaped groove pattern. Rhomboidal proximal crown outline. Buccal groove possibly ending in buccal pit. Buccal ridge
Height of contour: Buccal: cervical third; Lingual: middle third
Mesial and distal contact: Junction of occlusal and middle thirds
Distinguishing right from left: Distal cusp smallest with sharp cusp
Root features: Two roots more divergent and larger than second. Root trunks, furcations, and proximal root concavities

Mandibular Left Second Premolar (Three-Cusp Type)

Universal Number: #20 **International Number:** #35
Eruption: 11-12 **Root completion:** 13-14
General crown features: Occlusal table with marginal ridges and cusps with tips, ridges, inclined planes, grooves, fossae, pits.
Specific crown features: Larger than first. Almost square crown outline. Usually three cusps with Y-shaped groove pattern or two cusps with H- or U-shaped groove pattern. Increased supplemental grooves. Rhomboidal proximal crown outline. Buccal ridge
Height of contour: Buccal: cervical third; Lingual: middle third
Mesial and distal contact: Just cervical to junction of occlusal and middle thirds
Distinguishing right from left: Distal marginal ridge more cervically located with more occlusal surface observable from distal
Root features: Single root. Oval or elliptical on cervical cross section. Proximal root concavities

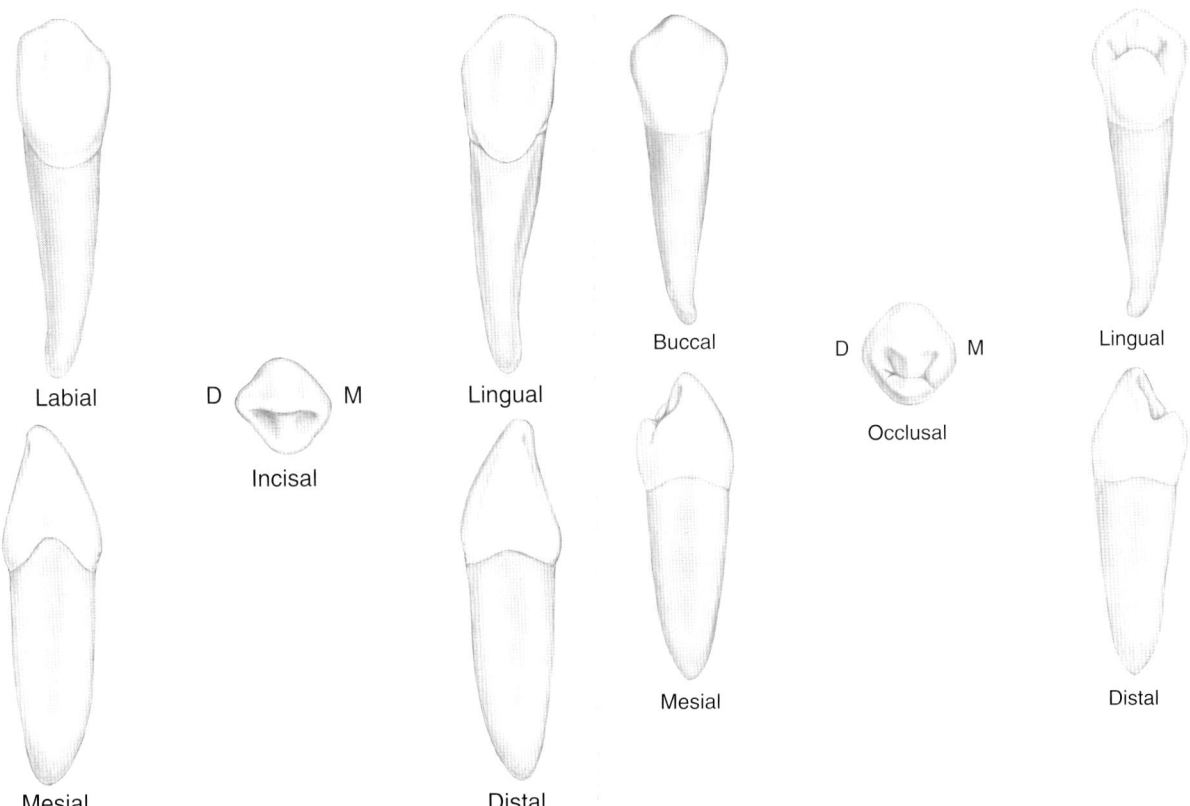
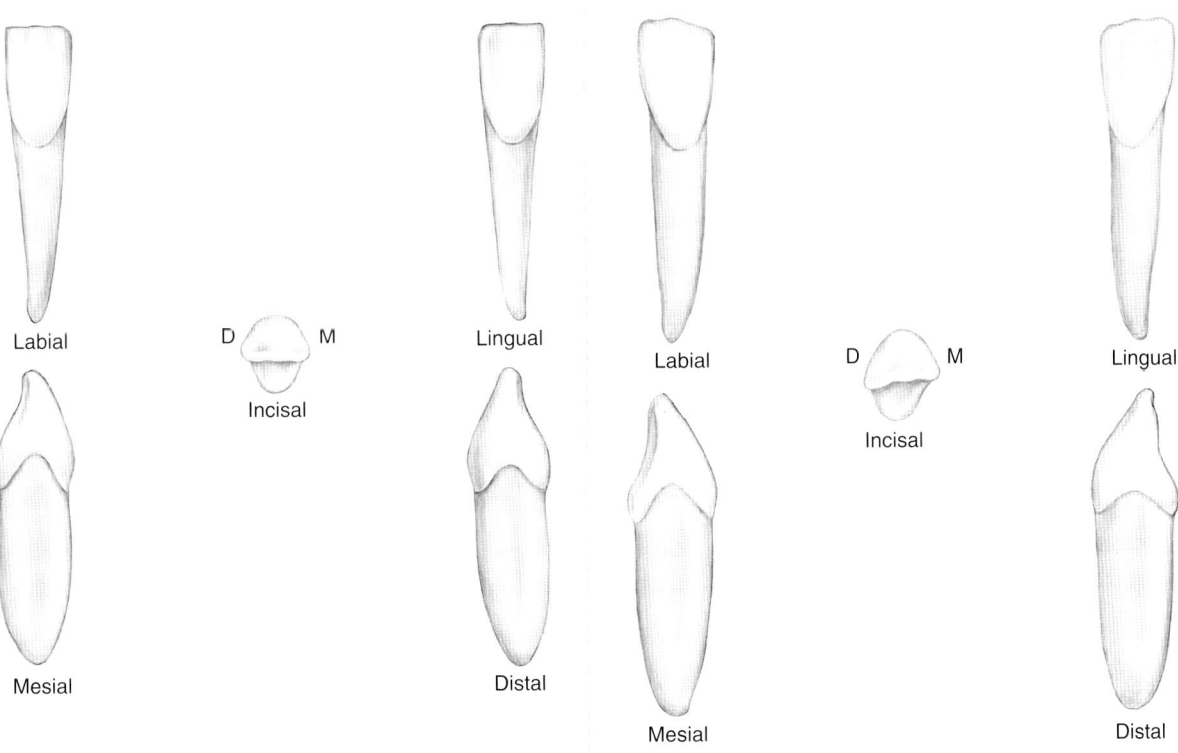

Mandibular Left First Premolar

Universal Number: #21 **International Number:** #34
Eruption: 10-12 **Root completion:** 12-13
General crown features: Occlusal table with marginal ridges and cusps with tips, ridges, inclined planes, grooves, fossae, pits
Specific crown features: Smaller than second. Diamond-shaped occlusal crown outline. Smaller lingual cusp of two cusps. Distinct mesial surface features. Rhomboidal proximal crown outline. Buccal ridge
Height of contour: Buccal: cervical third; Lingual: middle third
Mesial and distal contact: Just cervical to junction of occlusal and middle thirds
Distinguishing right from left: Shorter mesial cusp slope than distal and with distinct mesial surface features: deeper mesial CEJ curvature and mesiolingual groove
Root features: Single root. Oval or elliptical on cervical cross section. Proximal root concavities

Mandibular Left Canine

Universal Number: #22 **International Number:** #33
Eruption: 9-10 **Root completion:** 12-14
General crown features: Single cusp with tip, slopes, labial ridge, cingulum, lingual ridge, marginal ridges, lingual fossae
Specific crown features: Longest tooth in arch. Less pronounced lingual surface. Less sharp cusp tip
Height of contour: Labial: cervical third; Lingual: middle third
Mesial contact: Incisal third **Distal contact:** Junction of incisal and middle thirds
Distinguishing right from left: Shorter mesial cusp slope than distal with more pronounced mesial CEJ curvature. More cervical contact on distal. Shorter and rounder distal outline than mesial on labial with shorter mesial slope than distal
Root features: Long thick single root. Oval on cervical cross section. Proximal root concavities with developmental depressions on mesial and distal giving tooth double-rooted appearance. Pointed apex

Mandibular Left Lateral Incisor

Universal Number: #23 **International Number:** #32
Eruption: 7-8 **Root completion:** 10
General crown features: Incisal ridge, incisal angles, cingulum, marginal ridges, lingual fossa
Specific crown features: Like larger mandibular central. Not symmetrical. Appears twisted distally. Small distally placed cingulum with mesial marginal ridge longer than distal. More pronounced marginal ridges and deeper lingual fossa
Height of contour: Cervical third
Mesial and distal contact: Incisal third
Distinguishing right from left: Sharper mesio-incisal angle and rounder disto-incisal angle. More pronounced mesial CEJ curvature
Root features: Single root. Elliptical on cervical cross section. Root longer than crown. Pronounced proximal root concavities can give double-rooted appearance

Mandibular Left Central Incisor

Universal Number: #24 **International Number:** #31
Eruption: 6-7 **Root completion:** 9
General crown features: Incisal ridge, incisal angles, cingulum, marginal ridges, lingual fossa
Specific crown features: Smallest and simplest tooth. Symmetrical. Small centered cingulum with less pronounced marginal ridges and less deep lingual fossa
Height of contour: Cervical third
Mesial and distal contact: Incisal third
Distinguishing right from left: Sharper mesio-incisal angle and rounder disto-incisal angle. More pronounced mesial CEJ curvature
Root features: Single root. Elliptical on cervical cross section. Root longer than crown. Deeper proximal root concavities can give double-rooted appearance

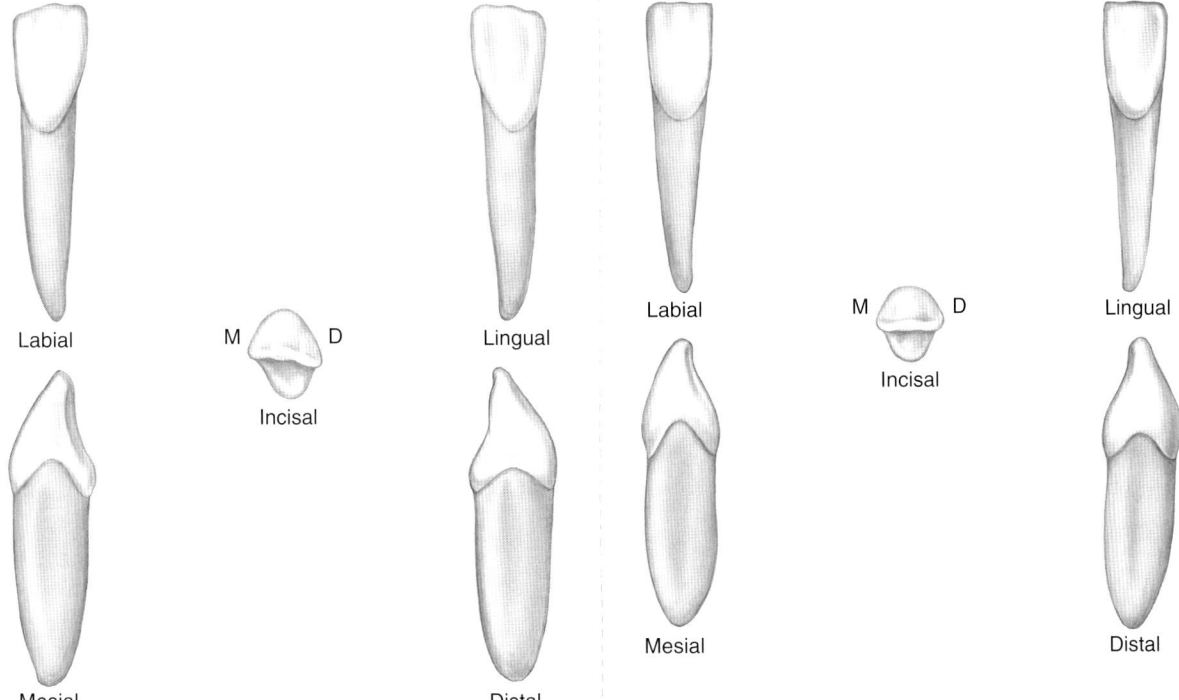
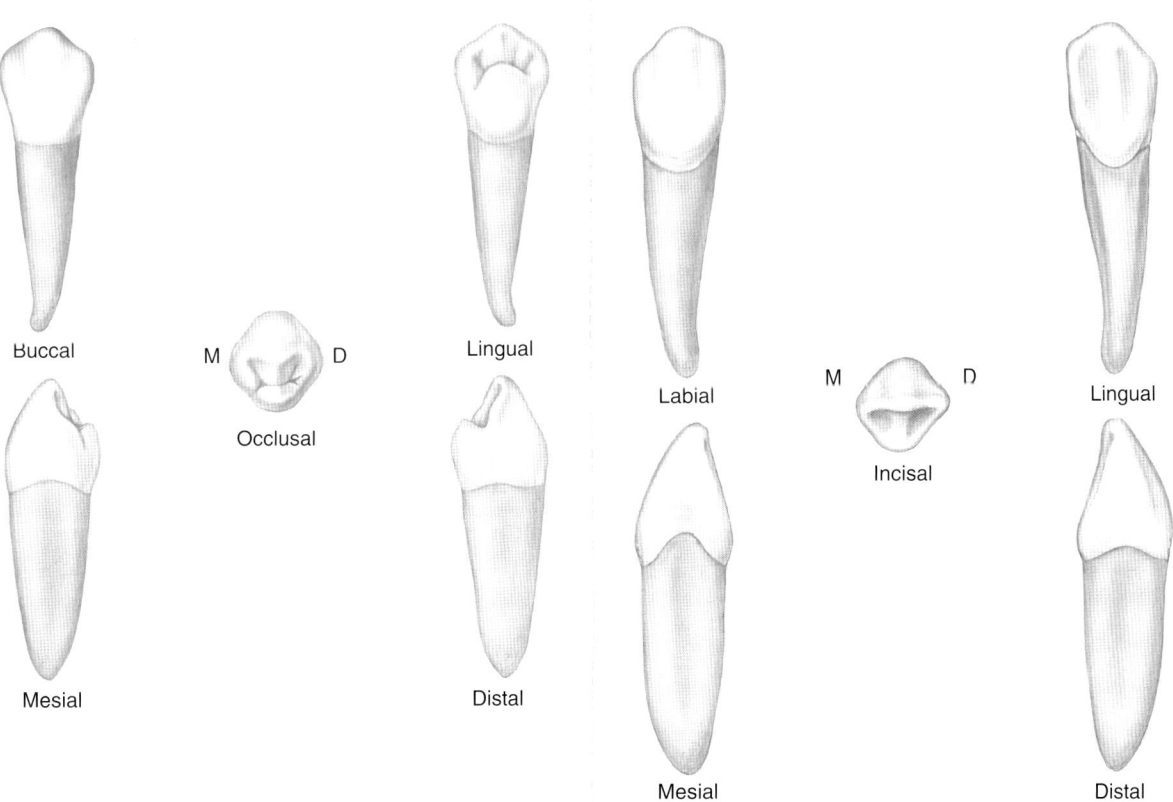

Mandibular Right Central Incisor

Universal Number: #25 **International Number:** #41
Eruption: 6-7 **Root completion:** 9
General crown features: Incisal ridge, incisal angles, cingulum, marginal ridges, lingual fossa
Specific crown features: Smallest and simplest tooth. Symmetrical. Small centered cingulum with less pronounced marginal ridges and less deep lingual fossa
Height of contour: Cervical third
Mesial and distal contact: Incisal third
Distinguishing right from left: Sharper mesio-incisal angle and rounder disto-incisal angle. More pronounced mesial CEJ curvature
Root features: Single root. Elliptical on cervical cross section. Root longer than crown. Deeper proximal root concavities can give double-rooted appearance

Mandibular Right Lateral Incisor

Universal Number: #26 **International Number:** #42
Eruption: 7-8 **Root completion:** 10
General crown features: Incisal ridge, incisal angles, cingulum, marginal ridges, lingual fossa
Specific crown features: Like larger mandibular central. Not symmetrical. Appears twisted distally. Small distally placed cingulum with mesial marginal ridge longer than distal. More pronounced marginal ridges and deeper lingual fossa
Height of contour: Cervical third
Mesial and distal contact: Incisal third
Distinguishing right from left: Sharper mesio-incisal angle and rounder disto-incisal angle. More pronounced mesial CEJ curvature
Root features: Single root. Elliptical on cervical cross section. Root longer than crown. Proximal root concavities can give double-rooted appearance

Mandibular Right Canine

Universal Number: #27 **International Number:** #43
Eruption: 9-10 **Root completion:** 12-14
General crown features: Single cusp with tip, slopes, labial ridge, cingulum, lingual ridge, marginal ridges, lingual fossae
Specific crown features: Longest tooth in arch. Less pronounced lingual surface. Less sharp cusp tip
Height of contour: Labial: cervical third; Lingual: middle third
Mesial contact: Incisal third **Distal contact:** Junction of incisal and middle thirds
Distinguishing right from left: Shorter mesial cusp slope than distal with more pronounced mesial CEJ curvature. More cervical contact on distal. Shorter and rounder distal outline than mesial on labial with shorter mesial slope than distal
Root features: Long thick single root. Oval on cervical cross section. Proximal root concavities with developmental depressions on mesial and distal giving tooth double-rooted appearance. Pointed apex

Mandibular Right First Premolar

Universal Number: #28 **International Number:** #44
Eruption: 10-12 **Root completion:** 12-13
General crown features: Occlusal table with marginal ridges and cusps with tips, ridges, inclined planes, grooves, fossae, pits.
Specific crown features: Smaller than second. Diamond-shaped occlusal crown outline. Smaller lingual cusp of two cusps. Distinct mesial surface features. Rhomboidal proximal crown outline. Buccal ridge
Height of contour: Buccal: cervical third; Lingual: middle third
Mesial and distal contact: Just cervical to junction of occlusal and middle thirds
Distinguishing right from left: Shorter mesial cusp slope than distal and with distinct mesial surface features: deeper mesial CEJ curvature and mesiolingual groove
Root features: Single root. Oval or elliptical on cervical cross section. Proximal root concavities

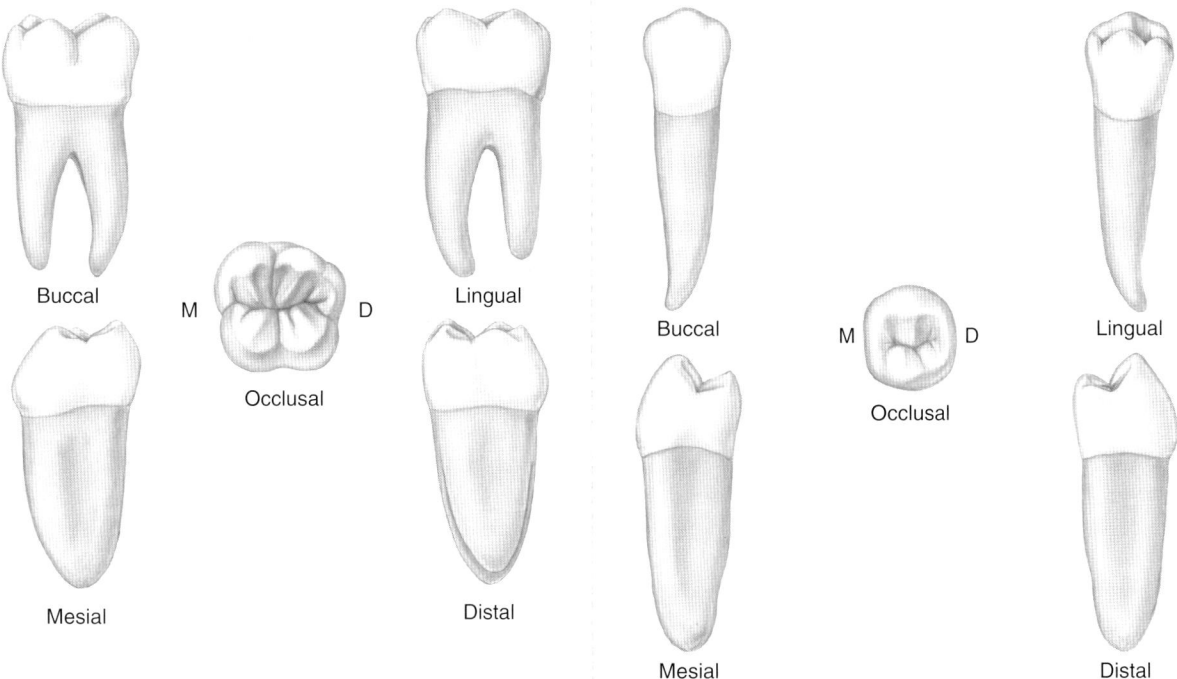

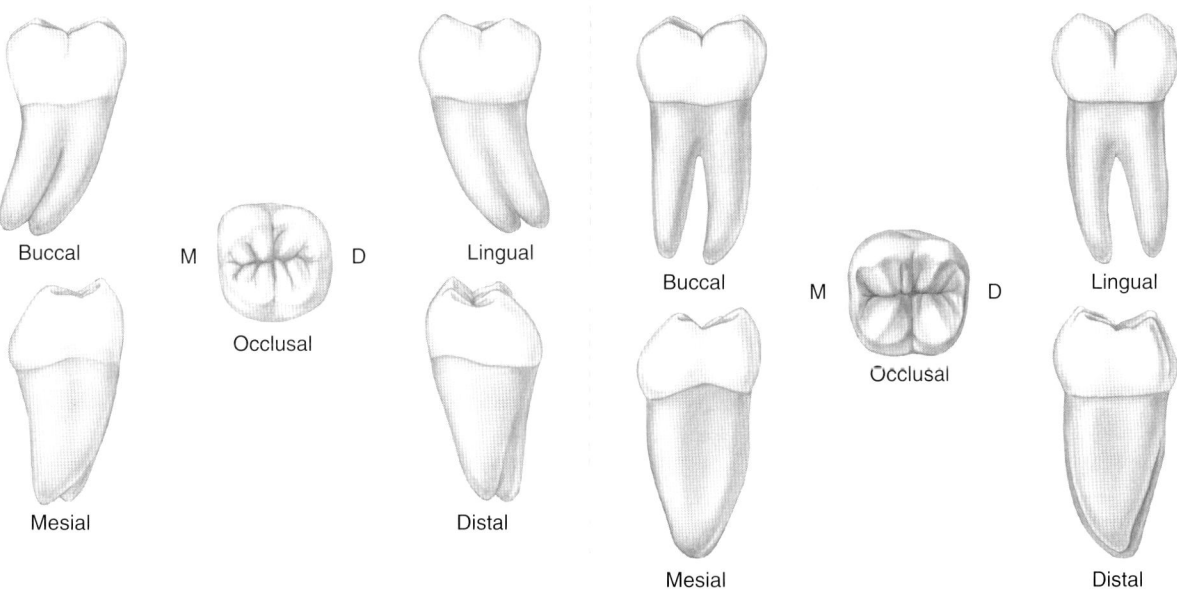

Mandibular Right Second Premolar (Three-Cusp Type)

Universal Number: #29 **International Number:** #45
Eruption: 11-12 **Root completion:** 13-14
General crown features: Occlusal table with marginal ridges and cusps with tips, ridges, inclined planes, grooves, fossae, pits
Specific crown features: Larger than first. Almost square crown outline. Usually three cusps with Y-shaped groove pattern or two cusps with H- or U-shaped groove pattern. Increased supplemental grooves. Rhomboidal proximal crown outline. Buccal ridge
Height of contour: Buccal: cervical third; Lingual: middle third
Mesial and distal contact: Just cervical to junction of occlusal and middle thirds
Distinguishing right from left: Distal marginal ridge more cervically located with more occlusal surface observable from distal
Root features: Single root. Oval or elliptical on cervical cross section. Proximal root concavities

Mandibular Right First Molar

Universal Number: #30 **International Number:** #46
Eruption: 6-7 **Root completion:** 9-10
General crown features: Occlusal table with marginal ridges and cusps with tips, inclined planes, ridges, grooves, fossae, pits
Specific crown features: First permanent tooth to erupt. Widest crown mesiodistally of dentition. Pentagonal occlusal crown outline. Five cusps with Y-shaped groove pattern. Rhomboidal proximal crown outline. Buccal groove possibly ending in buccal pit. Buccal ridge
Height of contour: Buccal: cervical third; Lingual: middle third
Mesial and distal contact: Junction of occlusal and middle thirds
Distinguishing right from left: Distal cusp smallest and has sharp cusp
Root features: Two roots more divergent and larger than second. Root trunks, furcations, and proximal root concavities

Mandibular Right Second Molar

Universal Number: #31 **International Number:** #47
Eruption: 11-13 **Root completion:** 14-15
General crown features: Occlusal table with marginal ridges and cusps with tips, inclined planes, ridges, grooves, fossae, pits
Specific crown features: Smaller crown than first. Rectangular occlusal crown outline. Four cusps with cross-shaped groove pattern. Rhomboidal proximal crown outline.
Height of contour: Buccal: cervical third; Lingual: middle third
Mesial and distal contact: Middle third
Distinguishing right from left: Difference in height of contour for buccal and lingual from each proximal surface and wider on mesial than distal
Root features: Two roots less divergent and smaller than first. Root trunks, furcations, and proximal root concavities

Mandibular Right Third Molar

Universal Number: #32 **International Number:** #48
Eruption: 17-21 **Root completion:** 18-25
General crown features: Occlusal table with marginal ridges and cusps with tips, inclined planes, ridges, grooves, fossae, pits
Specific crown features: Smaller crown than second. More oval occlusal crown outline. Rhomboidal proximal crown outline. Buccal ridge
Height of contour: Buccal: cervical third; Lingual: middle third
Mesial contact: Cervical third **Distal contact:** None
Distinguishing right from left: Wider buccolingually on mesial than on distal
Root features: Two roots fused, irregularly curved, with sharp apices